The CHANGING IMAGE of the NURSE

Philip A. Kalisch PhD
Professor of History, Politics, and
Economics of Nursing
University of Michigan

Beatrice J. Kalisch RN, EdD, FAAN
Principal and Director
Nursing Consultation Services
Arthur Young
Detroit, Michigan

ADDISON-WESLEY PUBLISHING COMPANY
Health Sciences Division, Menlo Park, California
Reading, Massachusetts • Don Mills, Ontario • Wokingham, UK
Amsterdam • Sydney • Singapore • Tokyo • Madrid
Bogota • Santiago • San Juan

To Philip and Melanie

Sponsoring Editor: Nancy Evans
Production Supervisor: Judith Johnstone
Designer: Ken Scott
Copyeditors: Brian Jones, Ira Kleinberg
Indexer: Steven Sorensen

Library of Congress Cataloging-in-Publication Data
Kalisch, Philip Arthur.
    The changing image of the nurse.
    Bibliography: p.
    Includes index.
    1. Nursing—United States—Public opinion.
2. Public opinion—United States.   3. Nurses in
mass media—United States.   I. Kalisch, Beatrice J.,
1943–   II. Title.   [DNLM: 1. Mass Media.
2. Nursing.   WY 16 K145c]
RT4.K35   1986   362.1'73'0973   86–3494

0-201-11655-3

CDEFGHIJ-HA-8987

Addison-Wesley Publishing Company
Health Sciences Division
2725 Sand Hill Road
Menlo Park, California 94025

PHOTO CREDITS

52b *The Splendid Sinner,* Goldwyn, 1918. Copyright © 1918 by Goldwyn.

53 *Adele,* United Pictures, 1919. Courtesy of Academy of Motion Picture Arts and Sciences Stills Archive.

54 *The Light,* Fox, 1919. Copyright © 1919 by Fox Film Corporation. All rights reserved.

56 *Flight,* Columbia Pictures, 1929. Courtesy of Columbia Pictures.

57 The Library of Congress.

58 Nursing and Hospital Archives, University of Michigan.

59 The Library of Congress.

60a Nursing and Hospital Archives, University of Michigan.

60b The Library of Congress.

61a Nursing and Hospital Archives, University of Michigan.

61b The Library of Congress.

62 Nursing and Hospital Archives, University of Michigan.

64 *Flight,* Columbia Pictures, 1929. Courtesy of Columbia Pictures.

67 *The New Commandment,* First National, 1925.

69 *Recompense,* 1925. Courtesy of Academy of Motion Picture Arts and Sciences Stills Archive.

72 *The Patent Leather Kid,* First National, 1927.

76 *The Storm,* Universal Pictures, 1938. Copyright © 1938 by Universal Pictures, a Division of Universal City Studios, Inc. All rights reserved. Courtesy of MCA Publishing Rights, a Division of MCA Inc.

77 National Archives, General Services Administration.

78 U.S. Department of Agriculture Archives.

79a U.S. Department of Agriculture Archives.

79b Nursing and Hospital Archives, University of Michigan.

82 *Night Nurse,* Warner Bros., 1931. Copyright © 1931 by Warner Bros. Pictures Inc. Renewed 1958 by Associated Artists Productions Corp.

83 *The White Parade,* 20th Century-Fox, 1934. Copyright © 1934 by Fox Film Corporation. All rights reserved.

88 *Vigil in the Night,* RKO, 1940. Copyright © 1940 by RKO Pictures, Inc. All rights reserved.

93 *The Great Hospital Mystery,* 20th Century-Fox, 1937. Copyright © 1937 by 20th Century-Fox Film Corp. All rights reserved.

95 U.S. Department of Commerce Archives.

97 *The Storm,* Universal Pictures, 1938. Copyright © 1938 by Universal Pictures, a Division of Universal City Studios, Inc. All rights reserved. Courtesy of MCA Publishing Rights, a Division of MCA Inc.

99 U.S. Office of War Information.

100 U.S. Office of War Information.

101 U.S. Office of War Information.

103 *Don Winslow of the Navy,* Universal Pictures, 1942. Copyright © 1942 by Universal Pictures, a Division of Universal City Studios, Inc. All rights reserved. Courtesy of MCA Publishing Rights, a Division of MCA Inc.

104 *To the Shores of Tripoli,* 20th Century-Fox, 1942. Copyright © 1942 by 20th Century-Fox Film Corp. All rights reserved.

106 *Parachute Nurse,* Columbia Pictures, 1942. Courtesy of Columbia Pictures.

107 *So Proudly We Hail,* Universal Pictures, 1943. Copyright © 1943 by Universal Pictures, a Division of Universal City Studios, Inc. All rights reserved. Courtesy of MCA Publishing Rights, a Division of MCA Inc.

108 *So Proudly We Hail,* Universal Pictures, 1943. Copyright © 1943 by Universal Pictures, a Division of Universal City Studios, Inc. All rights reserved. Courtesy of MCA Publishing Rights, a Division of MCA Inc.

112 *They Were Expendable,* MGM, 1945. Copyright © 1945 by Loews Incorporated. Renewed 1972 by Metro-Goldwyn-Mayer Inc.

113 *Lifeboat,* 20th Century-Fox, 1944. Copyright © 1944 by 20th Century-Fox Film Corp. All rights reserved.

114 *Since You Went Away,* United Artists, 1944. Copyright © 1944 by United Artists Studio. All rights reserved.

119 Nursing and Hospital Archives, University of Michigan.

120 Nursing and Hospital Archives, University of Michigan.

124 *Battle Circus,* MGM, 1953. Copyright © 1953 by Loews Incorporated. Renewed 1980 by Metro-Goldwyn-Mayer Inc.

125a Federal Security Agency.

125b U.S. Department of Agriculture Archives.

127 Nursing and Hospital Archives, University of Michigan.

128 The Library of Congress.

131 *Homecoming,* MGM, 1948. Copyright © 1948 by Loews Inc. Renewed 1975 by Metro-Goldwyn-Mayer Inc.

132 *The Hasty Heart,* Warner Bros., 1950. Copyright © 1950 by Warner Bros. Pictures Inc. All rights reserved.

133 *Pinky,* 20th Century-Fox, 1949. Copyright © 1949 by 20th Century-Fox Film Corp. All rights reserved.

135 *The Snake Pit,* 20th Century-Fox, 1948. Copyright © 1948 by 20th Century-Fox Film Corp. All rights reserved.

137 *Not As A Stranger,* United Artists, 1955. Copyright © 1955 by United Artists Studio. All rights reserved.

139 *Battle Circus,* MGM, 1953. Copyright © 1953 by Loews Incorporated. Renewed 1980 by Metro-Goldwyn-Mayer Inc.

140 *Hellcats of the Navy,* Columbia Pictures, 1957. Courtesy of Columbia Pictures.

141 *South Pacific,* 20th Century-Fox, 1958. Photograph from *South Pacific.* Courtesy of Rodgers and Hammerstein. Copyright © 1958 Estate of Richard Rodgers and Estate of Oscar Hammerstein II. Copyright renewed.

143 Nursing in the Mass Media Archives, University of Michigan.

144 Nursing in the Mass Media Archives, University of Michigan.

151 *Dr. Hudson's Secret Journal.* Courtesy of Nursing in the Mass Media Archives, University of Michigan.

155 *The Hospital,* United Artists, 1971. Copyright © 1971 by United Artists Studio. All rights reserved.

160 Nursing and Hospital Archives, University of Michigan.

162 *Catch-22,* Paramount, 1970. Copyright © 1970 by Paramount Pictures Corporation. All rights reserved.

163 *Carry on Nurse,* Governor Films, 1959. Courtesy of Governor Films, Inc.

165 *Carry on Nurse,* Governor Films, 1959. Courtesy of Governor Films, Inc.

167 *I, A Woman,* Audubon Films, 1965.

168 *Deep Throat,* 1972. Courtesy of Museum of Modern Art Stills Archive.

169 Advertisement for *Night Call Nurses,* New World Pictures, 1972. Copyright © 1972 by New Horizons.

171 *The Honeymoon Killers,* 1970. Photograph courtesy of Warren Steibel.

173 *The Hospital,* United Artists, 1971. Copyright © 1971 by United Artists Studio. All rights reserved.

174 *One Flew Over the Cuckoo's Nest,* Fantasy Films, 1975. Copyright © 1975 by United Artists Studio. All rights reserved.

179 Nursing and Hospital Archives, University of Michigan.

182 *Marcus Welby, M.D.* Copyright © 1971 by Universal Pictures, a Division of Universal City Studios, Inc. All rights reserved. Courtesy of MCA Publishing Rights, a Division of MCA Inc.

183 *St. Elsewhere,* MTM Studios. Courtesy of NBC.

188 Nursing and Hospital Archives, University of Michigan.

192 Nursing in the Mass Media Archives, University of Michigan.

193 Nursing and Hospital Archives, University of Michigan.

CONTENTS

PREFACE

When lay people are asked to evaluate the role of nurses in health care, they usually rely on information acquired from the mass media. These printed and electronic images are both persuasive and elusive. Each day, scores of images of nurses and nursing speed past readers and viewers, leaving only a diffuse awareness of their impact. These fleeting images rarely elicit prolonged contemplation or critical analysis. What symbolic worlds of nursing have these images produced? What beliefs about nurses do they communicate?

The 1979 federal report, *Social Indicators of Equality for Minorities and Women,* revealed the results of an occupational-prestige study that showed nurses ranking 91 out of 122 professions. Physicians ranked highest, yet registered nurses were surpassed by such professionals as social workers, clergy, school teachers, physical therapists, librarians, and dental hygienists. Nurses *did* score just ahead of embalmers. In a recent Gallup poll asking the public which occupations each sex was better suited for, both males and females overwhelmingly (99 percent) agreed that women were better nurses than men. This occupationally linked sex-role stereotype was stronger for nursing than for any other field, including secretarial work and truck driving.

THE DANGER INHERENT IN A NEGATIVE IMAGE

Modern health care involves complex technology and unquantifiable nursing actions, both often dimly perceived and misunderstood by the public. Thus the mass media substantially influence public perceptions of the delivery of health care, particularly nursing care.

Nurses with a strong degree of professional commitment unanimously agree that the popular image of nursing in the mid-1980s is weak, fuzzy and unrealistic. While some nurses find the conventional and frequently degrading images of their profession simply annoying, many see a danger in the continued negative portrayal of nurses. Nursing as a profession is maturing due to increased education, technological advances that have created new roles and responsibilities, and a complex of other social and political developments. Today's generation of nurses has both the motivation and the capacity to participate in a variety of expanded health care roles: nurses are increasingly making decisions that were once made only by physicians.

Nursing's goal is to improve the quality of life by meeting specific human needs. Misunderstandings about the nature and extent of nursing raise major obstacles to achieving this goal. Much of this misunderstanding is the legacy of an outdated ideology of nursing. Yet these public beliefs, attitudes, and interpretations of nursing are extremely powerful forces in determining actions. Once an ideology has taken hold, it expresses itself not only in clinical practice, but also at the highest levels of health care services' organization and structure. Its manifestations can be traced through analyses of messages, symbols, values and occupational relationships.

THE NEED TO COMMUNICATE A REALISTIC IMAGE

Reshaping an image is a long and arduous process; thus nursing must begin to educate various publics about the realities of its practice and its potential. The mass media can make nurses look "smaller than life" or "larger than life." The media can act as both mirrors and lamps, reflecting the reality of professional contributions, and lighting the way to new contributions. How the mass media portray nursing affects the politics of human resource allocation, development and utilization. Mass-media portrayals of nursing also influence public opinions and desires, which in turn influence the course of nursing. An informed public can contribute to the advancement of the nursing profession and, by so doing, promote the nation's health. Thus it is essential for the future of health care in this nation that the mass media begin to light the way for nurses and nursing.

THE OPPORTUNITY TO PROMOTE A NEW AND IDEAL IMAGE

The Changing Image of the Nurse attempts to foster debate on strategies to promote a fuller understanding of the powerful relationship between media portrayals and the public image of nursing. Enhanced awareness of the power of this relationship will encourage positive action to reduce the gap between inaccurate beliefs and scientific knowledge.

This book was written expressly for students and faculty in nursing education programs for use in professional issues, trends, and history of nursing classes, and for nurses in practice, administration, and research who are concerned about the advancement of nursing as an attractive professional career for the future.

Chapter 1 establishes a basic framework for the book by focusing on concepts and theories concerning the image of the nurse, mass communications, and the socialization process. Seven individual chapters explore the five dominant images of the mass media nurse since nursing's establishment as a profession in the mid-nineteenth century: the nurse as Angel of Mercy, Girl Friday, Heroine, Wife and Mother, and Sex Object. Chapter 9 identifies a new and ideal dominant image for the future—the nurse as Careerist—and suggests approaches to developing this new image.

ACKNOWLEDGEMENTS

A diverse group of individuals gave us important support toward the completion of this book, especially in the form of provocative discussions about the image of the nurse, what it has been and what it should be: Mary Anderson, LaCrosse Lutheran Hospital, LaCrosse, Wisconsin; Coy Baker, Iowa Methodist Medical Center, Des Moines; Rachel Booth, Assistant Vice President and Dean, Duke University; Connie Baker, Dean, School of Nursing, University of South Carolina; Jane Bailey, Puget Sound Health Cooperative, Seattle, Washington; Doris Bloch, Chief, Research Support Section, Division of Nursing, U.S. Public Health Service, Washington, D.C.; Gaye Bruce, Coordinator for Marketing and Recruitment, Stanford Hospital and Medical Center; Bonnie Bullough, Dean, School of Nursing, State University of New York at Buffalo; Sheila Burke, Deputy Staff Director, U.S. Senate Committee on Finance; Glenda Lee Butnarescu, Associate Professor of Nursing, University of Texas, San Antonio; Harriet Carroll, Research Support Section, Division of Nursing, U.S. Public Health Service; Michael Carter, Dean, College of Nursing, University of Tennessee, Memphis; Luther P. Christman, Dean, College of Nursing, Rush University; Olga Church, Associate Professor, College of Nursing, University of Illinois; Alice Clarke, Editor, *Nursing Publications,* Hillsdale, New Jersey; Joyce C. Clifford, Vice President for Nursing, Beth Israel Hospital, Boston; Jacque Clinton, Associate Professor, School of Nursing, University of Wisconsin, Milwaukee; Carol E. Colter, Nurse Recruiter, Kaiser Foundation Hospitals, Los Angeles; Mary E. Conway, Dean, School of Nursing, Medical College of Georgia; Connie R. Curran, Vice President, American Hospital Association; Leah L. Curtin, Editor, *Nursing Management,* Cincinnati, Ohio.

Others who facilitated our work included: Carolyne K. Davis, former Administrator, Health Care Financing Administration, Health and Human Services; Rheba de Tornyay, Dean, School of Nursing, University of Washington; Donna Diers, Professor, School of Nursing, Yale University; Barbara A. Donaho, Corporate Director of Nursing, Sisters of Mercy Health Corporation, Farmington Hills, Michigan; Florence S. Downs, Associate Dean and Director of Graduate Studies, School of Nursing, University of Pennsylvania; Janet Dunphy, Executive Director, Massachusetts Nurses' Association, District Five, Bedham, Massachusetts; Elaine Dyer, Dean, School of Nursing, Brigham Young University; Shirley H. Fondiller, Executive Director, Mid-Atlantic Regional Nursing Association; Louise M. Fitzpatrick, Dean, College of

Nursing, Villanova University; Teresa Fitzpatrick, Grant Hospital, Chicago; Juanita W. Fleming, Professor, College of Nursing, University of Kentucky; JoAnn Forrest, Assistant Professor of Nursing, Brigham Young University; Carol Gino, Amityville, New York; Laurie Glass, Associate Professor, School of Nursing, University of Wisconsin, Milwaukee; Irma E. Goertzen, Administrator, University Hospital, Seattle; Marilyn Goldwater, Legislator, Maryland House of Delegates, Annapolis; Susan R. Gortner, Associate Dean, University of California, San Francisco; Susan Haecker, Head Nurse, Santa Rosa Medical Center, San Antonio.

Others included Clifford H. Jordan, Executive Director, Association of Operating Room Nurses, Denver; Patricia Kane, Director of Professional Development, Riverview Hospital, Red Bank, New Jersey; Marguerite R. Kinney, Professor, School of Nursing, University of Alabama, Birmingham; Madeleine M. Leininger, Director, Center for Health Research, College of Nursing, Wayne State University; Mary Lohr, Dean, College of Nursing, Clemson University; Margaret L. McClure, Executive Director of Nursing, New York University Medical Center; Mary McHugh, Nurse Researcher, St. Joseph's Hospital, Ann Arbor, Michigan; Barbara B. Minckley, Executive Director, Midwest Alliance in Nursing, Indianapolis; Pam Maraldo, Executive Director, National League for Nursing, New York; Marie L. O'Koren, Dean, School of Nursing, University of Alabama; Irene S. Palmer, Dean, School of Nursing, University of San Diego; Deanna Pearlmutter, Massachusetts General Hospital; Nola J. Pender, Professor of Nursing, Northern Illinois University; Thomas P. Phillips, Chief, Advanced Nursing Training, Division of Nursing, U.S. Public Health Service, Washington, D.C.; Nancy E. Reame, Associate Professor, School of Nursing, University of Michigan; June S. Rothberg, Dean, School of Nursing, Adelphi University; Virginia Saba, Professor, Georgetown University, Washington, D.C.; Pat Scearse, Dean, College of Nursing, Texas Christian University; Rozella M. Schlotfeldt, Dean Emeritus, Case Western Reserve University; Nancy Sharpe, Nurses' Association of the American College of Obstetricians and Gynecologists, Washington, D.C.; Elizabeth Sharp, Professor of Nursing, Emory University; Roy Simpson, Manager, Nursing Systems Information Systems, Hospital Corporation of America, Nashville, Tennessee; Julie Sochalski, Northville, Michigan; Roxane B. Spitzer, Associate Administrator of Nursing Services,

Cedars Sinai Medical Center, Los Angeles; Ruth F. Stewart, Associate Professor of Nursing, University of Texas, San Antonio; Ora L. Strickland, Doctoral Program Evaluator, University of Maryland; Duane D. Walker, Vice President, The Queen's Medical Center, Honolulu; Doris L. Wagner, Chief Nurse, Division of Public Health, Indianapolis; Carolyn A. Williams, Dean, College of Nursing, University of Kentucky; Pat Winstead-Fry, Director, Division of Nursing, New York University; Alma Wooley, Dean, School of Nursing, Illinois Wesleyan University, Bloomington, Illinois.

The following national organizations provided us with the opportunity to present some of our study findings and discuss their implications with members: American Academy of Ambulatory Nursing Administration, American Academy of Nursing, American Association of Colleges of Nursing, American Association of Critical Care Nurses, American Association of Nephrology Nurses and Technicians, American Nurses' Association, American Society for Hospital Public Relations, American Society of Post Anesthesia Nurses, Association of Operating Room Nurses, Emergency Department Nurses' Association, National Association for Practical Nurse Education and Service, National League for Nursing, National Association of Nurse Recruiters, National Association of Orthopaedic Nurses, National Association of Pediatric Nurse Associates and Practitioners, National Kidney Foundation, National Student Nurses' Association, Nurses' Association of American College of Obstetricians and Gynecologists, Registered Nurses' Association of Toronto (Canada), and Sigma Theta Tau.

We also had the opportunity to present our work at the following regional, state and local organizations: The Chicago Hospital Association; Hospital Council of Northeastern Pennsylvania; Michigan Nurse Recruiters; New England Council of Higher Degree Programs in Nursing; New Mexico Society for Nursing Services Administration; Northeast Regional Assembly of Constituent Leagues for Nursing; Nursing Service Administrators of Iowa; Provincial Directorate, Calgary, Alberta, Canada; the Arizona, Chicago, District of Columbia, Hawaii, Illinois, Maine, Massachusetts, Michigan, New Jersey, New York, Rhode Island, South Carolina, South Dakota, Vermont, Washington, and Wisconsin State Nurses' Associations; the Connecticut, Georgia, Maryland, Michigan, North Carolina, Pennsylvania, Tennessee, and Wisconsin Leagues for Nursing; and the California, Florida, and Michigan Student Nurses' Associations.

In addition, we are much indebted to Jill Coogan, who meticulously edited the manuscript, and to Susan Slaviero, who supervised the typing and assumed responsibility for many other tasks, usually under pressure. There is one person of whom it must be said, "Without her, this book might have never come into being"—Nancy Evans of Addison-Wesley, who encouraged us to transform our research findings into this work. Finally, we are especially grateful to our two-year-old son, Philip Peter, and one-year-old daughter, Melanie Jean, who patiently endured the completion of the book. The joy they have brought to our lives provided more than enough energy to see the project to completion.

Philip A. Kalisch
Beatrice J. Kalisch
Ann Arbor, Michigan
Autumn, 1986

CHAPTER ONE

MASS MEDIA NURSING: BASIC CONCEPTS

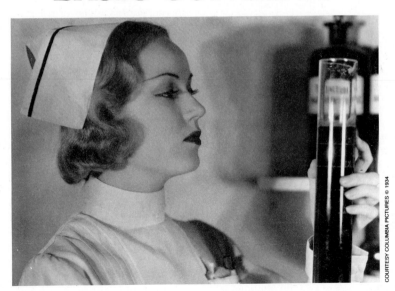

In an experiment conducted in the mid-1970s, a group of children saw a film of a child visiting a physician's office to receive an injection. A male nurse prepared the child for the procedure and a female physician administered the inoculation. The children later agreed that they had seen a male physician and a female nurse.[1] In 1983, a Long Island, New York, nurse found that even six-year-olds considered nursing for women only.

> "How many of you would like to be nurses when you grow up?" I asked. I was visiting my daughter's kindergarten class and was there to tell about my profession.
>
> Seated before me were 20 sparkling six-year-olds, eager to get their hands on my stethoscope. The boys all sat together on one side and the girls on the other. The age-old imaginary dividing line still existed, as it had in my school days. As if to reinforce the separation, most of the girls raised their hands in answer to my question.
>
> "I do, I do!" they exclaimed. At the same time every one of the boys made grimacing faces at me, accompanied by much moaning and groaning.
>
> "Only girls become nurses," they informed me. One elaborated and told me, "Boys become doctors and girls *have* to be nurses." Some of the females in the group disagreed.
>
> "I was sick once and the doctor who took care of me was a girl," one child told us. I explained that not only could women become doctors, but men could also be nurses. Alas, the boys in the class would have none of it. . . .
>
> After my visit, I couldn't get the conversation out of my mind. I had asked this question of other groups of children and gotten a similar response. It bothered me that children this young had such definite ideas about what kind of work is suitable for men and women. I'm reasonably certain no one ever said to them, "Girls grow up to be nurses; boys don't." The message is much subtler than that, and it comes from all directions. Television, movies and books contribute, and kids, like sponges, absorb everything.[2]

The children's assumptions that a male nurse had to be a physician because he was a man and that only women could pursue nursing careers exemplify the power of one aspect of the nursing image—that all nurses are female. Many pieces of cultural conditioning lay beneath the children's insistence that the scene with the female physician and the male nurse involved a male physician and a female nurse: the presumption of sex-role specialization overpowered the evidence before them. Their inability or refusal to recognize an exception to the usual patterns of sex-role specialization indicates the tenacity with which these stereotypes twist people's perceptions.

IDEOLOGY AND IMAGE

Nursing's ideology may be defined as the combination of beliefs that surround important nursing symbols, myths, and rituals. Ideology tends to portray its objects as natural, inevitable, and devoid of developmental history. The ideology of nursing has sought to confine the behavior and identity of half of humanity within strict limits—the supposed nature of woman. Ideology uses the fabrication of images and the processes of representation to persuade us that nurses are who and what they are because that is who and what they should be.

To see where we are going, we must remind ourselves of where we are coming from. Traditional sex roles constitute our starting point. In the United States, as in most other societies, traditional roles required women to nurture, care for, and provide affection for their families—first as daughters, later as wives and mothers. Their place was in the home. Their duties included homemaking, nursing, child care and education, and aiding their husbands. Satisfactory performance of these roles was regarded as incompatible with other roles. The traditional expectation was that these roles were appropriate for all women and would be performed within the family. The few alternative roles traditionally available to women outside the family—nursing, elementary school teaching—required similar skills and feelings.

The term *image of nursing* may be defined as the sum of beliefs, ideas, and impressions that people have of nurses and nursing. The literature concerning the image of nurses indicates that, while our culture acknowledges nurses' contributions to society, it greatly undervalues those contributions. Nurses are regarded as social inferiors, knowledgeable and competent, but only within a limited scope, not nearly as knowledgeable and competent as physicians. At best, our culture casts nurses in the romantic and deeply feminine role of the self-sacrificing angel who ministers to her patient and to the physician's bidding. This image exerts a strong residual appeal among nurses themselves, many of whom were initially drawn to the profession at an impressionable age, when the image of the ministering angel was emotionally satisfying. Most nurses learn in the course of their education to find less romantic

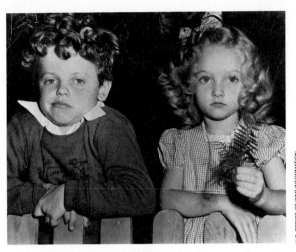

Our culutral traditions require that young females prepare themselves for nurturant roles.

U.S. OFFICE OF WAR INFORMATION

and more professional sources of satisfaction in their work, but the image of bedside care remains the cohesive element in the nurse's identity, and it appears to be rooted in the conception of nursing as a self-subordinating, giving, nurturing, quintessentially feminine activity. The professionalization of nurses—the movement away from this traditional image toward an image of individual achievement and personal autonomy—has met with much resistance and hostility, even among nurses themselves, largely because of the powerful residual appeal of the image of the self-sacrificing angel. One difficulty in supplanting this image is that we see the brusque, officious professional as the only alternative to the compassionate angel—Nurse Ratched instead of the Lady with the Lamp, something cold and masculine replacing what used to be warm and feminine.

OCCUPATIONAL STATUS

Socialization to the world of work begins in childhood and continues throughout life. In adult society the work role represents a primary source of identity, and occupational images are a major factor governing social interaction. Popular culture usually addresses some area of an individual's experience, however obliquely, and validates particular attitudes, beliefs, interests, fantasies, and identities.

It is important to understand the concept of *occupational status* and the perspectives from which it

may be viewed. The term *status* refers to social position; social positions may be defined along many dimensions. Wealth, education, sex, race, religion, and occupation are some of the more common dimensions for defining status in western society. Within a given society, some social positions are normatively valued more or less than others, and hence may be ordered in terms of their prestige or social value. This normative, hierarchical ordering gives rise to *status ranking*.

One of the most important sources of status ranking in American society is occupation. Since women have traditionally been unemployed, they often occupied a low status position in American society. As women acquired jobs outside the home, they altered their status and provided a means for differentiating among themselves.

MASS COMMUNICATIONS AND LEARNING

Nursing, like all other professions, rests on a cultural base. Every occupation must exist within some kind of structure, some kind of ordered world. Our culture provides clues about where nurses and nursing fit into the grand scheme of things. These clues may or may not be based on facts or truth. Communication theorists and social psychologists argue that mass media portrayals play a major role in shaping learned social behavior. Entertainment fare does more than merely entertain: it communicates information about the social structure and shapes attitudes about ourselves, others, and the world at large.

Research concerning the effects of motion pictures and television on viewers centers around the concept of *observational learning,* which states that the behavior of individuals is shaped and modified by exposure to the actions and values of others. Observational learning is a three-step process, involving (1) the observer's exposure to modeling cues (the observed behavior of others), (2) the observer's acquisition and recall of what was observed, and (3) the observer's acceptance of the model's behavior as a guide. Much important learning takes place vicariously. An individual observes the behavior of another and learns to imitate or in some way model that behavior. Individuals may also be influenced by models presented in more symbolic forms. Pictorial representations such as those in movie films and on television are highly influential sources of models.

By selecting out of the culture certain existing tendencies, patterns of behavior, attitudes, and values and by repeating them over and over again, television, motion pictures, and novels do not merely *reflect* the society but *shape* it by reinforcing those characteristics they select for attention. No mirror reflects without distortion. And every mirror produces some effect on the behavior of those who look into it.

SOCIALIZATION

Culture refers to the complex of values, ideas, attitudes, and meaningful symbols that a society creates to define and shape human behavior. A society transmits its culture from one generation to the next. Socialization is the process of learning basic values and orientations that prepare individuals to fit into their cultural milieu. Socialization occurs through the interaction of the individual with various agents in specific social settings. A socialization agent may be a person, such as a family member, friend, or teacher, or it may be a product of the mass media. These agents influence, on an on-going basis, the development of an individual's—and a society's—values and beliefs, even as new agents displace older ones. To understand the importance of the nurse's symbolic roles in the evolving health care system as well as the nurse's changing occupational prestige, we must examine how the image of the nurse has developed over time.

The assumptions underlying mass media presentations are often latent. They may not be immediately apparent to audiences and are often not recognized even by their creators. We can, however, identify these assumptions by analyzing the social structure and the patterns of social interaction that characterize the imaginary worlds that the mass media present. Mass media products explain social situations. Health care drama, as fiction, can provide the reader or viewer with a psychological portrait of a job incumbent—motives, attitudes, justifications, moral dilemmas, and so forth. Information of this type is rarely available firsthand, especially not to children and adolescents. Knowledge acquired through mass media fiction, once assimilated into a belief about a particular job, may remain as part of that belief until new information questions it. The media thus help indicate the elements which make for power, suc-

cess, and happiness in society and provide models for behavior.

Public opinion polls show that most of the new orientations and beliefs that adults acquire during their lifetime are also based on information supplied by the mass media. People do not necessarily adopt the precise attitudes and opinions that may be suggested by the media, but the media provide the basis for adjusting their existing attitudes and opinions to keep pace with a changing world. One must therefore credit the mass media with a sizable share of continuing socialization and resocialization about all aspects of nurses and nursing. The expressive nursing symbols, norms, values, and ideas that are part of our culture do not simply indicate or reflect current health care industry conditions. Ideas about nurses arising in one historical epoch are being transformed and, in turn, influence individuals and groups within a changed historical setting. Various forms of cultural expression provide resources of meaning that can be reinterpreted and adapted to new circumstances. Mass media drama is characterized by several features less common in firsthand, face-to-face contexts: (1) learning is more likely to be incidental than purposeful, (2) roles are stereotyped for recognizability, and (3) psychological motives are clear and unambiguous.

THE HEALTH CARE GENRE

A genre approach to entertainment mass media portrayals of nurses provides an effective means for understanding the nurse image formation process. A genre is a conventional system for structuring cultural products. Popular writers, directors, producers, and performers employ genres in the form of conventional formulas. These formulas provide standardized settings, situations, characters, and patterns of action. Such conventional systems in turn reflect patterns of games, rituals, dreams, symbols, and myths in the present and past of the larger cultural system.

The health care genre may be defined as encompassing all print and nonprint works that share a sufficient number of health care motifs, conventions, themes, stereotypes, and archetypes pertaining to nurses, so that they can be readily identified as products of this particular type. Taking into account not only the entrepreneurial and aesthetic aspects of the production of novels, feature films, and television series, but also the various other cultural aspects, the genre approach views the production of these entertainment products as a dynamic process among the publishing, film, and television industries, their audiences, and the nurses of the real world.

The argument that people consume these mass media health care messages as part of entertainment-seeking behavior is satisfactory as far as it goes, but it does not explain why certain forms like the health care genre persist, why others rise and fade, why both males and females respond equally to the health care genre but not to such alternatives as the gangster genre or the romance genre. Novel, film, and television health care genres occupy much of our entertainment time, yet little attention has been devoted to what this means for the public, for nurses, and for the health care industry. The health care genre can be thought of as a public dream. Like most dreams, its meaning is not obvious. But close analysis of this genre could reveal important aspects of our culture's subconscious.

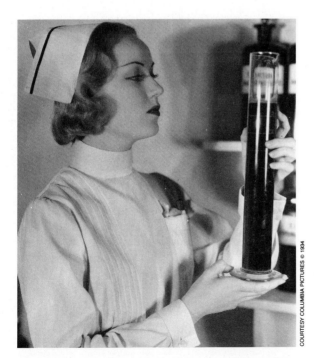

Analysis of mass media portrayals of nurses can bring to the surface ideas that are buried in our culture's subconscious.

The health care genre has both cultural and universal costs. A television series of today is related to archetypes of past centuries, folk tales, and myths. For example, the sexual division of labor that prevails in health care has deep roots in modern history and even reaching back to ancient and medieval times. It is interwoven with many other structural and functional characteristics of the present social organization, ingrained in attitudinal and behavioral patterns.

STEREOTYPES

The popular image of nursing at any given time is the result of a cluster of nurse stereotypes our culture uses to construct a symbolic reality. Stereotypes occur in day-to-day life as well as in mass media portrayals. Stereotyping is part of the normal process of developing categories, which enables people to impose a structure and meaning on events and objects. A stereotype, in addition to being familiar, also implies rigidity. But the type need not be identical each time. As long as certain aspects of the characterization are present, the audience supplies the rest. Sociologists consider stereotypical thinking necessary for society to create role models.

Stereotypes are a very simple, striking, easily-grasped form of representation but are nonetheless capable of condensing a great deal of complex information and a host of connotations. Some stereotypes may be false and have no objective behavioral data to support them. Other stereotypes may contain elements of truth but not take into account the individual differences in traits occurring within groups or the degree of overlap between groups. Stereotypes invoke consensus. They proclaim, "This is what everyone thinks members of such-and-such a social or occupational group are like." Stereotypes express a general agreement about a group, as if that agreement arose before, and independent of, the stereotype. Yet for the most part, it is *from* stereotypes that we derive ideas about social and occupational groups —not the other way around.

Shared myths and fantasies form part of the collective consciousness of modern societies. Contending groups may appropriate existing myths and symbols and utilize them for their own purposes. The stereotype- and archetype-laden health care genre is a social ritual that contributes to what might be called the contemporary American health care mythology. Much of this process is facilitated by mass media products that use the genre's visual coding of the narrative. Consumers distinguish between characters who are directly associated with positive health care outcomes and those who are not, those who are fairly autonomous problem solvers and those who are nearly always in dependent roles, those who are usually male and those who are overwhelmingly female. These distinctions reflect the thematic conflicts inherent in plots that are generally acted out in the form of a recital. Because visual coding involves narrative and social values, in nonprint media it also extends to such nonvisual aspects of production as dialogue, music, and even casting.

ICONOGRAPHY

In addressing the inherent meaning or intrinsic significance of objects such as the physician's lab coat, the nurse's white uniform, or the hospital's operating room table, we are considering the health care genre's iconography. Analysis of the genre's iconography involves the process of narrative and visual coding that results from the repetition of a ritualistic story. These objects are significant, in the same way that a white hat in a western or a top hat in a musical are significant, because they have come to serve a specific symbolic function within the narrative.

The health care genre's iconography reflects the values of our culture. The genre's implicit system of health care values and beliefs—its ideology or world view—has determined its cast of major and minor characters, its most important problems, and the preferred solutions to those problems. In short, the health care genre may be defined as a socioeconomic problem-solving enterprise. It repeatedly confronts ideological conflicts (opposing value systems) within the life and death confines of the health care arena, suggests various solutions through the actions of the major characters, and ultimately presents triumphs of life over death, good over evil, science over ignorance, or technology over faith. Thus the health care genre's problem-solving function affects its distinct formal and conceptual identity.

The nurse has come to form a substantial image in our culture, and an awareness of the symbolic role of the nurse in the evolving health care system reveals much about the nurse's changing status. To represent with images is to symbolize—a basic form

of communication. The mass media have an enormous impact on the formation of images. Kenneth Boulding calls the image the basis for human behavior in order to emphasize that it is "a subjective knowledge structure," not necessarily reflecting actuality in all of its components. Images are mental representations that influence how people see all aspects of life, including nurses and nursing. Images help people to achieve tangible goals, make judgments, and express themselves. Public images are "the basic bond of any society" and are produced by "sharing messages." Persons exchange images between each other by using symbols in both interpersonal and mass communication. According to Boulding, "behavior depends on the image," and in his view, messages change images, which in turn change behavior.[3]

Consumers are constantly developing symbolic conceptions about the health care world. Through language, science, art, and myth, for example, humans structure their health care world in mean-

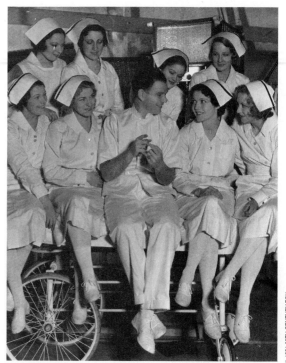

Through language, science, art, and myth, people structure their health care world in meaningful ways.

ingful ways. These attempts to objectify a reality embody subjective intentions implicit in the specific symbols used. Humans do not always acquire knowledge and understanding of the world through objective, external evidence; we often attempt to understand our world through essentially subjective processes. It is futile, therefore, to deplore the texts of the health care genre for their omissions, distortions, and conservative affirmations. We must instead strive to understand these texts and to let their very omissions and distortions tell us of the contradictions and fears they conceal.

The images found in popular culture are closely linked to political, economic, and social exigencies and provide a barometer of public opinion. Mass media products seethe with myths and heroes. They guide decisions, inform perceptions, and provide examples of appropriate behavior. Most Americans' current image of health care owes its origins to the heroic and self-perpetuating media messages about the miracles of modern medicine of the 1930s and 1940s: doctors at places like the Mayo Clinic could perform near miracles—mending broken bones, restoring lost eyesight, curing patients with otherwise fatal infections. Nurses know that these miracles are largely mythical. Life expectancy is not the longest in the country with the most advanced biomedical research or the greatest per capita expenditures on medical care. General health, morbidity rates, and life expectancy are influenced more by genetic, life-style, and environmental factors than by the advances of modern medicine. Yet the myths remain powerful, influencing occupational prestige as well as the allocation of scarce financial resources within the health care industry.

STUDY METHODS

The research methodology we used to study the image of the nurse in the mass media was content analysis, which is an application of scientific methods to documentary evidence. By objectively and systematically identifying characteristics of media depictions of nurses and nursing from 1850 to the present, inferences about the evaluation of the image emerged. As with all scientific inquiry, content analysis requires objectivity, a systematic approach, and the ability to generalize.

We used both quantitative and qualitative analysis methodology. By alternating between these approaches, we were able to gain a greater understanding of our subject: the qualitative analysis provided new insights that guided the quantitative analysis, and vice versa. In an effort to make this account useful to the widest group of nurses, we have not reported extensive statistical results. For readers who are interested in the more technical results of our research, we have included in the bibliography references to published journal articles that contain this information.

To conduct both the qualitative and quantitative content analysis, we employed three tools developed specifically for this project—the *Unit Analysis Tool,* the *Nurse Character Analysis Tool,* and the *Physician Character Analysis Tool.* The *Unit Analysis Tool,* used to study the overall dimensions of nurse characters, included items measuring overt actions of a group of characters, subjective impressions conveyed by the narrator's comments, behavior and attitudes of other characters toward nurse characters, and the situational contexts in which nurse characters were presented. (For the purposes of our study, a *unit* was the generic term used to describe an individual product of the mass media—a novel, a movie, or a television episode.) The *Nurse Character Analysis Tool,* used to study individual nurse characters, included items measuring the centrality and importance of a character in the plot, demographic profile data, general personality traits, and multiple aspects of a character's professional competence and conduct in the nurse role. The *Physician Character Analysis Tool* also contained demographic, personality trait, and professional competence profiles, as well as an assessment of the character's attitudes toward nurse characters, the nature of professional involvement with them, and preconceptions about nursing. The qualitative assessment concentrated on the character qua physician—its primary purpose to establish and evaluate the nature of his or her relationship with the unit's nurses.

Criteria were developed to guide the selection of units for the study. Novels were identified through a comprehensive examination of book reviews published between 1896 and 1982 in *The New York Times Book Review* and the reviews and notices appearing in *The Bookman* (1895–1933) and *Publisher's Weekly* (1912–1982). Motion pictures were identified by review of the cumulative reprints of the *New York Times Film Reviews, Variety Weekly Film Reviews,* the *American Film Institute Catalog of*

Motion Pictures, and through personal contact with public and private film archives. Prime-time television series with nurse characters were identified by a review of each weekly issue of *TV Guide* (New York City edition) published from 1950 to 1982. A 20 percent sample of the episodes was randomly selected from each series so that the representativeness of any given series in the sample corresponded to its duration on television. The total sample comprised 216 novels, 212 motion pictures, and 351 television episodes. A total of 726 nurse characters and 478 physician characters were analyzed.

The three analysis tools were applied by a group of coders recruited and trained specifically for the project. Intrarater reliability—the consistency with which a coder rated different units—was determined by having 5 percent of the sample coded twice several months apart by the same coder. Intrarater reliability across all coders and all items was 93.1 percent for motion pictures, 87.1 percent for novels, and 88.4 percent for television episodes. Interrater reliability—the consistency with which different coders rated the same units—was determined by having all coders analyze 20 percent of the units in the medium they were working on. Interrater agreement among all coders was 91.6 percent for motion pictures, 88.3 percent for novels, and 90.2 percent for television episodes.

Content validity was established by an inductive and additive process of classifying all aspects of the image of the nurse that were found to exist in the entertainment mass media until all categories of new phenomena were exhausted. The analysis tools were then reviewed by a panel of experts and modified before being used. Convergent validity was estimated by testing the ability of certain measurement items in the analysis tools to predict others in an expected or hypothesized fashion. For example, 92 percent of units coded as hospital dramas were also coded as showing nurses working in a hospital setting. One hundred percent of the nurse characters who stated that nursing constitutes a patriotic service were also coded as appearing in military drama or comedy. It was also found that nurses shown in administrative roles were also portrayed as having power and influence over others ($r = .54, p < .01$). There was a significant association between the extent to which nurse characters were seen helping patients and the degree to which they provided emotional support to patients and families ($r = .54, p < .01$).

PREVIEW OF THE FOLLOWING CHAPTERS

The experiment in which the children assumed that the man acting as a nurse had to be a physician exemplifies the power of sex-role stereotypes. What the children saw—a female physician and a male nurse—interfered with their normal cognitive patterns, so they refused to see it. The nurse has occupied a position of some emotional resonance in the public mind—a resonance based on the coming together of occupational and sexual stereotyping in the profession of nursing.

We initiated the study of the image of the nurse in the mass media in search of the symbols that express the evolving social perception of the nurse and of the profession of nursing. We have regarded the products of mass media as cultural indicators of the commonly accepted themes, symbols, concepts, styles, and sentiments associated with nursing in the mass society of the past century and a half. What emerged from our analysis were five dominant image types that are fundamentally characteristic of five successive periods of time: (1) the Angel of Mercy, 1854–1919; (2) the Girl Friday, 1920–1929; (3) the Heroine, 1930–1945; (4) the Mother, 1946–1965; and (5) the Sex Object, 1966–1982. These images epitomize the mode of thought and feeling about nurses that was inherent in the prevailing mass media entertainment and information messages of the day and, as such, constitute the nurse stereotypes fundamentally characteristic of their particular periods.

NOTES

1. Frank Mankiewicz and Joel Swerdlow, "Sex Roles in TV: Co-Opted Liberation," *Television Quarterly* 14 (Winter 1977–78):7.
2. *Newsday,* August 4, 1983.
3. Kenneth E. Boulding, *The Image: Knowledge in Life and Society* (Ann Arbor, Michigan: University of Michigan, 1956), p. 6.

CHAPTER TWO

ANGEL OF MERCY:
THE NINETEENTH CENTURY

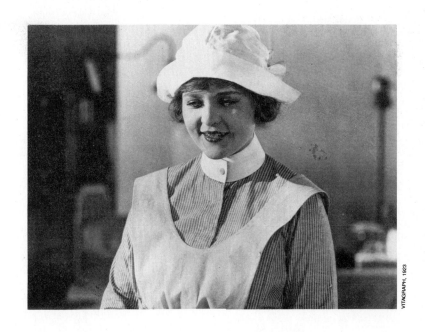

In colonial America and well into the nineteenth century, a woman had no legal existence except through her father or husband. She herself was devoid of both individual rights and responsibilities, with no legal control over her person, her property, or her own children. Moreover, formal education beyond the most elementary levels was closed to women. Only the wealthy and enlightened few provided their daughters with tutorial training at home, and it was almost impossible for a woman to acquire a formal college education. The vacuous but viable image of the genteel lady predominated. The prescriptive literature of the mid-nineteenth century told women that they should embody four critical qualities: piety, purity, submissiveness, and domesticity. Not all women manifested these four virtues, but the conventional wisdom was that they should strive to attain them.

THE VICTORIAN LADY

In the early- and mid-Victorian years, literature of advice directed at adolescent girls was emphatically explicit about one central feature of the adult role:

being a Victorian lady meant accepting limits and restraints and recognizing male superiority. In adolescence, the testing ground for adulthood, girls were to accept that they must keep a tight rein on both their aspirations and their behavior. Whereas adolescent boys were encouraged to develop their independence, adolescent girls were encouraged to accept dependence on the male as a natural and inevitable part of the female condition, and were prepared for a subordinate position in relationship to males.

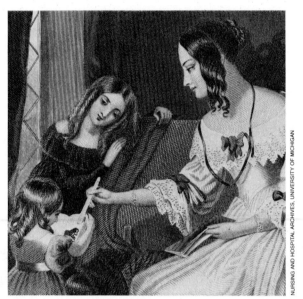

The Victorian middle-class girl was supposed to be preparing herself for the adult roles of wife and mother.

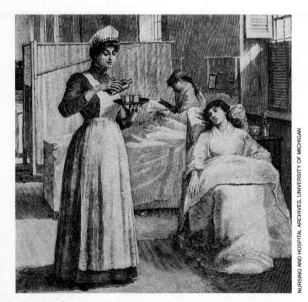

The Victorian sentimentalization of femininity coincided with the professionalization of nursing in the late-nineteenth century and led to the prevalent image of the nurse as ministering angel.

The adult role for which the Victorian middle-class girl was supposed to be preparing herself was that of wife and mother. The innate qualities of women supposedly suited them for their place in the home— and nowhere else. Within the home a woman performed a spiritual function, ennobling the characters of her husband and sons so that they went out into the world as better, finer persons than they otherwise would have. As for her daughters, a woman prepared them to become high priestesses in their turn by training them in all that was "truly womanly."

Even in the early- and mid-Victorian decades, it was acknowledged that a girl would need some education to provide her home with the refinements of intellectual culture. But early- and mid-Victorian advice books took pains to emphasize that girls should always keep in mind the ultimate purpose of their education: to make them pleasant and useful companions to men and responsible mothers to their children. (When the first women's college, Vassar, opened in 1865, its administrators were sternly warned by a host of doctors of the dangers associated with attempts to educate women as if they were men. Since women's bodies were generally seen as a battleground between the uterus and the brain, one doctor concluded that educating women would lead to the atrophy of the uterus.) The ideal Victorian lady spoke at least one foreign language, preferably French, and spiced her conversation with foreign words, could recite and discuss popular poetry, and could play the piano for the entertainment of family and friends. In addition, true ladies wept copiously at any pathetic, emotional, or embarrassing moment, and fainted when the emotion was too taxing.

A further source of frustration for Victorian women was the elaborate and constricted courtship procedures, based on the assumption that women must be protected unceasingly and strenuously from the advances of men who might have less than honorable intentions. In practical terms, these procedures only increased the difficulties of women's attaining the one goal, marriage, that was acknowledged to be rightfully theirs. Indeed, it was not maidenly to admit, even to themselves, that this was their goal. And the urgency of marriage for women was cloaked by the highly romanticized convention that men were overwhelmed by their good fortune in winning one of these pure, beautiful, angelic female creatures. Moreover, the flowery posturings of adoration and respect men paid to woman provided poor preparation for the emotional and physical realities of marriage. Emma Bovary flourished in America as well as in France, with as unhappy if not always as dramatic results.

Victorian clothing both identified gender and defined gender roles. Men were serious, so they wore dark colors and little ornamentation; women were frivolous, so they wore light pastel colors, ribbons, lace, and bows. Men were active, so their clothes allowed them movement; women were inactive, so their clothes inhibited movement. Men were strong, so their clothes emphasized broad chests and shoulders; women were delicate, so their clothing accentuated tiny waists, sloping shoulders, and a

softly rounded silhouette. Men were aggressive, so their clothing had sharp, definite lines and a clearly defined silhouette; women were submissive, so their silhouette was indefinite, their clothing constricting.

Beyond the incommodious encumbrances of crinolines and trains, the restraining fetters of tight skirts and sleeves, the item of clothing that directly and graphically disciplined women to their submissive role was the corset. The wearing of the laced corset was almost universal in England and America throughout the nineteenth century. It was designed to change the configuration of the body to accord more closely with the feminine ideal of the small waist that haunted the period. It exaggerated the differences in male and female anatomy by constricting the waist and enlarging the hips and bust. It also constricted the diaphragm, forcing women to breathe from the upper part of the chest—thus the peculiarly feminine heaving of bosoms so lovingly

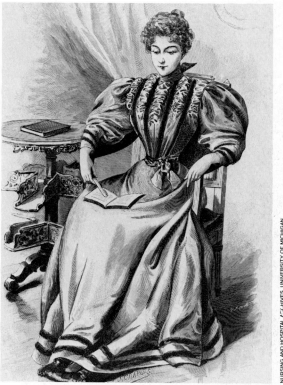

The degree of physical debility caused by the corset depended on how tightly it was laced.

described in popular novels. The degree of physical debility caused by the corset depended on how tightly it was laced. And this varied throughout the century according to the changing proportions of waist size, sleeves, and skirt that defined the fashionable silhouette.

Society in general did not know that there was cause for unhappiness among women. Women seemed better off than they had ever been: life was certainly easier for them than it had been under pioneer conditions. The image of the genteel lady, of the woman radiating love and spirituality within her home, was not without its seductions. It was safe, unchallenging, and comfortable. The genteel lady was guided by spiritual and religious precepts in all her activities and did her duty as these precepts demanded. The unmarried woman remained within the protection of her home, meeting only the people her family considered appropriate. Her finer moral constitution made her shrink from contact with the sordid aspects of the world outside her quiet hearth. Men owed her beautiful, almost holy innocence the homage of shielding her from those sordid aspects. Moreover, her frail physical constitution rendered her incapable of dealing with the rough hustle and bustle of that outside world. She shunned employment outside her home because it was fraught with the dangers of meeting unprincipled people and endangered her person and her status as a lady. She was not strong enough to enter public life, to vote, to hold a job, or to be too highly educated.

DEFICIENCIES IN HEALTH CARE

One hundred fifty years ago, the best nursing care consisted of commonsensible, supportive home nursing carried out by relatives who basically facilitated nature's own cure. For the ordinary citizen, the comfort of one's own family was the normal recourse in times of accident or sickness. The art of medicine could do little but set bones, amputate limbs, pull teeth, vaccinate against smallpox, and assist with childbirth. The few drugs physicians prescribed were nonspecific and often given in debilitating dosages. And the nineteenth-century custom of drawing blood and purging bowels harmed the sick more than it helped them.

Medicine had struggled along for centuries on sheer guesswork and the crudest sort of empiricism. Virtually anything that could be thought up for the treatment of disease was tried at one time or another—and often used for decades before being given up. It was, in retrospect, the most frivolous and irresponsible kind of human experimentation, based on nothing but trial and error, and usually resulting in precisely that sequence. Not only bleeding, purging, and cupping, but also the administration of every known plant, solutions of every known metal, every conceivable diet including total fasting—most of these treatments based on the strangest imaginings about the cause of disease, concocted out of nothing but thin air—this was the heritage of medicine in the mid-nineteenth century.

The larger cities like Philadelphia, New York, and Boston established hospitals to care for those outside the ministrations of family nursing: migrants, sailors, the elderly, the mentally ill, and the sick poor. As custodians of the homeless and castoffs, these early hospitals provided nursing care that fell far short of contemporary home care standards. Except in the few hospitals staffed by Catholic orders, nurses were women of the lowest status with little opportunity for other employment—they were retired prostitutes or former felons. Hospital funds were always short, rooms overcrowded, and the environment unsanitary. In the absence of special operating and treatment rooms and anesthesia, the screams of the patients echoed through the wards. Under such conditions, alcohol, then a major hospital remedy, was perhaps the most humane prescription.

The nominal heads of the untrained nursing staffs in voluntary hospitals were the matrons. Some had been upper servants in the households of persons connected with the hospitals, through whom they obtained their posts. They were essentially chief housekeepers, who hired and were supposed to supervise all the nurses and other hospital servants. The head nurses assumed such domestic duties as caring for the linen and supervising the cooking in their wards. They also accompanied doctors on their daily rounds to receive orders regarding treatment and medicines and were thus directly responsible for the care of patients. In addition to tending their patients, staff nurses scrubbed and cleaned the wards and bathrooms, made beds, cleaned utensils, washed bandages, cooked for the patients and hospital staff, and washed the dishes. Head nurses were usually on call at all times and slept in rooms adjacent to their wards. Staff nurses served for fourteen or fifteen hours at a stretch and slept in basement rooms or in cupboards on the stairs or sometimes even in the wards.

The best hospital matrons tried to select as head nurses and staff nurses women of good character, preferably with some hospital experience. But the difficulty of attracting applicants was usually so great that women had to be accepted without any testimonials. Ordinary nurses were for the most part rough, dull, unobservant, and poorly educated women. It was not uncommon to see nurses returning late at night from the public houses to the hospitals, drunken and rowdy. Nurses often smuggled supplies of spirits into hospitals in defiance of the strict rules against the practice, or simply appropriated for themselves the supplies then prescribed in considerable quantities to patients. An equally grave and very common charge against nurses was sexual promiscuity. Nurses came into daily contact with male physicians, surgeons, medical students, and patients, who were generally presumed to be both a corrupting influence on them and easy prey to unprincipled and immoral women.

Such women were hardly noted for their kindly attentiveness to patients. Indeed, they often took their patients' pillows, blankets, and food for their own use. Under these circumstances, families, friends, and even doctors of patients frequently bribed nurses with money and drink to insure that their charges received good care.

People entering hospitals for the first time were often overcome with nausea because of the so-called "hospital smell," then considered unavoidable but actually the result of unsanitary conditions. The wards were bare and gloomy, poorly heated and ventilated, crammed with beds that were sometimes dirty and vermin-infested, peopled by patients of the poorest classes who were sometimes drunk and disorderly, and periodically swept by epidemics that killed large numbers of both patients and nurses. The mid-nineteenth-century hospital not only failed to provide diagnoses or treatments that were significantly better than those available at home, but also exposed patients to the added danger of infections generated within its walls. With infectious diseases rampant and hospital epidemics unchecked, going into the hospital seemed and often was the equivalent of a death sentence. Hospitals deserved their popular reputation as places where shiploads of sick immigrants were dumped and where the poor went to die.

Taking all of these factors into account—family nursing, the undeveloped science of medicine, and the presence of unsanitary hospitals staffed with untrained nurses—existing health care presented a highly tenuous response to accident and disease. In 1985 the national death rate stood at about eight per thousand inhabitants. In 1900 it was seventeen and in New York prior to the Civil War, records indicate that it fluctuated between twenty-six and forty-one. Infants and children were in the greatest jeopardy, suffering about two-thirds of each year's deaths. Yet the public was not concerned about the high rate of child mortality and morbidity or even the major causes of adult death and sickness—tuberculosis, typhoid, and dysentery. People simply accepted these diseases as necessary hazards of life.

SAIRY GAMP: EPITOME OF AN UNTRAINED NURSE

In the mid-nineteenth century, two opposing conceptions of the nurse image were epitomized by two media-created nurses: Sairy Gamp, the alcoholic hag immortalized by Charles Dickens in *Martin Chuzzlewit,* and Florence Nightingale, the real-life heroine immortalized by reporter William Howard Russell in his articles in the *London Times.* Indeed, both figures contributed to the rapid revision of nursing's public image in the 1850s: Florence Nightingale's service to the profession, which will be dealt with in the next section, and the caricature of Sairy Gamp, which helped clear the way for Nightingale's seminal contribution to nursing. S. Squire Sprigge, a physician-author of Dickens's own day, noted that

> With regard to the nurses, Dickens . . . helped in a very pronounced degree to rescue society from the ministration of the hopeless class into whose hands the calling of nursing was committed. Society owes Dickens a double debt, for having buried the nurse-hag under inextinguishable laughter.[1]

Sairy Gamp epitomized the nurses of the day who lived and worked in appalling surroundings, whose work was considered a particularly repugnant form of domestic service for which little or no education or special training was necessary, and whose living

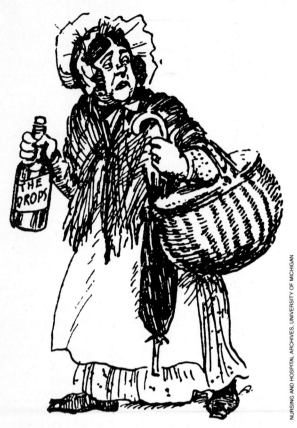

Sairy Gamp epitomized the nurses of the day, who lived and worked in appalling surroundings and whose work was considered a particularly repugnant form of domestic service for which little or no education or special training was necessary.

NURSING AND HOSPITAL ARCHIVES, UNIVERSITY OF MICHIGAN

enjoys a lying-in or a laying-out equally: "And it is precisely this indiscriminate 'zest and relish' that makes her both so funny and so frightening."[2]

DICKENS FOSTERS NURSING REFORM

As the most popular novelist of his age, Charles Dickens did much to influence the public's attitude on matters of health care and social reform. Through his satirical punches at inept government bureaucrats, Dickens uncovered the corruption and stagnation of nineteenth-century English politics. During the nineteenth century, effective sanitation and health measures were slowly being developed by nontraditional physicians and other experimental scientists. But these measures could not be implemented without government support, and consistent aid was almost impossible to obtain, for it was a heroic task even to attract the government's attention.

Dickens's essay, "The Nurse in Leading Strings," published in *Household Words,* begins with a comparative study of the use of the word *nurse* in various European languages. All the major European languages use some term equivalent to the English *nurse* to represent the woman who suckles, or nourishes, a newborn infant. Once an infant has been weaned, however, a different noun is used in certain languages to describe the governess or caretaker of a young child—for example, in French a *nourrice* becomes a *bonne.* In English, however, governesses are also known as nurses. In addition, English transfers the idea of nursing an infant to the broader meaning of nursing the sick, as Dickens explains: "We transfer our homely word with its fond meaning to the occupation of those who should cherish and sustain the sick by their good offices; we talk of nursing the sick." The Germans, on the other hand, speak of "waiting to perform their duty by [the sick]," while the French "watch over" their sick. Linguistically, English also makes use of the verb *nurse* in such contexts as nursing a cough, a grudge, or even a beverage. Obviously, the word *nurse* has great significance for English-speaking people. According to Dickens, the occupation of the hired nurse had caused the otherwise sacred significance of the word to suffer: "We English people, be that as it may, have among us the best nursing for love and the worst nursing for money that can be got in Europe, though our women are all nurses born."[3]

was meager indeed. Motivated by the desire to make money rather than by affection or self-sacrifice, these nurses drank and took snuff, were personally unclean and untidy, lacked delicacy, discretion, tact, and concern for their patients, and were generally unreliable and abusive. Sairy Gamp holds a patient's nose in order to pour medicine roughly down his throat, and having provided herself with her favorite food and drink—gin, tea, and cucumbers—steals his pillow to make herself comfortable for the night, which she spends sleeping instead of watching over him. Falsely sentimental, gossipy, and as uncultivated in her speech as in her person, she is at her most sinister as a "performer of nameless offices about the persons of the dead." Minimally acquainted with and meddling in the mysteries of birth and death, she

Following this linguistic exercise, Dickens reviews a pamphlet written by Florence Nightingale discussing the role of the nineteenth-century woman. Entitled *Cassandra,* this pamphlet is a passionate protest against the constraints to which early-Victorian girls and young women of the middle and upper classes were subjected.

> What form do the Chinese feet assume when denied their proper development? If the young girls of the "higher classes"... were to speak, and say what are their thoughts employed upon, their *thoughts* which alone are free, what would they say?[4]

Nightingale was already in her early thirties when she wrote *Cassandra,* but her status was still that of a girl. She was still restricted by the demands of her family, still "chained to the bronze pedestal," as she herself put it. For Florence Nightingale, the family and its demands were a pernicious force, sapping her strength, time, and talents.

> The family uses people, *not* for what they are, nor for what they are intended to be, but for what it wants

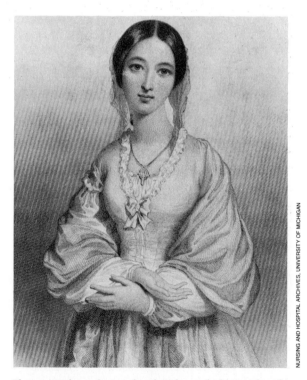

Florence Nightingale was already in her early thirties when she wrote Cassandra, *but her status was still that of a girl.*

NURSING AND HOSPITAL ARCHIVES, UNIVERSITY OF MICHIGAN

them for—its own uses. ... If it wants someone to sit in the drawing-room, *that* someone is supplied by the family, though that member may be destined for science, or for education, or for active superintendence by God, i.e., by the gifts within.[5]

According to Nightingale, all women desired to participate in some purposeful activity. Most women regarded marriage, home, and family as the preferable means of living an active life. For those who chose not to marry, Nightingale pointed out that, historically, caring for the sick and the poor has been considered women's natural vocation.

Dickens relates how nurses first began receiving systematic training by summarizing in his article the work of Pastor Fliedner, in Kaiserwerth, Germany, who wanted to help released women prisoners learn some useful occupation. In 1834 Fliedner opened an infant school that provided teacher training and established a hospital with a nurse training program. It was here that Florence Nightingale received her training. Like the Kaiserwerth Institution, the London training school for nurses, Saint John's House at Westminster, was also associated with a church, in this case the Church of England. The hospital had a strict hierarchical structure, and nurses were expected to cultivate patience, skilled observation, a sense of duty, and "strict military obedience." It seemed quite clear to Dickens that as women began to be paid for their work as nurses, the community fathers scrutinized them more closely. Nursing was no longer seen as a natural vocation, but as a socially necessary occupation.[6]

Dickens's discussion of comparative linguistics illustrates the unique and complex emotions associated with the terms *nurse* and *nursing* in the English language. Because nursing was associated with maternity care, women were expected to show the same love and devotion to complete strangers that they naturally showed to their own children. Because many hospitals were first staffed by Catholic nuns who had taken vows of poverty, all nurses were expected to work not for monetary gain, but from some sort of religious inspiration. This strict literal and historical interpretation of the term *nurse* was unfair. Florence Nightingale and Pastor Fliedner had proved that women were not born nurses but that nursing was an acquired skill.[7]

During the Christmas season of 1855, Dickens published an essay in the popular journal *Household Words* discussing the etymology of the words *hospi-*

tal and *hospitality,* along with the history of hospitals for the sick in Europe from their beginnings through the nineteenth century. The Latin *hospes* signified a guest. *Jupiter Hospitalis* was the patron of all such guests. In a Roman house the guest chamber was called the *hospitale.* According to the ancient Greeks, a guest ought to be received warmly because he or she might actually be a visiting god. The first hospital for the sick was established at the temple of Aesculapius at Epidaurus, for it was there that the sick regularly clustered—and died. The early hospitals were places of prayer and frequently were located at healing springs, such as the pool of Bethesda in Jewish tradition.[8]

The philosophy of Christian hospitality can be traced back to the Book of Acts of the Apostles, in which the early Church established procedures to care for widows, orphans, the sick, and the poor. At first food and alms were distributed from one large building so that many persons could be helped at once. Soon, however, bishops and saints, such as St. Basil and St. John Chrysostom, founded other hospitals to care not only for the poor but also for travelers. By the eleventh century, monasteries took over the care of the sick, and specialized hospitals were established to care for lepers, foundlings, and wounded soldiers.

In Victorian England, hospitals received a small endowment from government funds but were in the main supported by charitable contributions. Dickens applauded the work of the hospitals and gave special praise to those members of the medical profession who directed them. He announced that Florence Nightingale had offered to serve the London poor in the same capacity as she had once served the wounded soldiers in the Crimean War. Her ambitions were to train other women to become nurses and to supervise a hospital. Instead of simply pointing out that most nurses were inadequate and clumsy at their trade, Dickens drew a correlation between such inadequacy and the poor pay that nurses received. He suggested that London establish a training school for nurses under Nightingale's direction. As an advocate of social reform, Dickens recognized the value of having Florence Nightingale—an acknowledged heroine—direct a nurse training school. His timing for the publication of the essay and the plea—the Christmas season and the proximity of the Crimean War—was politically astute.

FLORENCE NIGHTINGALE

No one contributed as much to the development of nursing care as Florence Nightingale. She actively campaigned for and nearly single-handedly developed and implemented an educational program for nursing, thus raising nursing from a loathsome, ill-regulated occupation to a respected profession composed of educated women specifically qualified to practice nursing. No other nurse—perhaps no other woman—has so quickened the imagination and gratitude of a people as did Nightingale.

Nightingale's accomplishments loom all the larger in view of the great difficulties under which she labored. The original plan in 1854 was for her to take a party of forty nurses to the British military hospitals of the Crimean War. But in all of Britain only thirty-eight suitable women could be found who were willing to go—ten Catholic nuns, fourteen Anglican sisters, and fourteen hospital nurses—and Nightingale considered only sixteen of them really efficient. Other nurses later joined the original number, so by the end of the war Nightingale had had a total of 125 nurses under her supervision. The members of the religious orders acquitted themselves well on the whole, but the hospital nurses, attracted only by the prospect of good pay, proved utterly unfit, and a number had to be sent home for insubordination, drunkenness, and immoral conduct.

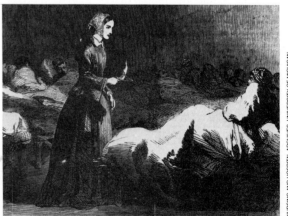

Nightingale gave to the nursing profession both an unprecedented degree of public respect and acceptance and a new and abiding symbol of excellence.

Nevertheless, Nightingale's achievements at Scutari Hospital during the Crimean War were astounding. Her later career, though somewhat less dramatic, was no less innovative or significant for the fields of nursing, health care, and hospital planning. Her effect upon the profession of nursing was immeasurable; indeed, her very name is still synonymous with the word *nurse.* Nightingale gave to the nursing profession both an unprecedented degree of public respect and acceptance and a new and abiding symbol of excellence.

THE ANGEL OF MERCY IMAGE IN POETRY

Unsurprisingly, Florence Nightingale often found herself a subject for creative artists, especially poets. Most of these poets wrote specifically about her, yet her influence was so pervasive that there is a close correspondence between the direct poetic image of Nightingale and the generally more implicit image of nursing. In 1857 American poet Henry Wadsworth Longfellow wrote a tribute to Nightingale in his well-known poem "Santa Filomena," published in the *Atlantic Monthly.* Here the poet speaks explicitly of the "lady with a lamp." Moreover, by identifying her with Saint Filomena, Longfellow makes use of the popular conception of Nightingale as the "saint of the Crimea."[9]

The poem opens with a statement of the inspiring and enlightening quality of noble deeds and thoughts. The presence, real or imagined, of "deeper souls" lifts the spirit from mean notions and superficial cares. This angelic imagery is emphasized by the reenactment of a scene that had been popularized for British readers through a celebrated newspaper account of Scutari Hospital.

> And slow, as in a dream of bliss
> The speechless sufferer turns to kiss
> Her shadow, as it falls
> Upon the darkening walls.

We are told here that she passed like a vision, as if a "door to heaven," left momentarily ajar, were suddenly shut. Longfellow calls Nightingale "A noble type of good,/Heroic womanhood"—a woman fit to carry the symbols once borne by Saint Filomena: the palm of peace, the lily of Christian love and mercy, and the spear of courage and determination. Longfel-

low's symbols of saintliness serve to reinforce the imagery of nobility, heroism, and self-sacrifice.[10]

Nightingale's "shadow" reappears, this time as the central image, in Elizabeth Stuart Phelps's poem "Her Shadow," published in the July 1906 issue of the *Atlantic Monthly.* This is really a poem within a poem, framed by a brief first-person introduction and a brief conclusion. In between lies a long descriptive poem entitled "Crimea," which differs from the framing sections in several important ways including point of view, for it has no self-conscious narrator.

The opening lines of the introduction tell us: "Old is the body of the tale; but, told anew,/Its fair elusive spirit floats from me to you." The "you" here is Florence Nightingale, not the reader. And it is Nightingale whom the speaker addresses in observing that it was a "dead wind which woke, and/slept, and blew/Our lives together, but to lash them straight apart." The "dead wind" that both unites and separates them is the Crimean War.[11]

The inner poem, "Crimea," now begins, and after a few words of introduction to the deplorably inadequate hospital conditions there (men were "shattered and bleeding and rent" and "mowed" and "heaped"), the poem introduces Florence Nightingale.

> Sweetest of women was she,
> First of the mild ministry
> Mercy of Heaven has sent
> Into the hospital tent.

This messianic imagery is reiterated a few lines later: those who were able, "worshiping, called after her." In an analogy particularly suggestive of her compassion, sensitivity, and humaneness, the poet equates Nightingale's suffering at Scutari to that of the wounded. "Gashed by the sight of that hell,/As flesh by the shot and the shell,/Spendthrift of mercy she gave."[12]

The intimation of religious faith in the lines "He went through a motherly land/Who passed with a hand in her hand" and "His face was the peacefulest there/Who died in the arms of her prayer" suggests again for Nightingale a saintly, even Christ-like image.[13] The following stanza brings her a bit closer to earth, however, for in it we read of the human limits of her work. Even Nightingale's tenderness and strength have bounds, and there are simply too many wounded. She is forced to ignore hundreds of them, a denial to which the men respond in the by now familiar way.

> Upon our pillows then we kissed
> Her shadow as it fell.
> She passed us by, and so we kissed
> Her shadow where it fell.[14]

The inner poem, "Crimea," now finished, the narrator/poet speaks again in several concluding lines. He—the speaker seems to be male—exclaims, "Dearest and lost!" and calls Nightingale the "eidolon" (phantom or ideal) of his every dream and the "sweetest" of his memories. This imagery suggests a love more amatory than spiritual and recalls the passionate quality of some biblical language. Indeed, an alternation between religious and romantic love suffuses this final section of the poem. The narrator describes Nightingale now as "Monarch uncrowned upon my soul's high, vacant throne," and in the next line as "Queen of royal joys to be unknown!"[15]

The final passages of "Her Shadow" explain what has gone before. The speaker reveals that he was once among Nightingale's wounded and that he once clasped her shadow as she passed. "Now," he tells us, "a warrior wounded and unhealed I lie;/Upon the empty pillow of my life I press/The shadow of a kiss. Trust in its sacredness." What is the reader to make of this? On a literal level, the narrator's wounds—including a strongly implied and well-known malady of the heart—have never healed. His life has been wasted by war, and Nightingale serves for him as a distant kind of spiritual ideal. And although she is "unconscious" of him and his feelings, the sense of a spirit (soul, eidolon, shadow, and so forth) is everywhere in these verses.[16]

However we read this poem, the image of Nightingale is clear: she is a savior worthy of worship, a saint characterized by mercy and tenderness, and, as the poet states, she is but the first of her kind. The imagery of saintliness used by Phelps and other poets is meant to illuminate both Nightingale and the modern profession of which she was and is the transcendent symbol. Interestingly, these poems attempt to equate the struggles and achievements of Nightingale and the Scutari Hospital nurses with heroism and sacrifice of the wounded men they served.

Victorian poet R. N. Cust's "Scutari Hospital" offers what seems to have been the conventional poetic image of Nightingale as angel while it also invokes her as a symbol for the best kind of nurse. Scutari's

nurses, he writes, can be seen "Flitting like angels/ From bed to bed" and "Wiping the clammy brows/ With tender hands." The wounded men are "Moaning in agony,/Writhing in pain," and their tears, in the standard cliché, pour "like rain." Yet the steady, compassionate work of the nurses elicits "Many a blessing,/Many a prayer . . . from rough lips for/Those angels there." While the poet here employs the familiar metaphors of angel or spirit (the nurse) and worshipper (the wounded soldiers), he also makes every effort to equate the earthly struggles and contributions of the two.[17]

PUBLIC REACTION TO FLORENCE NIGHTINGALE

Florence Nightingale had returned to England to find herself a heroine. But she never enjoyed her fame and disliked the sentimental reverence that her name inspired. The only testimonial she would accept was a fund, heavily subscribed to by the public and named in her honor, that she was to use to found the training school for nurses. Originally she hoped to establish an entirely new institution and direct its work personally, but ill health and the pressure of other business forced her instead to work through existing hospitals and other persons. Accordingly, she entered into negotiations that led in 1860 to the founding of the Nightingale School at St. Thomas's Hospital in London, under the direction of a committee nominated by her.

Florence Nightingale, in her *Notes on Nursing* (1859) and in a number of papers on sanitary reform submitted to the government, enunciated her philosophy of nursing and stated the rules under which the institution bearing her name should run. She denounced the prevailing notion that any woman, or at least any good woman, could be a good nurse. "Nursing is an art; and if it is to be made an art, requires as exclusive a devotion, as hard a preparation, as any painter's or sculptor's; for what is the having to do with dead canvas or cold marble, compared with having to do with the living body—the temple of God's spirit?" Under existing circumstances, Nightingale's most revolutionary proposal was that nurses should not be subject to the hospital directors, nor to the doctors, except in strictly medical questions. Instead, they should be under the absolute command and control of the hospital matron, who would both oversee their training and supervise their subsequent nursing work. Nursing was women's work, and women must reform it.[18]

An unsigned review in the *Saturday Review* of January 21, 1860, expressed undiluted praise for Nightingale's *Notes on Nursing* ("it is pervaded by power and wisdom and true goodness"), for her nursing work (her expedition to Scutari was "the single bright spot in one of our gloomiest national reminiscences"), and for her character (Englishmen will always remember "with pride and gratitude how the exigencies of a great crisis were bravely and successfully met by her genius, experience, and resolution").[19]

The language of *Notes on Nursing*—described here as "grave, earnest, and impetuous"—struck the reviewer as appropriate to one who had survived and helped others survive the innumerable sufferings of illness and war. In the process of giving "hints for thought to women who have personal charge of the health of others," Nightingale revealed the difficulty of the nurse's task. As to the specific matters of open windows, fresh air, and cleanliness, she endorsed opinions that, the reviewer hoped, were beginning to find general acceptance throughout Britain.

The review devoted perhaps half its length to a summary of Nightingale's theories on ventilation, pure water and good drainage, noise, interruption, visual variety, and bedside conversation. The reviewer observed that "it is in the petty management of the sick that Miss Nightingale's suggestions seem to us the most interesting"—an attitude that Nightingale herself would surely have found gratifying. Ventilation was "the first grand necessity. Children's nurseries and schoolrooms, close dormitories, crowded hospital wards, unaired cottages, are often mere hotbeds where the body is ripened for death, and slight forms of sickness are matured into worse." The reviewer further explained that carpets, musty paper hangings, and dark rooms were very often the real and ordinary causes of attacks customarily regarded as "mysterious visitations."[20]

Of all of Nightingale's topics, the matter of noises and interruptions received here the most extensive treatment. The reviewer remarked that Nightingale offered "a capital philosophy of noises, for which we are sure she is entitled to the eternal gratitude of every invalid." The good nurse avoided creaking, rattling, rustling, lingering, and surprise; she possessed

a firm hand and a light, quick step. The visitor to the sick "should neither fidget about the room, nor show symptoms of inattention, nor occupy a position where the sick man can only look at him by a painful effort."[21]

This same measure of thoughtfulness and attention should be observed in the decor of the sick room. Variety was the secret to cheerfulness and, to some extent, recovery. "The craving for variety in the starving eye," wrote the reviewer, "is just as keen a feeling as the craving of the starving body for food, and it is the greatest cruelty to refuse it indulgence." As monotony "is painful to the eye, so are chattering hopes and advices" to the ear. "Silly unadvised encouragement" will both exhaust the invalid and burden him or her with a sense of isolation. The best sympathy lies instead in the sharing of pleasant and practical information. The reviewer recommended *Notes on Nursing* to every hospital, workhouse, school, and nursery in the kingdom, suggest-

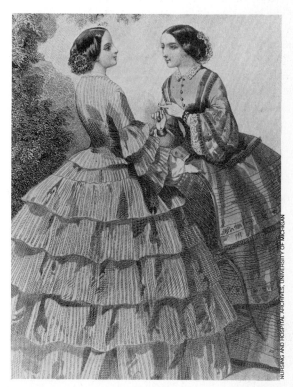

The best sympathy lies in the sharing of pleasant and practical information.

ing with some irony that "village girls" might more profitably study Nightingale than the infamously arcane schoolbook topics of history and geography. Even men, the reviewer concluded, had much to gain from a reading of *Notes on Nursing*.[22]

Florence Nightingale won a unique position during the Crimean War, and for the next forty years she used her great prestige as an adviser on matters of government health policy. She made nursing into a respectable profession that women could join without being taken for the drunken Sairy Gamp of Dickens's novel. She also made nursing scientific. At a time when doctors had very few drugs and anesthetics, nursing was even more important for patients' survival than it now is. "Nightingale nurses," instructed according to her principles, steadily raised hospital standards in England and in other countries. These nurses were still not well paid, however, partly because people thought of nursing as a way of life for devoted women with private means like Florence Nightingale herself, and partly because of the situation on the continent of Europe, where orders of nuns worked as nurses under vows of poverty.

PROFESSIONAL NURSING COMES TO AMERICA

Florence Nightingale's influence spread to the United States: in 1872 the New England Hospital for Women and Children offered a course in nursing, and the Bellevue Training School in New York City, the first American school organized on the Nightingale plan, admitted its first class in 1873. Nursing gradually ceased to be an occupation only for undesirables and members of religious orders. It matured instead into a suitable occupation for those educated middle-class and working-class women seeking independent roles in a society that had formerly offered them little work outside the factory, shop, school, or home.

"Training-Schools for Nurses," an unsigned eight-page essay, appeared in the December 1874 issue of the popular *Fraser's Magazine*. Writing in support of hospital-based training schools and homes for nurses, the author argued: (1) that there was a great need for trained nurses all over the world, (2) that this need could be met only by nurse training schools, (3) that such schools would provide not only proper training but many services and protec-

tions for both nurses and patients, and (4) that "the welfare of such training schools is worthy of the attention and liberality of the intelligent and benevolent"—in other words, that such schools deserved charitable contributions.[23]

This author suggested a number of reasons for the shortage of nurses, all of which could be remedied by the institution of nurse training schools. Nursing had been found variously repulsive, overly laborious (so taxing, in fact, that the average nursing career lasted no more than ten years), and miserably paid. Others had decided against a career in nursing because of the grim future awaiting the "so frequently incapacitated or superannuated nurse." Moreover, the work style of the average private duty nurse placed her, when out of an assignment, at the mercy of boardinghouse keepers who often required extra payment for the privilege (necessary for the private nurse) of surrendering lodgings at short notice.

By elevating nursing to the dignity of a profession, by providing enough hands to divide the labor, by making remuneration more secure, and by offering a year-round nurses' home for both active and retired nurses, the hospital training school would serve not only to attract women into nursing but to enhance the quality of nursing care.

Is it not a charity in the first place to see that the sick and suffering, whether rich or poor, are as well taken care of as the science and knowledge of the day will admit? Is it not a charity to furnish one way more for good, well-disposed women to earn their living honorably and usefully, when so many of them are now helpless and discouraged?[24]

While this author clearly recognized the importance of good nursing care, he or she evidenced a limited respect not only for the professional standing of nursing but for the character of women in general. The author defined nursing as "merely the care of the sick, and a nurse is a useful assistant when one is ill; a kind of servant under the doctor's orders." The author added that general opinion had altered of late, moving towards a definition of nursing as "an art, and the well-being of the nurse a public question."[25]

These latter concerns reflect fairly accurately the general tone of this article. The author of the essay wrote thoughtfully and with compassion of the concerns of the working nurse and seemed to be uncommonly and refreshingly sensitive to these concerns. Yet the quality that most often appears here in association with good nurses and nursing is *discipline*. "The greatest trial to many who would be nurses," wrote the author, "is the necessity of implicit obedience to the orders of superiors." Although these orders were "often arbitrary and peremptory," it was nevertheless not for the nurse to question them. Her place was "to do what she is told, and never complain or disobey." Furthermore, it was the quality of "implicit obedience to authority which proves the sincerity of purpose and abnegation of self essential in a good nurse."[26]

The author of "Sick Nurses," one M. Trench, shares with the author of the previous essay a humane concern about the shortage of nurses, but his emphasis lies less on the work and welfare of private nurses than on the proper training and performance of those nurses who serve in hospitals. Writing for the September 1876 issue of *MacMillan's Magazine,* Trench characterized nursing as a work "most blessed in itself," but "needing special watchfulness and thoughtful arrangements"—meaning thorough training. Contrary to much contemporary misapprehension on the subject of the necessity of training for nurses, Trench quoted Mr. Bonham Carter, Secretary of the Nightingale Fund.

> Whatever gift any one may have for nursing, it is utterly impossible that the requisite knowledge and experience can be acquired without a systematic training of considerable duration, and no such training can be afforded except in a properly conducted hospital. Good nursing does not grow of itself; it is the result of study, teaching, training, practice, ending in sound tradition, which can be transferred elsewhere.[27]

This evidence of a growing sense of the professionalism of nursing shows itself at other points in the essay, and the modern reader echoes Trench's declaration that

> it is certainly strange that while so much pains and skill were employed in training medical men, none should have been formerly given to the education of those on whose intelligence and fidelity in carrying out the doctor's directions the lives of their patients too often depended.[28]

Yet for all this emphasis on good nursing as a skill requiring careful training, the greater emphasis lay unmistakably on the need for close supervision. Trench elaborated three reasons why "special watch-fulness" should be required for hospital nursing: (1) because nursing was so often a matter of life and death, (2) because nurses of the old regime, through their notorious misconduct, proved themselves unable to function responsibly, and (3) because nurses were women. Much like the author of "Training-Schools for Nurses," Trench viewed women as easily discouraged, highly dependent, and particularly susceptible to the callousing effect of much suffering. He saw nursing as a work of compassion, charity, and Christian devotion—traits that were more commonly ascribed to women—indeed, he called nursing "the most womanly of women's work." Yet while he argued that the sensitivity of women suited them for nursing, he also argued that the innate weaknesses of women required them to be closely supervised.[29]

THE EVOLVING HOSPITAL

Meanwhile, during the late nineteenth century, an entirely new kind of institution, the voluntary general hospital, moved from the periphery to the center of health care in the United States. In the years after the Civil War, everything about the hospital changed. The discovery and perfection of techniques of asepsis and sanitary nursing practices made it a reasonably safe place to go for treatment for serious illness or severe accidents. As surgery became more reliable and effective and as biomedical science grew, the hospital became the center of scientific medicine. Only the large hospital could afford the expensive equipment and laboratories required for complicated techniques; only the large hospital could provide the variety of patients essential to quality nursing and medical education and research.

These science-based changes in the hospital engendered a new fusion—the union of nurse training schools, university medical schools, voluntary general hospitals, medical researchers and specialists, private practitioners, private duty nurses, and their middle-class clients. By 1880 there were 15 schools of nursing, 323 students, and 157 graduates in the United States. Twenty years later these figures had soared to 432 schools, 11,164 students, and 3,546 graduates. Moreover, the new hospitals proved so successful that they multiplied at exceptional rates in the late nineteenth and early twentieth centuries. In 1873 there were only 178 hospitals in the United

States; by 1909 there were 3,300; and by 1919 there were 7,000. Hospitals began to charge fees for their services, and these fees amounted to a major portion of their operating expenses. Although charity patients were subjected to crowded conditions, segregation in large wards and outpatient clinics, and poorer service than paying patients received, the new general hospital did give the poor access to health care of unprecedented quality.

THE ANGEL OF MERCY
IN LITERATURE

Once Florence Nightingale brought respectability to the nursing profession, a new image of the nurse began to appear. Nurses in late nineteenth-century novels were portrayed as noble, moral, religious, virginal, ritualistic, and self-sacrificing. A majority of late nineteenth-century authors contrasted the newer "trained nurse" with the older, discredited "Sairy Gamp" type of nurse. For example, *St. Bernards: The Romance of a Medical Student* (1887) contrasts a "born nurse" with a religious vocation, Sister Agnes, with a bad nurse of the Gamp type, who sides with the doctors in practicing new and experimental medical and surgical techniques on patients. Medicine is condemned—particularly the hospital whose primary functions are research and the training of medical students. But dedicated nursing, which is "a great work of love," is praised. Sister Agnes is a "knighterrant" who never grows weary or ill-tempered and looks out for the welfare of her patients. She and another humane person, a resident named Elsworth, rebel against the practices of the hospital and eventually leave it to set up an institution along Nightingale lines. The message is that not newfangled medicine but devoted nursing—consisting of kindness, good hygiene, and some technical competence—is best for healing patients.[30]

The new nurse, as well as the new hospital, was positively portrayed in *Hors de Combat, or Three Weeks in a Hospital* (1891), in which an upper-class patient injured in a carriage accident is taken to a charitable hospital. There he discovers a cheerful ward and has the best nursing and medical care available. Surgeon Matthews stresses the difference between "born" and trained nurses.

> "No, my dear fellow," interrupting a remark of mine, "you are wrong there; it is quite an old-fashioned idea

that a nurse, like the poet, must be 'born and not made.' In these enlightened days, one of these born nurses, whom you are so fond of talking about, would be quite useless in our infirmaries, unless she had undergone a thorough training."[31]

Sister Agnes and Nurse Graham, the trained nurses in *Hors de Combat*, are efficient, intelligent, hard working, and compassionate.

The "lady nurse" who is an "angel of mercy" appears in *Marcella* (1894) and *The Christian* (1897). *Marcella*, by Mrs. Humphry Ward, is the story of the maturation of a proud but noble-spirited idealist. Marcella Boyce is a beautiful young woman whose family, at the beginning of the novel, has recently been restored to the family estate, Mellor. Marcella captivates Aldous Raeburn, a very worthy, serious, and wealthy young aristocrat. Although she and Aldous become engaged, Marcella is chiefly interested in philanthropy. As his fiancée, she looks forward to being able to do much good for the poor people who live on her father's estate, on the Raeburn estate, and in the town nearby; otherwise, her future wealth embarrasses and depresses her. She meets an old acquaintance of Aldous, Harry Wharton, who is running for Parliament in the district, and becomes attracted to him for his exuberance and liberal ideas. Then a local man whose family she has been helping kills Aldous's gamekeeper on the same night that Harry Wharton confesses his passionate attraction to her and kisses her. Marcella helps the poor murderer's family through the trial and hanging, then breaks her engagement with Aldous and leaves home for London.[32]

Volume 2, which begins a year or so later, finds Marcella already a trained nurse, working as a district nurse among London's poor. She finds the work satisfyingly exhausting, and has matured considerably. She again encounters both Harry Wharton and Aldous Raeburn. With Harry she almost forms an alliance; the young man, now a member of Parliament, has gained much prominence for his work in liberal politics and has treated her with utmost respect since the night of the kiss. But it turns out that he has a passion for gambling and has run up considerable debts. He proposes to her to gain her fortune and support but also accepts a bribe to cease supporting a strike. Meanwhile, Marcella's father grows ill and she returns to Mellor to await his death. She realizes by this time that she loves Aldous after all, having finally come to appreciate his fine qualities, but feels that he will never forgive her for her careless treatment of him during their engagement. After she takes over the estate, she learns that he still loves her. She makes her love known to him, finally reaping the rewards she has earned—love, marriage, wealth, and social status.

Marcella Boyce only works as a nurse for about two years, but they prove to be the most significant years in her personal growth. Thus, nursing is central to her story, even though we only see her nurse two or three patients. The novel's image of nursing is almost wholly a product of Marcella and her experiences in nursing school and as a district nurse among London's poor. The image is certainly a positive one; nurse training apparently turns Marcella from a headstrong, idealistic, and often foolish (if very noble) young woman into a much humbler, more sensible, more respectful doer of good deeds.

Marcella's story suggests that the humbling aspects of nursing training and work were just what she needed to become a more humane person. Her work in school and in her district is presented as strenuous and often squalid, yet Marcella takes much satisfaction from it. Her friends don't support this view, however. Aldous thinks,

> Was this what her new career—her enthusiasm—meant, or might mean! Twenty-three!—in the prime of youth, of charm! Horrible, unpardonable waste! . . . let her leave the human brute and his unsavory struggle alone! It cannot be borne—it was never meant—that she should dip her delicate wings, of her own free will at least, in such a mire of blood and tears.

More crassly, Harry Wharton remonstrates with Marcella, "Why do you bury yourself in that nursing life? It is not the life for you; it does not fit you in the least. . . . you are wanted among your own class—among your equals. . . . It is absurd. You are masquerading." We are meant to see a grain of truth in these protests.[33]

Marcella eventually leaves her nursing after the incident that provokes Aldous's uncharacteristically violent thought, a brawl between a husband and a wife that leaves Marcella with an injured arm. But she isn't simply masquerading: her nursing career is a period of sackcloth and ashes that she must pass through on her way to maturity. We also see that she is a competent nurse: she stands up bravely to an alcoholic doctor who has been endangering a patient of hers, and she keeps her head in crises and delivers expert care. She demonstrates the possibility for nursing to seize and shape a young will into something useful, even if nursing takes her out of her "natural" element. As she explains it, "the enormous interest of the work seized me . . . and I ended [nurses' training] thinking the hospital the most fascinating and engrossing place in the whole world." And as the friend to whom she briefly narrates her experience in the hospital notices,

> How richly human the face had grown! . . . that look which had often repelled him in his first acquaintance, . . . as of a hard speculative eagerness more like the ardent boy than the woman, had very much disappeared. It seemed to him absorbed in something new—something sad and yet benignant, informed with all the pathos and the pain of growth.[34]

The principal problems and conflicts that nursing shows Marcella are poverty, suffering, and the frustration that very little can be done about them. These are realizations that one might expect from a nurse. They do not drive Marcella from her work or threaten her capacity to function as a nurse; rather, they enrich her capacity to feel. That Marcella drops her nursing when her father's illness worsens indicates that the author is saying that although nursing is all right for people like Marcella for a time, she must eventually get back to her *real* work, which is the chastened and now informed deployment of wealth in the service of good. Marcella can do even more good when she combines the talents she uses in nursing with the wealth and power she inherits from her father and shares with her husband. None of this diminishes the positive image of nursing in the novel—Marcella had the money and the position from the start but needed to "grow a soul," as she eventually comes to realize. And her nursing experience helped her to do just that.[35]

In *The Christian,* by Hall Caine, Glory Quayle, an orphan and the granddaughter of a poor country clergyman, decides to become a nurse to escape her dull life. Her mentor, the young preacher John Strom, refers to nursing as "true woman's work . . . the purest profession in the world." But Glory is not serious or old enough for the work she has chosen. She has a busy, promiscuous social life and dreams of becoming an actress. She is dismissed from the hospital for loosening a patient's bandage without permission, allowing an unauthorized visitor into the wards, singing to the patients, and taking leave without permission. Her offenses are generally the result of an overly kind heart, but she is clearly unsuited to bear the rigors of hospital discipline. On the one hand, nursing is depicted as a profession with high standards. On the other hand, however, its representatives, such as Ward Sister Allworthy, are stereotyped as stern and inflexible, and Glory objects to the training that has failed to make her "a machine called Duty."[36]

Hilda Wade is a novel started by Grant Allen at the turn of the century and completed by the more famous Sir Arthur Conan Doyle after Allen's death. *Hilda Wade* appeared in serial form in the popular *Strand Magazine*. The novel begins with some very promising discussions of nursing and women in general, but ultimately succumbs to the need of the serial to serve up novelty, romance, and suspense on a monthly basis in order to sustain reader interest. In search of such audience bait, the authors of *Hilda Wade* send their characters from England to South Africa, Rhodesia (the serial was published around the

time of the Boer War), Tibet, and India, shipwreck them somewhere in the English Channel, and embroil them in quite a lot of violence along the way, including a race war in Rhodesia. Nevertheless, as might be expected, all of this turmoil is resolved in a romantic and happy ending.

The heroine, Hilda Wade, is a lovely, strawberry blonde nurse with amazing powers of insight and memory. Her story is told by a young physician, Hubert Cumberledge, who works with Hilda at St. Nathaniel's Hospital and is in love with her. They both work closely with the hospital's chief physiologist, Dr. Sebastian, whom everyone regards as a scientific genius. Hubert is Sebastian's most devoted disciple, but Hilda reveals that she has chosen to work at St. Nathaniel's in order to be near Sabastian for a different reason—he has done some wrong that she seeks to redress. Confiding in Hubert, she characterizes Sebastian as a fanatic interested in the acquisition of scientific knowledge for its own sake without any real concern for its effect upon human welfare, and her powers of insight are so impressive that Hubert cannot wholly reject her characterization despite his worship of Sebastian.

In the course of the novel, Hilda impresses and then intimidates Sebastian as he connects her with a figure in his past, Dr. Yorke-Bannerman, a colleague of Sebastian's earlier days, who had been accused of poisoning his uncle, Admiral Scott Prideaux, in order to benefit from his will, but who died of a heart ailment before his murder trial actually took place. Sebastian had provided the principal evidence against Yorke-Bannerman. Sebastian identifies Hilda as Yorke-Bannerman's daughter and tries to kill her, but Hilda's astuteness saves her, and she flees England. A lucky accident enables Hubert to follow her to South Africa and then to Rhodesia; Sebastian trails them and goes so far as to foment a race war in order to kill Hilda. His ploy fails and the young pair escape to the Indian subcontinent, where they attach themselves to a nouveau riche British couple for protection, functioning as attendant nurse and physician to the wife, who is desperately frightened at the prospect of catching some tropical disease.

Once again, Sebastian attempts to arrange their deaths, in this instance bribing a native guide to lead them into a hostile Tibetan monastery. But Hilda's knowledge of Buddhist customs saves them, and they inadvertently encounter Sebastian, who himself has contracted an unnamed tropical disease and has

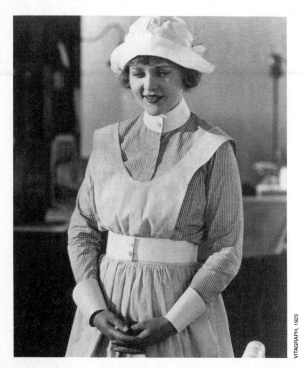

Glory Quayle, an orphan and the granddaughter of a poor country clergyman, decides to become a nurse to escape her dull life.

VITAGRAPH, 1923

sent for a doctor. In his delirium, Sebastian admits to Hubert that he has tried to kill them. Hilda tells Hubert that Sebastian must be brought back to England alive in order to clear her father's name, so the two of them nurse him back to health. They release Sebastian but book passage in the same ship to England, much to Sebastian's chagrin. When the ship crashes into an island off the English coast and sinks, Hilda bravely refuses rescue with the women and children, preferring to remain with Hubert and Sebastian in order to guarantee Sebastian's survival, upon which her mission to clear her father's name depends.

Eventually they are rescued, and, moved by Hilda's courage and tenacity, Sebastian manages to stay alive just long enough to confess before witnesses that he, not Hilda's father, had been responsible for the death of Admiral Scott Prideaux. Sebastian and Yorke-Bannerman had been experimenting with a new drug, and when Yorke-Bannerman's uncle, the admiral, contracted a rare disease, Sebastian urged his colleague to try the new drug on his patient. Yorke-Bannerman did so, but only in very conservative doses, which Sebastian bribed the pharmacist to magnify without Yorke-Bannerman's knowledge. When the admiral died of the treatment, Yorke-Bannerman was believed responsible. His heart couldn't stand the strain of the disgrace and he died. Sebastian admits all this then dies, leaving Hubert and Hilda to begin their new life together.

Had Hilda Wade not become a nurse, her abilities would have served her well in a number of fields. She has a prodigious memory and can quote at length from newspaper items she read casually years before. Despite her single-minded devotion to her mission, she manages to be interested in everything around her and to take a sophisticated interest in customs and culture. Just prior to the shipwreck off the coast of England, for example, Hilda had been holding forth on the relationship of Ibsenism to British culture. She is a keen interpreter of human temperament, solving several domestic mysteries in the course of the novel, and has an unerring eye for the smallest details. She reads physiognomy infallibly—in fact, she is infallible in all of her judgments. She is also beautiful, according to Hubert, her smitten chronicler.

> She looked about twenty-four, and had cheeks like a ripe nectarine, just as pink and just as softly downy.

> She smiled again, showing a row of semi-transparent teeth. . . . She was certainly most attractive. She had that indefinable, incommunicable, unanalyzable personal quality which we know as *charm*.

> Hilda Wade, when I first saw her, was one of the prettiest, cheeriest, and most graceful girls I have ever met—a dusky blonde, brown-eyed, brown-haired, with a creamy waxen whiteness of skin that was yet warm and peach-downy. . . . She was in the main a bright, well-educated, sensible, winsome, lawn-tennis-playing English girl. . . . But she was above all things wholesome, unaffected and sparkling—a gleam of sunshine.[37]

Hilda is characterized as a dedicated nurse, but her feeling for the profession of nursing is not entirely clear. One assumes that she became a nurse in order to fulfill her mission—that is, to force Sebastian to clear her father's name. Yet there are suggestions that she would have been drawn to nursing even if she had not dedicated herself to this mission. Her father had been a doctor and she resembles him in many ways. More important, she is deeply committed to humanitarian principles, although her dedication to her mission seems to take precedence over everything else. Fortunately, her humanitarianism does not conflict with her pursuit of Sebastian, but rather, one serves the other, since Sebastian is characterized as being anti-humanitarian.

The narrator, Hubert, gives the impression that most people of his time did not think as highly of the nursing profession as Hilda does. He cannot understand at first why Hilda, who does not need to support herself, has become a nurse and indicates that he finds nursing an unlikely, if not unfit, profession for her.

> She looked to me far too much of a butterfly for such serious work. . . . "Are you one of the ten thousand modern young ladies who are in quest of a Mission, without understanding the Missions are unpleasant? Nursing, I can tell you, is not all crimped cap and becoming uniform."[38]

And later, even after Hubert has acknowledged that Hilda is not a butterfly and takes nursing very seriously, he cannot fathom her commitment.

> "What can have induced a girl like you, with means and friends, with brains and . . . beauty, to take to such a life as this—a life which seems, in many ways, so unworthy of you!" . . . "And yet," she murmured . . . "what life can be better than the service of one's kind? You think it a great life, for Sebastian!" "Sebastian! He is a man. . . . But

a woman! Especially *you,* dear lady, for whom one feels that nothing is quite high enough. . . ."[39]

Hilda is a remarkably gifted woman and therefore a remarkably gifted nurse. She provides a stunningly positive image of a nurse, yet, at the same time, we are aware that she is unique and not typical: we cannot apply all of her qualities to nurses in general. However, it is safe to infer that Allen is showing us what he conceives to be nursing at its very best in Hilda, who combines absolute dedication and a brilliant mind with "the deepest feminine gift—intuition" and a tender sympathy for her patients. Early in the story Hilda quickly impresses the lofty Sebastian.

> He not only allowed that she was a good assistant, but he also admitted that her subtle knowledge of temperament sometimes enabled her closely to approach his own reasoned scientific analysis of a case and its probable development. "Most women," he said . . . "are quick at reading *the passing emotion;* they can judge with astounding correctness from a shadow of one's face, a catch in one's breath, a movement of one's hands, how their words or deeds are affecting us. . . . But underlying character they do not judge so well as fleeting expression. . . . Most men, on the contrary, guide their life by definite *facts*—by signs, by symptoms, by observed data. Medicine itself is built upon a collection of such reasoned facts. But this woman, Nurse Wade, to a certain extent, stands intermediate mentally between the two sexes. She recognizes *temperament*—the fixed form of character and what it is likely to do—in a degree which I have never seen equalled elsewhere. To that extent, and within proper limits of supervision, I acknowledge her faculty as a valuable adjunct to a scientific practitioner."[40]

From the events of the novel, it seems reasonable to assume that the author intended for his readers to go beyond Sebastian's rather condescending assessment of Hilda. Clearly, she is superior to all the other characters in the novel, whether male or female, nurse or physician: she directs Hubert and outsmarts the tenacious genius Sebastian. Nevertheless, readers are meant to accept Sebastian's characterization of Hilda as combining the male and female mental complements as an expression of the author's point of view. Furthermore, these comments imply something about Allen's view of the healing professions, for both Hubert and Sebastian fail in their pure "masculine" rationality to respond sensitively to patients and to understand the workings of the human heart to the extent that Hilda does. In one

case, Hilda enables a young woman to recover from a dangerous operation, after both men have given up on her, by treating her tenderly and gently reminding her that she must live in order to see her lover again. In a telling detail, both physicians consistently refer to the patient as "Number 14"—her bed number—while Hilda makes a point of using the woman's name.[41]

Once Florence Nightingale brought respectability to the nursing profession, there began to appear, in the latter part of the nineteenth century, a new portrayal of the nurse. Novelists generally characterized the new breed of nurses as refined young ladies who were "angels of mercy," rather than educated, skilled professionals. These fictional nurse characters were successful nurses not because of their education and training but because of their breeding and social class, and their tenure in the profession was often only temporary.

NOTES

1. S. Squire Sprigge, "The Medicine of Dickens," *The Cornhill Magazine* 35 (1877):258–267.

2. Charles Dickens, *The Life and Adventures of Martin Chuzzlewit* (Boston: Dana Estes & Company, 1849), p. xxviii.

3. Charles Dickens, "The Nurse in Leading Strings," *Household Words* 17 (June 12, 1858):602–606.

4. Ibid., pp. 603–604.

5. Ibid., p. 605.

6. Ibid., pp. 605–606.

7. Ibid., p. 606.

8. Charles Dickens, "Hospitals," *Household Words* 12 (December 15, 1855):457–471.

9. Henry Wadsworth Longfellow, "Santa Filomena," *Atlantic Monthly* 1 (November 1857):22–23.

10. Ibid., p. 23.

11. Elizabeth Stuart Phelps, "Her Shadow," *Atlantic Monthly* 49 (July 1906):371.

12. Ibid.

13. Ibid.

14. Ibid., pp. 371–372.

15. Ibid., p. 372.

16. Ibid.

17. R. N. Cust, "Scutari Hospital," *Notes and Queries* 9 (August 25, 1908):337.

18. Florence Nightingale, *Notes on Nursing: What It Is and What It Is Not* (London: Harrison, 1859).

19. "Notes on Nursing," *Saturday Review* 11 (January 21, 1860):84–85.

20. Ibid., p. 84.

21. Ibid., p. 85.

22. Ibid., pp. 84–85.

23. "Training-Schools for Nurses," *Fraser's Magazine* 10 (December 1874):706–713.

24. Ibid., p. 707.

25. Ibid., pp. 709–710.

26. M. Trench, "Sick Nurses," *MacMillan's Magazine* 34 (September 1876):423.

27. Ibid., p. 423.

28. Ibid., p. 422.

29. Ibid., p. 429.

30. Edward Bersoe, *St. Bernard's: The Romance of a Medical Student* (London: Swan, Sonnerschein, Lowery and Co., 1887), p. 273.

31. Gertrude Southam and Ethel Southam, *Hors de Combat or Three Weeks in a Hospital* (London: Cassell & Co., 1891), p. 63.

32. Mrs. Humphry Ward, *Marcella* (New York: Macmillan, 1894).

33. Ibid., Vol. 1, p. 233.

34. Ibid., Vol. 1, p. 145.

35. Ibid., Vol. II, p. 8.

36. Hall Caine, *The Christian* (New York: D. Appleton and Co., 1897).

37. Hilda Wade, *A Woman With Tenacity of Purpose* (New York: G. P. Putnam's Sons, 1900).

38. Ibid., p. 41.

39. Ibid., p. 68.

40. Ibid., p. 207.

41. Ibid., p. 193.

CHAPTER THREE

THE ANGEL OF MERCY
AFTER THE TURN
OF THE CENTURY

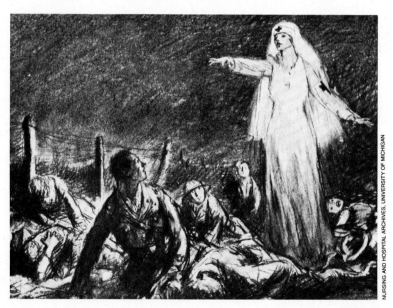

Industrialization and urbanization changed the status of women more than revolutionary ideology and protest. The first hints of the acceleration of living that has characterized this century were in the air. The sounds of the early twentieth century were still fairly quiet, but noise was on the way. Horse-drawn buggies were being replaced by Henry Ford's "Tin Lizzie." Motoring was a rattling, bouncing, wind-blown adventure, as these new creations traveled at a reckless 25 miles per hour over dirt roads. In its early stages, such travel necessitated veils to protect the women's hats and faces, and goggles and visored caps for men.

THE NEW WOMAN

As the straitlaced Victorian morality of the first decade of the century gradually gave way to a more relaxed and carefree approach to life, the clothes people wore reflected these psychic changes. When women abandoned boned corsets around 1912, and soon thereafter some men stopped wearing stiff, starched shirt collars, the entire country began quite literally to breathe and move more freely. The female silhouette, which had been characterized by an S-curve since the 1870s—the bosom thrust out in front and the derriere thrust out behind—now reversed itself and became the opposite curve. As the painfully restricting corsets of the Victorian era were discarded and the lines of the figure relaxed and straightened, the prevailing stance became the "debutante slouch," with shoulders sloping, chest dropped, hips slung forward, and knees (in more pronounced cases) slightly bent.

Conventions in manners, dress, and amusements were changing rapidly. By 1912, changes in women's dress were so drastic that they had become the subject of sermons, jokes, cartoons, and headlines. Women were discarding corsets, camisoles, petticoats, and ankle-length skirts. Shirtwaists and blouses had become peekaboo, and knees were openly exposed to public censure or approval. By 1914, the "hobble skirt" was generally if not widely worn in the suburbs as well as the cities, sanctioned by Paris styles the experts pronounced "the most daring in a hundred years." The new skirt led to other adjustments. Its tightness revealed any unbecoming lumps underneath, so underclothes were therefore shortened or eliminated altogether. For

women in tight skirts to walk at all, a slit or slash nearly to the knee was required.

During the summer, the furor mounted as women began appearing in bathing suits their mothers called scandalous. Shopgirls at Rockaway Beach, middle-class teenagers at Asbury Park, and socialites at Newport were all discarding the voluminous black bloomers and cotton stockings hitherto regarded as essentials of bathing propriety. The one-piece, black neck-to-toe bathing suit featured by the expert swimmer Annette Kellerman in the popular movie *Neptune's Daughter* became the new fashion.

Press photographers had a field day. Harried police chiefs and town councils from Maine to Florida were faced with problems of morality and law enforcement they had never anticipated. They wanted to follow public opinion, yet it was difficult to determine what majority opinion really was on slit skirts and bathing suits. One section of their constituents insisted loudly that public morals should be strictly enforced by public officers; others approved the disrobings, or at least said they should not be curbed by ordinances and arrests.

Nearly every wife and daughter was asserting herself in some way. During the late-nineteenth century in the cities of America, thousands of women left the home to work in factories and shops. In 1880 women constituted 15 percent of the American labor force, but by 1900 this figure had reached 20 percent. Mechanization created jobs that required less physical strength, jobs as suitable for women as men, and women were willing to work for less money. The growing importance of service industries and communications also created thousands of jobs for women as nurses, retail clerks, and telephone operators. Most women worked in industry a relatively brief period of time. In 1900, 49 percent of working women were under twenty-five years old, and 71 percent were under thirty-five.

The average working woman at the turn of the century was young and single. Some of the changes in female lifestyle first began to appear among younger women. Single, middle-class women found their way in increasing numbers into the array of jobs that opened up to women during the early-twentieth century. Young, middle-class women did not generally view work as oppressive drudgery but rather as an avenue toward independence and increased social contact. Moreover, even for those

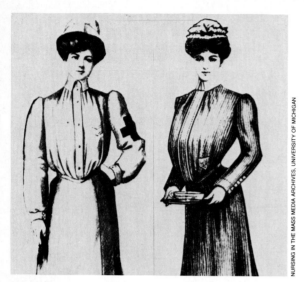

NURSING IN THE MASS MEDIA ARCHIVES, UNIVERSITY OF MICHIGAN

The female silhouette, which had been characterized by an S-curve since the 1870s—the bosom thrust out in front and the derriere thrust out behind—now reversed itself and became the opposite curve.

who were not working, the idea of a career loomed as an exciting, desirable opportunity. Thus young women who in earlier, more sheltered generations would have almost without question accepted the confines of marriage were coming of age during an era when the idea of a career was increasingly acceptable. However, since it was still generally unacceptable for women to combine marriage with a career, most women had to decide between the two. Although the ultimate choice of most women might be a home and family, many expressed discontentment with the limitations that decision implied.

But the formulation of a character structure that would enable women to function both comfortably and effectively in the two quite different spheres—the business-industrial-professional arena and the circle of home and family—was to prove extremely difficult. Each sphere demanded very different qualities. As a worker a woman was expected to be efficient, self-reliant, intelligent, logical, unemotional; to succeed she had to be determined and competitive. But these were not the qualities that the culture prized in women or that were associated with their role in the home. The desirable wife was still gentle, loving, emotional, passive, dependent, unassertive—and, if possible, pretty and not overly intellectual.

The ideal of femininity presented to a growing girl did not fit her for the competitive activities of the business world. Her education, if she went on to college, only served to increase her discontent if she married and restricted herself to the home. And despite all the sentimental tributes the home-oriented woman received, society did not really place a high value on that function. For, in fact, she lived in a culture that stressed productive achievement as the measure of individual worth—meaning a tangible contribution to the material output of a predominantly technological economy. To be truly feminine, as the culture defined femininity, was to place herself outside the mainstream of American life, but to be a functioning member of society was to run the risk of destroying her womanliness.

The convinced feminist of the turn of the century often spurned marriage. To the woman interested in realizing her human capabilities, marriage in the nineteenth century was not an opportunity but a dead end. And it was indeed a minor scandal of the time that many women did reject marriage. This conscious rejection was most pronounced among highly educated women, many of whom felt strongly their obligation to serve society through careers. Around 1900 more than one-quarter of the women who graduated from college and more than half of the women medical doctors never married.

After 1900 increased vocational opportunities began to effect slow but inexorable change in societal attitudes not only toward working women but toward the roles of women in general. Higher education was becoming more available to women; more of the professions were admitting them; property and divorce laws were slowly being reformed in their favor; between 1889 and 1896 four of the western states (Wyoming, Colorado, Utah and Idaho) had granted women suffrage and, though the struggle was to remain a bitter and difficult one, the winning of suffrage on a national level was clearly only a matter of time.

The growing acceptance of a woman more independent and active than her mid-nineteenth-century predecessor was perhaps best epitomized by the arrival of the Gibson Girl as the feminine ideal of the 1890s. Between the mid-1890s and World War I, the Gibson Girl symbolized the standard of the ideal woman. She was the creation of artist Charles Dana Gibson, whose drawings of her first appeared in *Life* magazine, and she was a national sensation by 1894, when the first folio edition of Gibson's work was published. Though her skirts were long and blouses prim, the Gibson Girl displayed a healthy vitality whether she golfed, played tennis, swam, or just walked along the seashore. Staring coolly into the distance, only rarely gazing at her reader or pictorial admirer, she conveyed a mysterious elegance. Her physical presence not only dominated Gibson's drawings but literally dwarfed her male counterparts. Statuesque, long-limbed and -necked, her physical bearing conveyed authority; her thrown-back, upright carriage and lowered eyelids projected power and control over self and others.

Nursing was the only occupation identified with this lofty female ideal, attesting to the acceptability of the profession for well-bred women in a time when women working outside the home was viewed negatively and as solely for misfortunates who did not have men to take care of them. Positive imagery surrounding trained nurses contributed to the rapid growth of the profession, and the census bureau found that the 1,500 professional nurses of 1880 grew to 4,600 by 1890; climbed to 11,800 by 1900; and soared to 82,000 by 1910. The characterization of nursing during this era emphasized the noble, self-sacrificing angel of mercy—the quintessence of femininity. Thus, at a time when the masculine professions were all but closed to women, entry into the profession of nursing represented an attractive step toward emancipation from the confinement of the domestic sphere and well-intentioned but often ineffectual good works.

The ranks of nurses came to represent a good cross section of society. Women of the lower classes flocked into nursing, for they could obtain higher pay and do less menial work than if they had entered domestic service—and also move up the social ladder. At the same time, women of the better classes entered the field in large numbers when they realized that they could lead an independent life in respectable company and that the work was no longer a menial occupation but involved the training and exercise of their intelligence.

THE NEW WOMAN IN LITERATURE

The working woman began to appear as a heroine in American literature at a critical point in American history—during the rapid growth and consolidation of industrial capitalism around the turn of the century. The novels with working women heroines do not represent the whole spectrum of the work experiences of real women; in fact, writers were highly selective in their choices of which professions and jobs to portray. The transformations that were occurring in women's lives during the early-twentieth century were reflected in the changing image of what contemporaries believed to be commendable characteristics for a woman to possess and appropriate activities for her to engage in.

Justine Brent, the nurse in Edith Wharton's famous novel *The Fruit of the Tree* (1907), is one of the first professional nurses used as the main character of a full-length, serious, literary novel. Justine is initially described as a professional—expert, cool, observant, steady, and authoritative rather than cajoling. She leads a "crowded yet lonely life," made more interesting by mental classification of people. She wears a dark blue linen dress with an apron and cap when working as a surgical nurse in the hospital or on private duty. Her nursing activities include supportive comfort measures (straightening pillows, wiping a patient's forehead), technical procedures (administering medication, monitoring vital signs, assisting the physician in applying emergency measures to stabilize the condition of a dying patient), psychological support and education (answering a patient's inquiries about his prognosis), night watching, and consulting with the physician about a patient's condition.[1]

During the time that she works more as a companion than nurse to a wealthy but bored and sickly woman, Bessy Westmore, she also manages the household (supervising servants, writing letters, organizing social functions) and sometimes acts as governess to Bessy's daughter. She is at ease in this upper-class environment, but her social status is somewhat uncertain. Well-educated and well-connected, she is nevertheless stigmatized within this group by having to work for a living. Her own preference is to live independently and disassociate herself from any social group. Not only social issues but also professional ones, like confidentiality and euthanasia, are raised in the novel from the beginning. Justine breaks her vow of confidentiality by discussing a patient injured in a factory accident and also conjectures, during this discussion, that "the professional instinct to save would always come first," but later events alter her views.

John Amherst is the assistant manager of the factory owned by Bessy Westmore. He is driven by the desire to improve the lives and working conditions of the mill workers, and his marriage to Bessy quickly sours when he discovers that she does not share his aims. Bessy is childish, selfish, indolent, and impulsive: it is while riding her favorite horse, Impulse, on an icy day that she has a near-fatal accident. Her spine injury is likely to cripple her and make her suffer a slow and agonizing death. Justine, after considerable deliberation, gives her an overdose of morphine that quickly kills her. Justine opposes Christianity, conventional morality, and the blind dedication to science and self-advancement that made the attending physician continue to employ extraordinary measures to keep Bessy alive when all hope seemed lost. She feels further justified in her decision because Bessy was in terrible pain and had pleaded to die, and because she felt from reading John's books and from past conversations with him that he would agree with her decision.

He does agree, in principle, but he does not learn about Justine's action until after he has married her. The physician, whom she had refused to marry and who had subsequently become a morphine addict, blackmails her. She is about to reveal the truth to her husband when the physician does so. Her husband's trust in her is irrevocably shaken because she had not spoken earlier, and she decides that the only way to save his social position, which Bessy's relatives largely control, is to leave him. She confesses the truth to Bessy's father but disguises her real motive for leaving John. Only after a year, when he has discovered that she left only to protect his reputation and not because she didn't love him, does he seek her out.

The biblical allusion in the title and numerous authorial comments indicate that Justine, like Eve, has been punished for yielding to the temptation to usurp divine powers. Like Eve, she is driven out of paradise, represented by the happy marriage that never fully recovers from the blow of her terrible secret. "The tie between them was forever stained and debased." Justine's conscience remains clear, since her motives were purely selfless, but Wharton judges her act of euthanasia as antisocial.

> Not till that morning had she seen those consequences in their terrible, unsuspected extent, had she understood how one stone rashly loosened from the laboriously erected structure of human society may produce

remote fissures in that clumsy fabric. She saw that, having hazarded the loosening of the stone, she should have held herself apart from ordinary human ties, like some priestess set apart for the service of the temple. And instead, she had seized happiness with both her hands, taken it as the gift of the very fate she had herself precipitated! She remembered some very old Greek saying to the effect that the gods never forgive the mortal who presumes to love and suffer like a god. She had dared to do both, and the gods were bringing ruin on that deeper self which had its life in those about her.[2]

Having ignored the conventions by which society protects itself, she cannot expect to find happiness within the very structure she has violated.

Wharton implicitly condemns euthanasia, but Justine remains the most moral character in the novel nevertheless: consistent, pure, truthful, unselfish, and courageous. Justine Brent's strengths also include intelligence, warmth, wit, compassion, perception, an ability to listen to people and to give constructive advice and encouragement, true composure, and steadfastness in moments of crises. One mistake in judgment has fatally flawed the happiness she had otherwise deserved, but she is able to expiate her sin by an exhausting year of hospital nursing. "Justine had paid . . . to the utmost limit of whatever debt toward society she had contracted by over-stepping its laws. And her resolve to discharge the debt had been taken in a flash, as soon as she had seen that man can commit no act alone, whether for good or evil." Thus, nursing serves as expiation even for a nonreligious person.[3]

AN ANGEL OF MERCY'S CRISIS

Realism, broadly defined, also plays a part in the opening chapters of *The White Linen Nurse* (1913), "probably the most talked-of novel of the present book season," according to *The New York Times Review of Books*. For the first sixty or so pages of this novel, the major theme is nursing—why young women decide to enter nursing school, what nurse training does to different people, what being a trained nurse means. The narrator describes three very different roommates, each about to graduate from nurse training.

> So the three faces foiled each other, sober city girl, pert town girl, bucolic country girl,—a hundred fundamental differences rampant between them, yet each fervid, adolescent young mouth tamed to the same monoto-

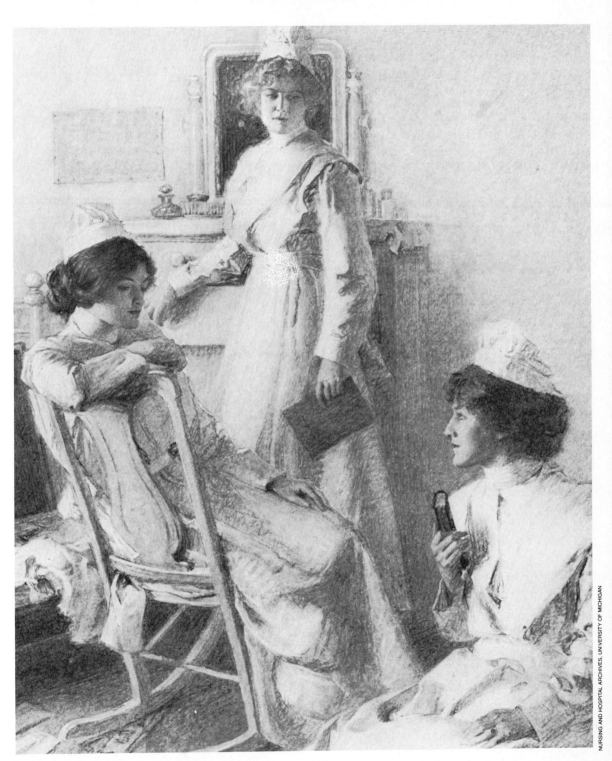

In The White Linen Nurse *(1913), the narrator describes three very different roommates, each about to graduate from nurse training.*

nous, drolly exaggerated expression of complacency that characterizes the faces of all people who, in a distinctive uniform, for a reasonably satisfactory living wage, make an actual profession of righteous deeds.[4]

It would seem from this passage that the narrator shares the point of view of the protagonist, Rae Malgregor, more than that of the other young women, who receive only about two pages each to explain why they entered nursing school and give some sense of what they hope to do as trained nurses. In contrast to their firm convictions that they want to be trained nurses, Rae finds the creature "trained nurse" a monstrosity—an automaton in the guise of a human being. The message seems to be that nurses are necessary to tend the sick, but that there is something inhuman about the ability of the nurse to dole out care and compassion automatically, to become automatically noble—being invested with all kinds of virtue by the world for simply doing her job, just as any other worker does a job—to inspire admiration and even love for doing what she's getting paid to do, to minister to needs that other women cannot meet as competently, to be a "holy chorus girl"— that object of male fantasy that impossibly combines pure physicality with pure spirituality by dispassionately comforting the body while mechanically cheering the soul.[5]

The idea that a trained nurse is a kind of machine is further developed in a scene with the senior surgeon, when he tells Rae:

> "Gad! . . . What a hand! You're a wonder! Under proper direction you're a wonder! It was like myself working with twenty fingers and no thumbs! . . . Excuse me for not recognizing you, but you girls look all alike."[6]

And a bit later, speaking of Rae to the superintendent of nurses, the senior surgeon says:

> "There goes my best nurse! Oh no, not the most brilliant one . . . but the most reliable! The most nearly perfect human machine that it has ever been my privilege to see turned out,—that one girl . . . has always done what she was told,—when she was told,—and the exact way she was told,—without questioning anything, without protesting anything, without supplementing anything with some disastrous original conviction of her own."[7]

Early in the novel, Rae undergoes what seems to be a temporary breakdown from the strain of her last few weeks of training—she has lost several patients in a row, through no fault of her own, and has slept very little. The following excerpts characterize her state of mind.

> The White Linen Nurse was so tired that her noble expression ached. Incidentally her head ached and her shoulders ached and her lungs ached and the ankle bones of her feet ached. . . . But nothing of her felt permanently incapacitated except her noble expression. Like a strip of lip-colored lead suspended from her poor little nose by two tugging wire-gray wrinkles, her persistently conscientious sickroom smile seemed to be whanging aimlessly against her front teeth. The sensation certainly was very unpleasant. . . .

> Dizzily with her stubby fingertips prodded deep into every jaded facial muscle that she could compass, she staggered towards the air . . . and sat staring blankly out across the monotonous city roofs that flanked her open window,—trying very, very hard for the first time in her life, to consider the General-Phenomenon-of-Being-a-Trained-Nurse.[8]

Rae can't accept the professionalism she has been trained for; she can't accept her ability to care for people competently but automatically and to do noble things not because they are good or noble but because they're her job.

> "Is there any woman from here to Kamchatka who doesn't look upon a trained nurse as her natural born enemy? . . . Look at the impudent jobs we get sent out on! Quarantined upstairs for weeks at a time with their inflammable diphtheritic bridegrooms—while they sit downstairs—brooding over their wedding teaspoons! . . . Snatching their new-born babies away from their breasts and showing them, virgin-handed, things perfectly—flippantly—*right*—for twenty-five dollars a week—and washing—that all the achin' love in the world don't know how to do right—just for love!"[9]

Later on Rae pours out more of her confusion and resentment at being turned into something against her grain.

> "My face is all worn out trying to 'look alike'! My cheeks are almost sprung with artificial smiles! My eyes are fairly bulging with unshed tears! My nose aches like a toothache trying never to turn up at anything! I'm smothered with the discipline of it! I'm choked with affectation! I tell you—I just can't breathe through a trained nurse's face anymore. . . . I want to look like *myself!* I want to see what life could do to a silly face like mine—if it ever got a chance! When other women are crying, I want the fun of crying!"

> "I haven't got any judgment! I've never been allowed to have any judgment! All I've ever been allowed to have is

the judgment of some flirty young medical student—or the House Doctor—or the Senior Surgeon. . . . Oh, what am I going to do," she begged, "when I am way off alone—somewhere . . . and something happens—and there isn't any judgment around to tell me what I ought to do?"[10]

The points that Rae makes are appealing, if incoherent, and her protest against being-a-trained-nurse is a particularly intriguing one. She later walks away from this dilemma by accepting the senior surgeon's offer of a "position of general heartwork" to him and his motherless, crippled daughter. The natural role of women, it is implied, is to care for men and children. For this reason, the surgeon expresses his marriage proposal as a job offer. The nurse redecorates the house, plays with his daughter, and works like a drudge while the doctor takes a vacation in Canada and then returns in a bearish mood. She fights his black mood, as he undergoes a last bout with alcoholism, with sublime and serenely good-natured submissiveness, repelling his repeated verbal abuse with kindness and going so far as to sleep on the threshold of his study. Her angelic devotion transforms him, and he apologizes and takes her on a honeymoon. It is as a wife and mother, a born nurse, that the White Linen Nurse acts as an angel of mercy.[11]

ARISTOCRATIC NURSES

In *Alice-for-Short* (1907), William De Morgan makes a similar statement in his depiction of a well-born woman trained as a nurse. Contrasting Alice with Mrs. Gaisford, who has nursed in an insane asylum for eighteen years, the novel implies that without angel of mercy qualities, nursing hardens a woman. The angelic Alice is more sensitive and compassionate than Mrs. Gaisford. Although the attending physician respects Mrs. Gaisford's opinion on diagnosis and treatment in a difficult case of amnesia, the patient herself reacts with hostility to the nurse's authoritative, cool, and detached manner and tone and only opens up to Alice. Alice's superiority, from the author's point of view, is inherited—she is the daughter of a nobleman, as she discovers only after she has married the benefactor who rescued her from the street when she was six. Like the White Linen Nurse, she renounces professional nursing to

become a wife and mother to her husband's boy, whom she had nursed through smallpox.[12]

The aristocratic nurse is also the winner in love in the 1914 novel *The Night Nurse,* by J. Johnston Abraham. Nora Townsend, "the Duchess," and Moira Otway compete for Dr. Fitzgerald ("Fitz") in a light-hearted story of doctor-nurse flirtation that becomes increasingly serious after Nurse Sheila dies as a result of her affair with a resident. The novel depicts the conflict between sexual instinct and social convention, which required that sexual desires be submerged, disguised, and delayed. For example, the costumes of nurses make them more attractive to men, according to Dr. Fitzgerald, but nurses are trained "into a nun-like unconsciousness of men." Nurses supposedly expect physicians to flirt with them, but hospital rules forbid social relationships, and marriage between nurses and physicians is impractical for several reasons. In addition, the author holds that nurses have "a knowledge of the hidden things of life . . . that made the ordinary barriers of convention futile, a knowledge absolutely undreamt of by the sheltered unmarried woman of their outside acquaintance." This knowledge gives nurses more power and equality with men in flirtation and courtship.[13]

Men are obviously the real heroes of this story, which is told from the male point of view. They play more active roles, except in the final scene, and are shown rowing and playing tennis. Nora is idealized by Fitz as a princess, angel of mercy, madonna, goddess, and saint. She is, however, particularly cold and aloof, and misunderstandings that arise after their engagement drive Fitz to become engaged to Moira. But when he falls ill with typhus, Moira, realizing that he really loves Nora, sacrifices her own love and asks Nora to come to him. The restoration of his first love saves his life.

Nora and Moira both act as angels of mercy because each sacrifices her love—Nora for honor (she insists that Fitz keep his promise to Moira) and Moira for Fitz—but only Nora is idealized as such. Moira represents the class of nurses who are like "a third sex"—"useful accessories" and "companions" but not objects of reverence. Nora is portrayed as an exception to the rule that independently wealthy, young, and beautiful women do not long survive the drudgery of nursing. Fitz thinks she may have entered the hospital only to have an affair with a doctor, but when she arrives at the fever ward to

nurse the dying Sheila, his worship of her is intensi-
fied, and his love is revived when she is knocked
unconscious after chasing a delirious patient.

Like *The White Linen Nurse, The Night Nurse*
reflects a changing view of women. Nora finds sex,
marriage, childbearing, and the stereotype of "old
maids" old-fashioned and says she will never marry.
Moira, on the other hand, typifies the "flapper," who
is actively interested in men and pursues several at
once. But although *The Night Nurse* demonstrates
that a lady can be an excellent nurse, it lacks the
courage of its radical convictions at the end, where
nature triumphs, as it had in *The White Linen Nurse,*
over the highly artificial system of training that tries
to make nurses out of upper-class women, who will
supposedly always revert to their natural feminine
role in the home.

The White Sister (1909) presents the conflict
between nursing and marriage most clearly. The
aptly-named Angela, thinking her fiancé, Giovanni, is
dead, becomes a nursing nun in order to work at
something useful and to support herself, since a
spiteful aunt has cheated her out of her inheritance.
She becomes the best surgical nurse in the convent
hospital and refuses to forsake her vows when Giovanni returns, but he ultimately coerces her into
seeking a dispensation from Rome so that they can
be married. The White Sister is idealized as untiring
and perfect: "The modern trained nurse is a
machine, and a wonderfully good one on the whole;
when she is exceptionally endowed for her work she
is quite beyond praise." Like the aristocratic nurses
of *Alice-for-Short* and *The Night Nurse,* Angela is consistently depicted as strong, disciplined, and confident, with a high standard of honor that goes beyond
the loyalty and discretion expected of a nurse.[14]

MARY ROBERTS RINEHART, NURSE-AUTHOR

As far as the study of the image of nursing is concerned, Mary Roberts Rinehart is doubly important.
Aside from being an extremely popular author who
focused her novels and short stories on the nursing
and medical professions, the young Mary Roberts
was herself a nurse. Those of her works that feature
major nurse or physician characters show nursing
through the eyes of an author familiar with her
subject.

For almost the entire first half of this century,
Rinehart's mystery and romance novels remained
firmly lodged on the best-seller lists. Indeed, Irving
Harlow Hart, in his 1946 article in *Publisher's Weekly,*
placed Rinehart in first position for the entire 50-year
period from 1894 to 1944, because eleven of her
best sellers were in the annual top ten list during
that period. It was not until the late 1940s, after
social mores had been dramatically altered by World
War II, that Rinehart lost her footing. Until that time,
her novels and short stories were so popular and
her output so enormous that she was able to amass a
multimillionaire's fortune.[15]

Rinehart was an extraordinary and, in some ways,
a curious woman. Brilliant and innovative in her
writing though she was, biographical and autobiographical accounts of her views suggest that she was
often intellectually and politically naive and bewil-
dered. Although her opinions were not always rigid,
they often filtered through into her stories as strong
convictions. In her stories about nursing and medicine, her views on both professions are clearly
stated, and these do remain fairly consistent; but they
are by no means always favorable to the profession
of nursing. Her strongest sympathies lay with conservative politics and conservative thinking. Therefore, although she admired the nursing profession,
she was not always anxious to see it advance and
modernize.

Mary Ella Roberts was born on August 12, 1876, in
Allegheny, Pennsylvania, a middle-class suburb of
Pittsburgh that has since been absorbed into the
greater industrial city. Both her parents were of
Irish-Presbyterian descent. Though her father was
not a churchgoer, her mother and grandmother
were religious, and Mary was raised in a strict Christian environment that included tiresome, silent Sab-
baths. At the age of 16, she was "saved" at a revivalist
meeting, but though she remained religious all
her life, she was troubled by God's unkindness to
humanity. At first Mary's family lived in the same
house with her father's mother and her aunt and
uncle, but after some years they moved to a new
home on Arch Street, which later became the fictional setting for her novel *K.*

Mary Roberts did fairly well in high school and
was, for a time, editor of the school paper and a
member of the debating society. In 1892 she wrote
two stories for the *Pittsburgh Press* short story competition and, although she did not win first prize, she

did receive sufficient acclaim to have them printed in the newspaper. The first story, "Lord Ainsleigh's Heir," told of a young man's mistaken identity as a pauper and his eventual rehabilitation into the upper-class world. Significantly, many of her later stories dealt with people mistakenly relegated to the ranks of the poor but eventually reinstated to their proper station in life. The idea of escaping unpleasant family backgrounds seems to have haunted her ever since her childhood, which she spent in relative poverty.

Mary Roberts did not take writing seriously, however, and on learning that the new neighborhood medical doctor was a woman (Dr. C. Jane Vincent), she was determined to become a physician herself. Although her family would not take her aspirations seriously, this appears to have been her goal for some years. When she was graduated from high school in 1893, the 1890s depression had set in and her father was especially poor. The family had moved again, this time to Poplar Street, a less attractive neighborhood. Mary wanted to study medicine but her father was unable to pay the costs. Although Mary's generous Uncle John offered to pay, she discovered that at 16 she was too young to enter medical school. The local general practitioner had told her that she would make a good nurse, so she decided to ask him for more detailed advice—her intention being to enter the medical profession by way of nursing. When she arrived at the doctor's office, however, the older physician was away and it was none other than her future husband, young Dr. Stanley Rinehart, temporarily minding his colleague's practice, who advised her on how to become a nurse.

MARY RINEHART'S NURSING EXPERIENCES

Dr. Stanley Rinehart was critical of Mary's attitude toward nursing. He accused her of being a romantic. "You think it is nothing but smoothing pillows and stroking foreheads," he told her. But Mary succeeded in persuading him of her good intentions. He agreed to show her around the Pittsburgh hospital where he was an intern. Although Mary was only 16 when she applied for entry to the School of Nursing of the Homeopathic Medical and Surgical Hospital and Dispensary in Pittsburgh, she lied about her age, claim-

ing to be 17, and was thus accepted into the school as a probationer. Mary's mother was horrified by her daughter's chosen profession.

Mary herself was shocked by her experiences at the hospital. Like Sidney Page, the heroine of *K,* she now witnessed "life in the raw." The problems of typhoid, a seasonal disease resulting from the combination of summer droughts and bad sanitation, and the steel and coal mill accidents so often caused by the dreadful safety conditions in industry at the time, offered Mary a glaring look at the poverty and misery of the world. She was equally shocked by the more natural but nonetheless painful experience of childbirth. Like Katie Walters, a leading nurse character in her novel *The Doctor,* she loathed observing the experience, at least at first. Unlike Katie, Mary Roberts grew accustomed to the maternity ward and grew to enjoy the experiences of young and older mothers, many of whom were unmarried, or even prostitutes.[16]

Although the work of a probationer was very grueling and involved much menial labor, Mary Roberts survived her probationary months and, indeed, her three years as a nursing student. As a probationer, she had worn her own dresses in pretty prints, covered of course by large white aprons. As a student nurse, she could now wear the full nurse's uniform of a striped dress and white, voluminous apron and starched cap—a uniform that Mary found extremely glamorous. As a student, work was just as hard but demanded more responsibility. Students, like probationers and trained nurses for that matter, worked 12-hour shifts; unlike probationers, student nurses were often left in charge of wards at night. Regular prayer meetings and rigid rules of conduct, especially with respect to the physicians, were strictly adhered to.

Near the end of her period of training, Mary, like the other students, did a stint as a visiting nurse, going to the homes of families in the Pittsburgh area to care for those unable to get to the hospital. These patients were often poor and destitute, and again Mary witnessed "life in the raw"—the harshness of Pittsburgh industrial life and the trauma of typhoid. Although she later used many pieces of her nursing experience in her novels, Mary Rinehart claimed that she never wrote of the real horror of hospital work and the ordeal of the poor. She tended instead to transform painful experiences into comedy and romance.

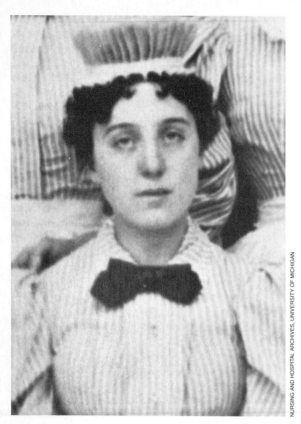

NURSING AND HOSPITAL ARCHIVES, UNIVERSITY OF MICHIGAN

Although the work of a probationer was very grueling and involved much demeaning labor, Mary Roberts survived her probationary months and, indeed, her three years as a nursing student.

Mary's experiences at the hospital were not all bad, however. She met some women who were to serve as models for engaging characters in her novels. The superintendent of nurses at the hospital, Marguerite Wright, was a pioneer in the profession, having been one of the first graduates of the Training School for Nurses at Bellevue Hospital in New York. With her black silk dresses and stern manner, Miss Wright became the model for the superintendent of nurses in *The Doctor,* Miss Nettie Simpson. The head nurse of Mary's first ward was also clearly a model for the head nurse in *The Doctor.* A good nurse, the head nurse was chiefly remembered by Mary for her too-high heels.

In addition to meeting interesting women at the hospital, Mary also regularly saw Dr. Stanley Rine-

hart. Stanley had been to Adrian College, Michigan, and then studied at the medical school in Hahnemann Hospital, Philadelphia. When Mary had first met him at Homeopathic Medical and Surgical Hospital, he was working on his internship there. Since Mary already knew him on a friendly basis, she asked him to teach her German, and the lessons blossomed into a romance. Nurses were not supposed to become involved with the doctors at the hospital and, when rumors began to fly about Mary and Stanley, Mary feared for her position. Stanley went before a board meeting, however, and, booming at his colleagues and superiors, very like Rinehart's fictional character Dr. Arden in *The Doctor,* told them that he had every intention of marrying Mary when they had both completed their courses. Both of them were permitted to remain.

Mary's world was rocked in October 1895, when she was completing her training as a nurse, by the sudden death of her father, Tom Roberts. She always claimed that she had loved him dearly and understood his rather frivolous nature, but she had also resented his lack of practicality, which was at least partially responsible for the family's lack of a steady income. In *K,* Rinehart tells us that Sidney Page, like Mary herself, inherits practicality from her mother but a vivid imagination from her father. Tom Roberts had once set up a sewing machine business that at first did rather well, but he was continually trying to patent new inventions that may have been clever but certainly never won him acclaim and, indeed, lost him a great deal of money. He persisted in his hopes and his patents, however, until he ran out of money altogether in paying for the renewal of some old patents.

When the family moved to Poplar Street, Tom Roberts became a traveling salesman in wallpaper, but he could not succeed even in this job. At this point the family took in a lodger, much to Mary's disgust, since it meant a certain loss of privacy and a lowered social status. In 1895 Roberts was dismissed from his salesman job because he was now drinking heavily. He was in a hotel room in Buffalo when he received the devastating news of his job loss, and he shot himself there, checking his aim in the mirror. The local newspaper publicized the suicide, and Mary was filled with horror. She often returned to this event in her fiction: the victim in her mystery novel *Miss Pinkerton,* for instance, is at first thought to have shot himself while looking in the mirror.

A whole new life awaited Mary now, however, as the wife of Stanley Rinehart. When they had both graduated, Mary and Stanley were married in a Presbyterian church in 1896. Practically the entire hospital nursing and medical staff attended the wedding. Mary was beautiful in a $100 dress of satin and tulle, paid for by Uncle John. The couple honeymooned in Bermuda—Mary's first trip outside Pittsburgh. On the honeymoon, Mary suffered her first bout of serious illness, which was to plague her continually for the rest of her life—by 1946 she had gone through fifteen operations. After an operation to remove her gallbladder, a psychiatrist suggested that Mary's numerous operations had been necessitated by psychosomatic disorders. Whatever the cause, she was sick for the major part of her Bermuda honeymoon.

MARY RINEHART BEGINS HER WRITING

Back in Allegheny again, Mary lived the busy life of a doctor's wife and became the mother of several children. Her first son, Stanley, was born in 1897; her second, Alan, in 1900; her third, Frederick (or Ted), in 1902. In 1903 Mary's mother came to live with them also, so the house was full and busy. Often ill herself and petrified by her children's illnesses—Ted was a particularly sickly child—Mary was nonetheless writing by 1904. The stock market crash of 1903 left the Rineharts heavily in debt, so to help with the family expenses, Mary wrote her first story. It sold immediately to *Munsey's,* a leading magazine of the day, for $34. She proceeded to write and sell 45 more short stories that year, earning $1,842.50, a fair sum at that time. *Munsey's* suggested she write a full-length mystery that they would serialize before book publication, and she wrote *The Circular Staircase,* published in 1908. She then scored a major hit with the serialization of her novel *The Man in Lower 10* in the magazine *All-Story.* The book was published in 1909 and was her first novel and the first American detective story ever to reach the top ten best-seller list. These two novels established Rinehart as an ingenious new mystery writer. In *My Story,* Rinehart tells us:

> To my astonishment I read that I had developed a new technique of the detective novel. In other words, that my simple device to keep up the interest by having the initial crime merely the forerunner of others to follow,

was the first advance in the technique of the crime novel since Edgar Allan Poe![17]

In 1910 there came a turning point in the Rineharts' lives as Stanley started to lose the use of his hands on account of arthritis. He had been a surgeon but now was unable to operate adequately, and he decided to specialize in something else instead, as so many physicians were then doing. He decided to go to Vienna to study, and in 1911 the Rineharts packed up and went to that prewar city for some months. Mary enjoyed her stay in Vienna, using the opportunity to practice her German and to discover the galleries and museums of that historically and academically rich European city.

Upon their return to the States, the Rineharts were now well-off from Mary's increasing literary output. She decided to buy a very expensive house a few miles out of Pittsburgh, in Sewickley. This rambling mansion was so in need of repairs and remodeling that its final cost of $90,000 was well beyond the price she had anticipated. To meet her financial burdens, Mary—as always—sat down and wrote. While enjoying gracious living in their beautiful home, Mary Rinehart increased her output and became a success. In 1912 she was invited to the prestigious William Dean Howell's birthday party, an event that marked her acceptance into the literary establishment.

"The Miracle" was one of Rinehart's first magazine stories, and it was her first story to include a nurse among the major characters. This short story was printed in the June 1912 issue of *McClure's* magazine along with charming drawings, including two of the nurse character. The story deals primarily with illegitimacy and an unwed mother's hostility toward her unwanted child. The subject is presented sympathetically and fairly realistically, but a secondary theme of romance and a happy ending to this particular mother's tale of woe contribute some cheer as well as comic relief to what could otherwise be a depressing matter.

The nurse character is head of the women's ward, where expectant and delivered mothers are all housed together, as was the practice at that time. The nurse is referred to only as "the nurse." Though young, she is obviously efficient, capable, and intelligent and succeeds in controlling her often troublesome patients and their babies. The illustrations show her to be dressed in a crisp nurse's uniform: a striped, full-length dress with white apron, collar, cuffs, and cap. Despite the starchiness of her uniform, her disciplined manner, and her lack of a personal name, the nurse does have a personality and private life; the secondary plot deals with her romance with a physician, "E.J."

In quiet moments the nurse sits at her desk, ostensibly reading her Bible but more often gazing wonderingly at a note she received that day from E.J. "At the top it said: Annie Petowski—may sit up for one hour. And below that: Goldstein baby—bran baths. And below that: I love you. E.J."[18] We only meet the young physician once when he visits the ward, but in that brief moment, in a restrained manner consistent with hospital discipline, the doctor and nurse openly confess their love for each other: "The nurse shook down a thermometer and examined it closely. 'I love you too!' she said."[19]

The story takes place on Easter Sunday, the day of the miracle. The only blot on the happy nurse's horizon is Claribel, the unmarried mother who has rejected her newborn child and is committed to a speedy suicide. Another patient, a seasoned mother called Liz, who helps the nurse with her job of watching over the mothers and babies, tries to snap Claribel out of her misery but to no avail. Claribel insists on staring darkly at the ceiling, even after the nurse has shown her her lovely little girl. When Liz suggests that things could get dangerous with Claribel, the nurse hits on a plan of action. She telephones Claribel's friend, Rosie Davis, a less-than-respectable women with a good heart who, importantly, knows the identity of Claribel's lover. With a little persuasion from the young nurse, Rosie agrees to seek out the irresponsible young man and haul him in to see his little girl.

Rosie's plain talk does the trick. Al, the sheepish father, is brought to a sense of paternal pride by Rosie's jabbering and eventually asks Claribel to marry him. Although Claribel is unhappy with this idea at first, she soon recognizes that Al is really in earnest and she cheerfully agrees. All's well that ends well. Despite the trite-sounding plot, the story is a good one. The characters are real and believable, and the tale is told with much wit and insight. The unwed girl's situation is treated sensitively. She has already tried to kill herself, and is shown to be deeply distressed. Having babies is shown to be a painful, exacting experience, and the state of motherhood

not always as wonderful as it may seem. There is a serious message behind the wit and comedy.

The image of the nurse in this story is compassionate, understanding, and tolerant: "It did not occur to the nurse to deprecate having to use an evil medium [Rosie] toward a righteous end. She took life much as she found it." She is also capable, womanly-wise, and efficient, despite her youth. She has an air of serenity about her that affects the whole ward. "How beautiful you are here, and how peaceful! Your ward is always a sort of benediction," says the lady from the House Committee. Called the "nurse-queen" who sits at a desk likened to a throne, the nurse has complete charge of her domain and is clearly an able decision maker, someone to be trusted.[20]

Although we only see the nurse for one day, she is involved in a variety of activities. She oils a new baby and cleans her eyes out, wheels a new mother from the operating room to the ward, gives orders to patients and orderlies, and constantly reprimands one mother for overfeeding her baby. When the doctor makes his rounds, she attends him and answers his questions about the patients' temperatures and pulses. Although she is apparently not supposed to, she brings Claribel her baby in an attempt to draw out Claribel's motherly love. And, of course, of her own volition and "with quick decision," she effects a reunion between Claribel and her lover, to the good of all concerned.

A NURSE NOVEL BECOMES A BEST-SELLER

It was her next novel, however, that really established Mary Roberts Rinehart as a major American author. In 1914, when war was in the air, Rinehart started on her first nonmystery novel, *K.* This was serialized in *McClure's* in 1914–15 and published in book form in 1915. The book was immensely popular and was made into two films, *The Doctor and the Woman,* in 1918, and *K—The Unknown,* in 1924. Not a traditional mystery, *K* is particularly important because it is partially autobiographical and has a strong health care theme.[21]

Sidney Page lives on "The Street"—a microcosm of life and its problems. As the story opens, Sidney is trying to cool her boyfriend's ardor for her, in anticipation of greater things than marriage. Her life is about to be changed but not altogether as she expects, and this change is heralded by the appearance of K. Le Moyne. "K," as he calls himself, is a young man who is to board at Sidney's home to help alleviate the family's financial troubles. Mr. Page is dead and Sidney's Aunt Harriet, who had been living with the Pages and helping to support them, has decided she wants to live on her own and start a sewing business. When the local physician, Dr. Ed Wilson, tells Sidney that she would make a good nurse, Sidney decides to take up this profession to attain independence.

Sidney goes to visit Dr. Ed to ask his advice, but like Mary Roberts before her, she finds a younger doctor in his office instead. The younger doctor in this case is Ed's brother, Max, a prominent surgeon in the hospital and clearly something of a ladies' man. Although Max suggests that Sidney is a little too young to be a nurse, she persuades him of her serious intentions and he agrees to show her around the hospital that very afternoon. Sidney leaves his office much impressed by him and his cooly efficient office nurse, Carlotta Harrison. But Sidney does not see the unprofessional flirtation that occurs between Max and Carlotta after she leaves.

Sidney returns home that evening full of excitement at her new career prospects and speaks of her joy to K, the new tenant. K is a mysterious character: we know nothing about him at this point, except that he works at the gas company office and dresses somewhat dowdily. He is a good listener, however, and glad of Sidney's new interest. When she finally leaves her home to become a nurse, he gives her a watch to take pulses with.

Work as a probationer is hard for Sidney and is made even harder by Carlotta Harrison, who turns up as head nurse of Sidney's first ward and treats her unkindly. Life is also made difficult by Sidney's boyfriend, Joe Drummond, who is still anxious to marry Sidney and extremely unhappy about her career aspirations. Sidney spends most of her free time at home talking with K, and Joe becomes jealous. It does not take long, however, before Joe (and the reader) realizes that Sidney is not in love with K but with Max Wilson.

Max Wilson, meanwhile, is flirting with Carlotta. Although she risks her position at the hospital by going out driving with Max, Carlotta is anxious to make a good match for herself in marriage, and she tries unsuccessfully to win Max's heart. Max has his eyes on the sweet and innocent Sidney, who clearly adores him like a god. After taking her out on a couple of occasions, Max asks Sidney to marry him. Sidney has been experiencing life at the hospital; she has mixed with unmarried mothers and prostitutes, and is not as naive as she once was. She has also seen the marriage of her close friend, Christine Palmer, turn sour on account of her husband's drunkenness and womanizing. Sidney knows of Max's reputation as a ladies' man, and she even knows that he has dated Carlotta more than once. She explains that she fears marriage to him, even though she admits she loves him.

Meanwhile, K and Joe Drummond watch Max and Sidney's developing relationship with some trepidation. We come to realize that K knows Max and Carlotta from the past and is all too aware that Max is not a dependable man. It is eventually revealed to us that K's real name is Dr. Edwardes. He had been an eminent surgeon, but he lost faith in his work after a series of mysterious surgery accidents led to the deaths, and near deaths, of a number of his patients. Max, who recognizes K and subsequently becomes the only person privy to his true feelings, tries to persuade him to return to his life's work. Max begins to use Dr. Edwardes's famous surgical techniques on his patients, with K's reluctant advice.

Max finally gets Sidney to agree to an engagement with the understanding that she should complete her training as a nurse before they formally announce it. However, Max cannot escape Carlotta, who is scheming to win him back for herself at any price. Things come to a head one evening when Max and Carlotta drive to a somewhat disreputable hotel and Carlotta, feigning illness, persuades Max to take her to a hotel bedroom. Joe, who has been jealously watching Max for some time, now thinks that Max is taking Sidney into the disreputable hotel. Incensed and armed with a gun, Joe storms the hotel and shoots Max.

The only thing that can save Max's life is the famous Edwardes operation, but only the elusive Dr. Edwardes himself can perform this difficult surgical technique. Carlotta, it so happens, used to work at Edwardes's clinic before it closed, and she too has recognized K. Anxious to save her lover's life, she breaks the news of K's true identity to the hospital staff. Reluctantly, K agrees to perform the operation and succeeds in saving Max. Sidney is totally confused by these events, but when she finally emerges from her dazed state, she knows she cannot marry a man who is so wont to be unfaithful to her. The engagement is broken, as is Sidney's heart. Sidney is also, of course, shocked to learn that K is actually the famous Edwardes.

K feels sorry for Joe, and helps him evade the police and get to Cuba, where he was thinking of going to work all along. K himself decides he will go to Cuba, for although he has saved Max's life, he still cannot restore his faith in himself. Carlotta is expelled from the hospital when it is learned that she was at the hotel with Max, and she leaves the United States to become a missionary nurse in Africa. Before she leaves, however, she sends a letter to K confessing her past sins. Apparently, Carlotta had been often reprimanded by Edwardes when she was a nurse at his clinic, and she became so angry with him that she devised a plan to discredit him. She put an extra sponge in various sponge bags so that sponges were left in patients' bodies, thus killing them. Since this letter explains the mysterious deaths, K's confidence is restored. The story ends when Sidney comes to the realization that she has been in love with K all along, and since he is, of course, in love with her, they agree to marry and to have Sidney become a nurse in his clinic.

RINEHART'S CREATIVE USE OF HER NURSING EXPERIENCES

Sidney's experiences as a nurse probationer are very similar to Rinehart's own. The probationer's work was menial and often nauseating. In *My Story,* Rinehart tells us how she worked a 12-hour day, or rather night, as both a probationer and student nurse.

> A probationer was a novice not to be trusted to, save with the most menial tasks. And although my stomach revolted at some of these tasks, and my pride at most of them, I somehow got through the day. It was not what I had dreamed.[22]

She tells us of her horror when she first cleaned out the operating room.

> The day of bloodless operations had not yet come. A blood vessel was cut, located by the spurting blood, and clipped. The result was that an operating room after a

series of operations looked like a shambles.... I was told to carry out a pail, and there was a human foot in it . . . I carried it out, and I was not sick.[23]

Like Sidney, Mary Roberts came into "contact with life as it is at its rawest and hardest," and she lost her illusions to reality, "stark and naked reality." As a student nurse, she had greater responsibility and no longer had to do menial work, but the 12-hour shifts of night duty were still the norm. Her only rest of the day came after work when the nurses congregated in the nurses' parlor for prayers.

Chapter nine of *K* is devoted to Sidney's first impressions of hospital life, and her accounts are similar to those given in Rinehart's autobiography, *My Story.*

> Sidney never forgot her early impressions of the hospital, although they were chaotic enough at first. There were uniformed young women coming and going, efficient, cool-eyed, low of voice. There were medicine closets with orderly rows of labeled bottles, linen rooms with great stacks of sheets and towels, long vistas of shining floors and lines of beds. There were brisk interns with duck clothes and brass buttons, who eyed her with friendly, patronizing glances. There were bandages and dressings, and great white screens behind which were played little or big dramas, baths or deaths, as the case might be. And over all brooded the mysterious authority of the superintendent of the training school, dubbed the Head, for short.
>
> Twelve hours a day, from seven to seven, with the off-duty intermission, Sidney labored at tasks which revolted her soul.... At twilight when, work over for the day, the night nurse, with her rubber soled shoes and tired eyes and jangling keys, having reported and received the night orders, the nurses gathered in their small parlor for prayers.... In a way, it crystallized for her what the day's work meant: charity and its sister, service, the promise of rest and peace. Into the little parlor filed the nurses, and knelt, folding their tired hands.[24]

The portrayal of nursing in *K* is, obviously then, an accurate one for its time—realistic, though not altogether appealing. Although Sidney works demanding 12-hour shifts, she only receives a uniform and $8 a month allowance, barely enough to buy her thermometers. At first Sidney considers giving up her nursing career to marry the great surgeon Max Wilson (just as the real-life Mary Roberts married Dr. Stanley Rinehart), but when she turns her affections to K/Edwardes instead, she commits herself to pursuing her profession, at least for a while. Never does

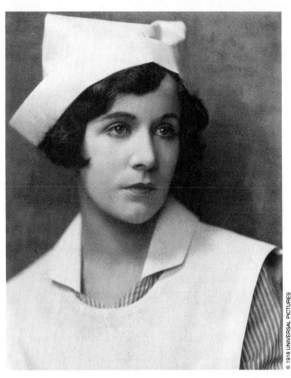

Although Sidney works demanding 12-hour shifts, she only receives a uniform and $8 a month allowance, barely enough to buy her thermometers.

Sidney complain that the hospital demands too much from her; it is up to her to knuckle under and do more than her best. Mary Roberts Rinehart in fact was physically worn out and ill after her stint of three years as a nursing student, but she does not show Sidney suffering any detrimental effects from her nursing experiences except extreme fatigue.

Sidney is characterized rather idealistically. Because one of the major themes of the novel is the importance of achieving a balance between service to humanity and clearheadedness in personal relationships, Sidney, like K, serves an important function in representing this happy medium. When the novel opens, Sidney appears to be particularly young and innocent, though determined. Through her exposure to "life in the raw," however, she gains a broader perspective on the nature of the world and on nursing, learning to cope with pain, dissatisfaction, and even tragedy. But more important, she learns to read people more accurately. Thus she can

say to Max at the end of the novel: "Now I know that I didn't care for you, really, at all. But I built up an idol and worshipped it. I always saw you through a sort of haze. . . . It's just that I never loved the real you, because I never knew the real you." It is hard to imagine a real-life human being making such a controlled statement of his or her feelings, and throughout *K,* Sidney's firm grasp on her life appears as unlikely, particularly when all around her are suffering deep inner anguish. Sidney seems charmed, sailing unconcernedly through life while people try to poison her patients, shoot her fiancé, and take advantage of her sweetness. Nonetheless, although Sidney does not come across as a totally realistic or complex character, she is human enough, and certainly has an engaging personality. She is honest with others and makes an attempt to be honest with herself. She has no pretensions and is capable, despite her seriousness toward nursing, of admitting her attraction to her uniform: "I am afraid just now I am thinking more of the cap than what it means. It *is* becoming!"[25]

Sidney personifies the ideal of dedication to a nursing career. While her view of the world undergoes some changes during the course of the novel, she remains convinced of the importance of providing service to the needy. In this respect she echoes Rinehart's own attitude toward the nursing profession, which she clearly saw as a noble service. In *My Story,* Rinehart writes:

> That night at prayers I had the beginnings of a sense of service, and of the joy of service. The tired women, their caps askew, their aprons soiled and stained, kneeling before those hard oak chairs, and humbly confessing their sins . . . my heart swelled. I would be good. I would work very hard and be very good.[26]

And Sidney Page's idealism is no different: she would not "forget the vow she had taken of charity and its sister, service, of a cup of water to the thirsty, of open arms to a tired child."[27]

Only one other nurse is characterized fully in *K,* and that is Carlotta. In a sense, Carlotta is the villain of the plot; it is apparent from the beginning that she is cunning and dishonest. On her first date with Max, she thinks:

> What an adventure! What a night. Let him lose his head a little; she could keep hers. If she were skillful and played things right, who could tell? To marry him, to

leave behind the drudgery of the hospital, to feel safe as she had not felt for years, that was a stroke to play for![28]

Carlotta's lack of interest in her job is apparent, and although she does not go out of her way to shirk her regular duties, she seems to barely tolerate caring for patients. Her responses to unpleasant situations within the hospital are occasionally downright appalling: she poisons one patient in order to try to discredit Sidney, of whom she is jealous, and she had sabotaged the sponge count at Edwardes's clinic in order to discredit him. Carlotta does have some conscience, however: after poisoning a patient, "her very soul was sick with fear of what she had done." In the end she commits herself to a life without sexual fulfillment in barbaric Africa, as a missionary nurse, as if to purge herself of her sins. "I am not going because I feel any call to work, but because I do not know what else to do," she writes K.[29]

Carlotta provides a sharp contrast to Sidney, who is both the ideal woman and the ideal nurse. Sidney is committed to her profession, interested in patients' welfare, warm, giving, and at all times rational and responsible. Carlotta's malpractice in hospital settings does not contribute to a poor image of the nursing profession, because it is clearly understood that she does not behave as a normal nurse (or person) would. She certainly contributes to an image of the nurse as a woman who enters the profession in order to catch a medical man for a husband, and this image is also enhanced by Sidney's marriage to K. But probably the strongest contribution to the image of nursing made by Carlotta is that same one contributed by Sidney: that nursing is a noble service. Being a bad person, Carlotta is unable to comprehend such an ideology, and she is thrown out of her nursing position at Edwardes's clinic and then at the hospital basically because of that. Though Carlotta has the opposite character traits of Sidney, she ends up contributing toward the same image of nursing.

The other nurses in the hospital are, in general, presented favorably. Background figures, they are depicted as busy, concerned, involved, and dedicated. Although they do not have the optimistic view of life that Sidney exhibits, "their philosophy made them no less tender." But Rinehart does, on occasion, emphasize the coldness of some of the older nurses.

"To them, perhaps just a little weary with time and much service, the banging cup meant not so much thirst as annoyance." To Sidney each patient deserves a personal commitment, and she refuses to ignore their calls: "To them [the older nurses], pain was a thing to be recorded on a report; to Sidney, it was written on the tablets of her soul."[30]

A significant problem with the image of the nursing profession in *K* comes from the relationship between the nurses and the physicians. Whereas the physicians are venerated by the nurses, no doctor openly admires or praises a nurse. Physicians are condescending in their attitude toward nurses. When Ed Wilson suggests to Max that Sidney start work as a probationer at the hospital, Max's immediate response is, "she used to be a pretty little thing. There is no use filling up the wards with a lot of ornaments; it keeps the interns all stewed up." And when Sidney explains to Max, "I am not in love with anybody; I haven't time to be in love. I have my profession now," Max trivializes her ambition: "Bah! A woman's real profession is love." Max asks the head nurse to have Sidney assigned to the operating room, and although the hospital is very busy and moving Sidney is a great inconvenience, the nurse readily complies. The reasons for the reassignment are totally unprofessional. Max "wanted her with him, and he wanted her to see him at work: the age-old instinct of the male to have his woman see him at his best." The interns seem to resent "the patronizing instructions of nurses as to rules," the implication being that although nurses may be better trained than recent medical school graduates, their display of superior knowledge is unwanted.[31]

The overall image of nursing in *K*, then, is a familiar one in fiction: it is a noble profession of service, demanding hard work but offering only vicarious rewards. This is a conventional image, one that Rinehart herself did not seek too hard to question and certainly did not seek to alter. The angelic image of nursing in literature continued to be effective in attracting better-class women to nursing at the turn of the century and beyond, although it was being tempered with realism, and a secularized, middle-class nurse, competent but still human, was beginning to emerge. Nursing had been accepted, along with the stereotype of noble, womanly work, as an occupation that could be exercised by the most respectable, educated women before marriage.[32]

THE ANGEL OF MERCY MOVES TO THE SCREEN

The commercial production and exhibition of movies began early in the twentieth century, first as peep shows and then with film projected on theater screens where many people could watch simultaneously. The first movies were primitive in technique, with inexperienced actors and directors. Shown in nickelodeons, these short films depicted familiar scenes of city life—the pool hall, the ghetto, the pawnshop, the police and fire departments in action. Crude though they were, the early films proved enormously popular. This attracted businessmen who built theaters and companies that produced hundreds of short films.

From 1896 to 1903, films were categorized into such loosely defined major classifications as "View," "New Events," "Vaudeville Turns," "Incidents," and "Magical Pictures." After 1903, however, with the introduction of the fictional or narrative film of ever-increasing length, these types began to proliferate and assume a more substantial form. In the period from 1903 to 1915, the film industry continued to standardize film production by devising the concept of the formula picture—dramas (or melodramas), romances, action pictures, westerns, and comedies were all reduced to certain fixed formulas that made these types of films the major staples on which movie producers depended for regular, consistent profits. By 1910 the nickelodeon had so captivated the public that 10,000 theaters were playing to total weekly audiences of 10 million.

D. W. Griffith, the first film director to use such modern film techniques as close-ups and fade-outs, remained firmly under the spell of late-Victorian dramatic conventions. Movie heroines were demure creatures with large luminous eyes and ringlets. Heroes were broad-chested stalwarts in white shirts and riding boots. Comedy films relied on nineteenth-century vaudeville traditions of knockabout.

When this comedy formula was applied to nursing, amusement most commonly arose from the antics of a nurse being pursued by an ardent admirer. In about a dozen films of the period, an erstwhile stranger sees a pretty nurse and immediately falls in love with her: this happens in *Hospital Hoax* (Kalem, 1912), *Billy's Nurse* (MinA, 1915), *Wanted—a Nurse* (AM&B, 1915), *Perkin's Pep Producer* (Selig, 1915),

Ham's Busy Day (Kalem, 1916), *Not What the Doctor Ordered* (Arrow Film Corp., 1916), the British *Nursie! Nursie!* (Klever Pictures, 1916), *The Nurse of an Aching Heart* (LKO, 1917), and *Red Cross Nurse* (World Film Corp., 1918).

In all these, the hero typically sees the nurse by accident (usually on the street) and then determines to inveigle himself into his dream woman's presence. In keeping with the inconsequentiality of early comedy—which rarely attempted to ascribe motivation—complete strangers were most commonly smitten with nurses. In *Good Morning Nurse* (Victor, 1917) and *Some Nurse* (Universal, 1917), however, the heroes are identified as the nurses' friends and hitherto-spurned lovers, eager to recapture their affection by drastic action. Would-be suitors, having selected the nurse of their choice, were prepared to endure all manner of inconvenience in order to achieve proximity to her. The usual ploy was to become a patient, either by feigning illness (as in *Billy's Nurse*) or by engineering a disability (as in *Good Morning Nurse,* where the lovesick hero pays someone to run him over).

As the feature-length film gradually replaced the two-reeler, the number of substantial dramatic films

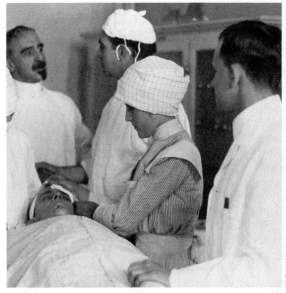

KALEM, 1912

Complete strangers were commonly smitten with nurses, as in the 1912 two-reeler, Hospital Hoax.

increased. Of these early films, 20 incorporated nursing into their main plots, either by having a nurse as the heroine or by associating the heroine with nursing in a thematically important way. Moral courage, professional dedication and objectivity, a capacity for heroic, selfless action and forgiveness, a strong sense of duty—such qualities recurred persistently in the nurse heroines who populated the dramas of the time. Romance continued to play a leading role, and in many nursing dramas that meant a token alignment with a convenient physician, as in *The Nurse at Mulberry Bend* (Kalem, 1913), *The Nurse and the Counterfeiter* (Kalem, 1914), and *A Man's Sin* (Thanhouser, 1916). These films are unusual in that they placed little emphasis on romantic interest. *The Nurse and the Counterfeiter,* for example, portrays a doctor-nurse partnership that, eschewing a hospital setting and professional concerns for the duration of the film, sets out to combat a couple of criminals. In this instance, suspense is far more important than romance, and both are more important than nursing.

The Promise Land (Essanay, 1916), however, does more with the doctor-nurse relationship, using the doctor's love as an ultimate reward that the previously ill-used and subsequently deserving heroine eventually obtains. The film depicts how once-poor, childhood sweethearts from a small town drifted apart. Both had originally had dreams about the "promise land" of the title, a place where all their ambitions would be achieved. But time deals with each quite differently. The boy becomes a distinguished surgeon, fulfilling his desires, but finds little satisfaction in his work. The girl marries an unreliable salesman who eventually deserts her, leaving her with a child. She becomes a nurse to support the child and then, one day, she and her childhood sweetheart are reunited over an operating table. Their patient is the woman's long-lost salesman husband, severely injured in an accident. Despite their combined efforts, however, the man dies. Then the couple realize that their dreams have been mere illusions and that they belong together in the small town where they were born. Accordingly, they return there to begin life together.[33]

The exceptional *Dr. Neighbor* (Universal, 1916) derives considerable drama from the interaction between doctor and nurse but without involving romance between them. In essence, the story tells how a wealthy young woman, severely injured in an accident, asks her nurse—who is also her devoted best friend—to end her agony by administering extra morphine. The nurse, harrowed by the sight of her friend's suffering, does as she is begged. Dr. Neighbor, the heroine's physician, finds the telltale bottle, deduces what has happened, and nobly claims responsibility for the young woman's death to clear the nurse from suspicion. When a jealous rival initiates an investigation, Neighbor is put on trial for his life. Unable to keep silent any longer, the nurse eventually admits her guilt, thus saving the physician from conviction as a murderer.[34]

The necessity, however, of including romantic interest was very strong. If, as in *Dr. Neighbor,* the physician does not attract the nurse character in a romantic way, another man usually does. In *The Nurse* (Edison, 1912), the nurse eventually marries the man she forgives for injuring her brother. In *The Regeneration of Margaret* (Essanay, 1916), the nurse falls in love with the doctor's son, whom she had once thought to be her own brother. In *When a Woman Sins* (Fox, 1918), Theda Bara is a private-duty nurse who eventually marries her patient's son.[35]

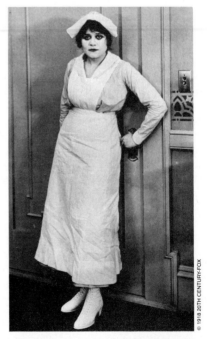

In When a Woman Sins *(1918), Theda Bara is a private-duty nurse who eventually marries her patient's son.*

© 1918 20TH CENTURY-FOX

Despite the domination of romantic interest in pre-World War I films, there were at least a few productions of a dramatic nature in which the emphasis was placed more on the courage and determination that professional commitment—not sentimentality—inspired. In 1913 *The Nurse at Mulberry Bend* portrayed an ambitious career nurse who, while supposedly convalescing from the results of excessive study, becomes deeply involved in helping a disadvantaged family. When an Italian woman comes begging at the heroine's door, she is alerted to the appallingly impoverished conditions under which the woman and her family have to survive. Subsequent visits to the family home compound the nurse's concern for the welfare of the woman's baby, whose safety seems threatened by a brutal and ignorant father. Although a doctor's help is required to rectify the situation, the film appears to have depicted its heroine as a young woman of strong character, dedicated to her profession, with a well-developed social conscience and a firm belief in the need for a public health service. At the end she decides to dedicate herself to working with physicians to alleviate problems in other poverty-stricken areas.[36]

In 1917 female director Lois Weber's *The Hand that Rocks the Cradle* (Universal), one of the most interesting nurse films of this period, was released with widespread publicity. Although apparently fictional, the story was suggested by events surrounding the case of Margaret Sanger, the New York nurse and social reformer whose controversial ideas on family planning Weber had bravely propagated in a documentary released a month earlier called, simply, *Birth Control* (Message Photoplay, 1917). Sanger's attempts to gather and disseminate birth control information among the poor of New York—whose desperate health, social, and financial conditions so often seemed to relate to unwanted pregnancies—aroused much wrath in the early-twentieth century. After setting up the nation's first birth control clinic in Brooklyn, she was sent to the workhouse for a month on the charge of creating a public nuisance. But her subsequent appeal and a supportive public outcry led to her release and permission for her work to continue.[37]

The Hand that Rocks the Cradle depicts Mrs. Sanger in the fictional character of Mrs. Broome, who is also a doctor's wife. As the film opens, Dr. Broome has just secured his wife's release from police custody by giving his word that she will stop disseminating birth control literature—an activity he just learned about and one of which he strongly disapproves. The Grahams, friends of the Broomes, tell them about their old nursemaid, Sarah, whose life is miserable because of too little money and too many children. Mrs. Broome, overwhelmed with compassion when Sarah calls on her for advice, sees that her duty lies in sharing her valuable knowledge. The Grahams themselves, however, adamantly refuse to benefit from the lesson of Sarah's story, even though Mrs. Graham has her own hands full with three children.

Despite being ostracized by her friends and condemned by society in general, Mrs. Broome determines to launch an all-out crusade to bring her knowledge to those like Sarah who need it most. In her campaign she is assisted by Sarah herself, the steadfast supporter who willingly accompanies her to prison after they are arrested for spreading propaganda in violation of state laws. As in the Sanger case, the women are pardoned and find consolation for the future in the words of an enlightened judge who considers that the only controversy about birth control relates to "how and by whom it should be exercised."[38]

NURSE EDITH CAVELL

When war broke out in Europe in August 1914, public sentiment in the United States favored strict neutrality. Most war films produced in the United States promoted pacifist themes, in keeping with the national mood. However, as news of German atrocities committed in Belgium filtered into American consciousness, gradually U.S. filmmakers began favoring the Allies and encouraging Americans to think in terms of preparing for possible war. British films were among the first pro-Allied propaganda tools to find a ready audience in the United States. One of the most publicized tales of German perfidy concerned the life and work of an English nurse working in Belgium, Edith Cavell, whom the German military authorities arrested for treason because of her assistance in getting wounded Allied soldiers out of Belgium. Her arrest and detention aroused the indignation of the Allied world and the United States. Despite efforts to obtain her release, the Germans executed her on October 12, 1915.

Edith Cavell's execution still chills the soul of whoever reads of her courage and nobility. The execution of a woman, particularly a nurse engaged in humanitarian work, before a military firing squad, confirmed many Americans' suspicions that accounts of German atrocities toward innocent civilians were quite true. Ironically, Cavell herself denied any chauvinistic purpose in her work and would undoubtedly have shuddered at the war-mongering uses for which her story worked so well. Yet within six months of her death, American audiences were able to see a film version, *Nurse and Martyr* (Midland Studio, 1916), produced in England and distributed throughout the world.[39]

Nurse and Martyr, which dealt with the "glorious passing of Nurse Cavell," preceded by only a few months an Australian version, *The Martyrdom of Nurse Cavell* (Australia Films, 1916), which set attendance records in several major cities. The popularity of these two films assured that after American entry into the war in 1917, U.S. filmmakers would

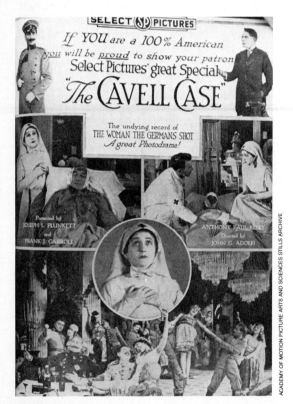

The film The Woman the Germans Shot *(1918) contrasted the self-sacrificial work of Nurse Edith Cavell with the licentious living of the Germans occupying Brussels.*

present their own versions. *The Woman the Germans Shot* (Select Films, 1918), a six-reel feature starring Julia Arthur, received high praise from New York critics, one of whom urged readers to see it "so that their sense of justice may be quickened." The film contrasted the self-sacrificing work of Cavell with the licentious living of the Germans occupying Brussels. Cavell always assumed saintly poses, eyes cast heavenward, while she comforted the afflicted or awaited her execution. The Germans swilled champagne and danced with loose women while Cavell bravely risked her life to help Allied soldiers. This film demonstrated that a nurse needed physical courage to save the lives of soldiers: she might even sacrifice her life.[40]

Two more Cavell films appeared at the time of the Armistice. Both *The Great Victory* (Metro, 1919) and *Why Germany Must Pay* (Metro, 1919) used Cavell's story to support demands for harsh punishment for vanquished Germany. In all of these films, the viewer's attention was focused on the barbarism of the German army in persecuting and executing a brave woman and nurse. The titles of the first two films left little doubt as to the association between nursing and saintliness during wartime.[41]

The transference of the strong emotional response elicited by Cavell's true-life story to fictional film melodramas was easily accomplished, partly because of the unsophisticated level of film criticism of both viewers and professional critics. Filmmakers during the war routinely staged recreations and passed them off as actual footage of historic events; a very fine, often invisible line separated fiction from fact in the early efforts of wartime propagandists. Thus fictional nurse heroines evoked in film audiences a ready sympathy, a sympathy built upon what was known of Nurse Cavell and her fate. The nursing identification served a variety of symbolic functions that sanctified and legitimized the actions of the heroine. Not only did the nurse character provide a ready foil to Germanic malevolence, but she also provided clear guidelines for approved female behavior during wartime.

IDEAL FEMALE WAR IMAGES

The war years gave a military flavor to costume as the populace turned its attention to sending soldiers overseas. Women served in several military departments during World War I. In general their uniforms consisted of ankle-length skirts and jackets similar to those worn by the men in service. The "Marionettes," or Women Marines, and members of the Women's Motor Corps wore khaki uniforms, with khaki blouses and ties, and wool overcoats to match. Those in the Army Nurse Corps, the Navy Nurse Corps, and the "Yeomanettes" wore navy blue uniforms, white blouses, blue ties, black shoes, and blue straw sailor hats with brims and overseas caps. The American Red Cross nurse wore an Oxford-gray uniform, white blouse, red scarf, white cotton gloves, gray overseas cap, and high-laced black shoes. A nurse on duty might also wear a white uniform, white cap or draped headpiece with a Red Cross insignia on it, and a navy blue cape with a red lining.

World War I saw the last glorious outpouring of the angel of mercy imagery that had persisted since the time of Nightingale. The nurse was the envy of all American women as rampant, media-inspired patriotism instilled the desire to play an active role near the fighting front. Hundreds of society women sought to pressure Congress to allow them to go overseas to serve as nursing aides at their own expense. In the media, nurses were consistently pre-sented as noble and heroic. An inspirational, saintly, other-worldly aspect to nursing the wounded was seen in countless portrayals. For example, several recruitment posters and magazine covers featured nurses imposing themselves between recumbent, wounded soldiers and the threatening, robed figure of Death lurking in the foreground. A typical draw-ing, inscribed, "The Angel of Life in the Valley of the Shadow of Death," featured an ethereal, illuminated nursing figure standing and pointing the way for a group of fallen soldiers in no-man's-land.

The typical World War I film told of how a young American male volunteered for service in the war, how his nurse sweetheart joined up to be near him, how he was wounded, and how, fortuitously, she found him and restored him to health. Furthermore, the strong propagandist attitudes of filmmakers usu-ally guaranteed that there would be a few scenes of a brutal and animalistic German officer threatening to rape the nurse.

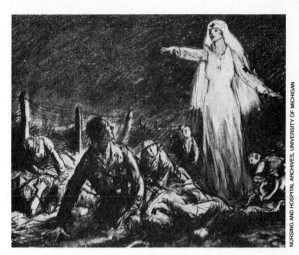

The Angel of Life in the Valley of the Shadow of Death.

VIRGIN NURSE AND GERMAN BEAST

In *The Heart of Humanity* (Universal, 1919), the deeply religious heroine, Nanette, is inspired by a vision of a Red Cross nurse bringing relief to refugee children. After joining the war effort, Nanette works in a small French village where she nurses and feeds homeless children. The urgent need for care of wounded soldiers brings Nanette to the battlefield. Accompanied by her faithful Red Cross dog, Nanette kneels over the stretcher cases in an effort to nurse the wounded. She tries to give a drink of water to a wounded German enlisted man, but the brute takes advantage of the opportunity to force himself upon Nanette. Fortunately, the Red Cross dog intervenes and quickly rips out the throat of Nanette's attacker. As the battle continues, Nanette, carrying a lamp like her famous predecessor, ministers to the dying and wounded.[42]

When the Germans are later closing in on the small town where Nanette's orphans are gathered, she tries to evacuate them. As the last truck of orphans and their nurses is moving out, Nanette hears the cries of one more infant and sets out to rescue it. She is seen entering the abandoned house by Erich, a nasty-looking German officer. He follows her upstairs, his intentions perfectly and horrifyingly clear. As the baby howls in its crib, Erich advances upon Nanette, rips her uniform to shreds, and attempts to pin down and rape the struggling nurse. The baby's cries interfere with Erich's perverse plea-sures, so he brutally tosses the child out the window. At this, Nanette flees into another room, where she regresses into her childhood, cradling a grotesque broken doll while Erich tries in vain to break through the heavy door. An American soldier appears on the scene just in time and shoots Erich before the brute reaches Nanette.

Nanette recuperates in a French hospital, where she is decorated by the authorities for her courage. After recovering, she returns home with several orphans, whom she distributes among families who have lost their sons. Eventually, the long war is over, and the Allies have triumphed—humanity has conquered the beast. The final scene shows Nanette reunited with family and friends.

Although Nanette is the only nurse character featured prominently in this story, other nurses appear in several scenes. In one sequence, a legion of volunteer nurses marches through the streets on their way to join the struggle. In this example of military organization, it was made clear that through nursing women could contribute to the fight against the evil Germans.

Nursing in this film commanded the audience's great admiration and respect. Nanette is brave, loving, and kind. She chooses nursing as a way to serve humanity; indeed her nursing activity qualifies her to symbolize the "heart of humanity." Association is made between religious feeling and the desire to nurse. Nanette's demeanor and attitudes toward her religion cast her in a Madonna-like role, thus raising nursing to the level of a divine calling. In a scene reminiscent of the experiences of Joan of Arc, Nanette sees visions and hears voices calling her to dress as a Red Cross nurse and to save the suffering children. The climax of the story comes when Erich threatens both her chastity and her maternal concerns. Although she is distressed by Erich's obscene advances, only when he tosses the child out the window does Nanette's mind snap, causing her to retreat into a childlike shell. Because of all these powerful and emotive associations, the German's deeds become even more loathsome. If anything could be worse than attempted rape, it would be attempted rape of the Virgin Mother, personified by Nanette— after first throwing the baby Jesus out the window.

In *Vive La France!* (Paramount, 1918), Dorothy Dalton plays a nurse named Jenevieve who, while working in New York, learns that her parents have been killed by the Germans. She hastens to her native village, where she finds her brother still alive, so she remains to nurse him. When the village is captured again by the Germans, her brother is killed.

A German attempts to overpower her, but she falls unconscious in the struggle against him. When she awakens she finds that she, like many other captured women, has been branded with the "cross of shame."[43]

Jenevieve begins to work as a Red Cross nurse in her native village. There she meets a wounded soldier, Jean, who happens to be an ex-actor and former colleague. She restores Jean to consciousness and bravely figures a way to smuggle him out of the hands of the Germans. Later, trying to escape the Germans herself, Jenevieve puts on the uniform of a dead German soldier. She is caught by the French and almost executed as a spy, until someone spots her "cross of shame." Jean returns to the village again months later, suffering from amnesia; again Jenevieve nurses him back to health, and at the end of the film, they acknowledge their love for each other.

This film contrasts the "cross of shame"—the symbol of sexual violation—with the Red Cross uniform worn by the heroine while she works among the wounded in her village. The nursing uniform negates the sullying mark of rape and allows the heroine to remain within her village and even to marry her beloved at the film's end. The restorative power of the nurse's uniform lets the filmmaker shock his audience with their worst fears for the young woman's safety and at the same time assure them that her suffering will be relieved. We see the woman not only returned to her prewar chastity by wearing the spotless white uniform, but also rewarded for her physical bravery with the love of a good man. The nursing identity in every way served as an amulet for the preservation of moral integrity in the midst of corruptive influences.

The Splendid Sinner (Goldwyn, 1918) starred Mary Garden in a war story that combined a good number of plot twists and character transformations noted in other war films. In this story, there is a triangle between a woman, a German-American lover, and an Allied rival; there is some spying activity by the nurse; there is a moral transformation of a fallen woman redeemed by nursing; and finally, there is an interesting ending that says a lot about the image of nursing. The story follows the attempts of beautiful Dolores to change the direction of her life. As the movie begins, Dolores is the rich and pampered mistress of a German-American, Rudolph von Zorn. She has tired, however, of the empty friendships and

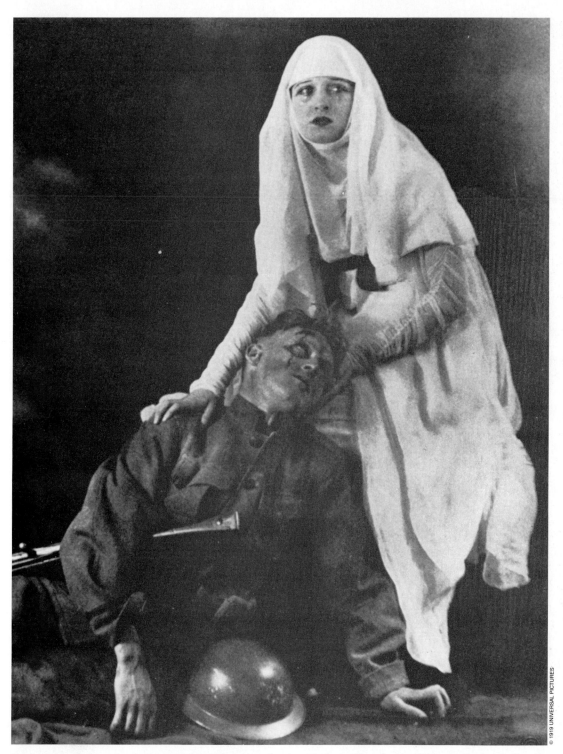

© 1919 UNIVERSAL PICTURES

Nanette's demeanor and attitudes toward her religion cast her in a Madonna-like role, in which nursing was raised to the level of a divine calling.

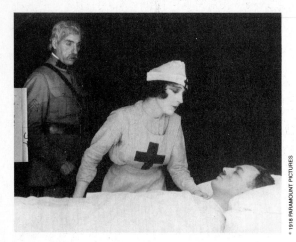

Vive La France! *(1918) contrasted the "cross of shame"—the symbol of sexual violation—with the Red Cross uniform worn by the heroine while she works among the wounded in her village.*

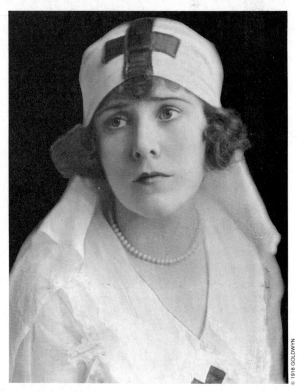

In The Splendid Sinner *(1918), German General Von Zorn offers Dolores a chance to escape execution by becoming his mistress once more. Ennobled by her recent reunion with her husband, Dolores refuses and is executed in her Red Cross uniform.*

humiliating bondage to an unattractive but wealthy man. So she leaves von Zorn and escapes into the country to restore herself. There she meets Hugh Maxwell, a young American physician, and marries him without telling him of her past. Although she loves her new husband, she does not enjoy his relative poverty, and she slips back into her loose morals. Eventually Hugh learns of her past and abandons her to enlist in the Canadian army. Dolores becomes a Red Cross nurse in order to atone for her misdeeds and works in a hospital that has come under the control of the Germans. One of her patients is none other than her wounded husband; they are reunited in their love for each other. Her husband asks her to smuggle a message across the German lines, but she is discovered and arrested as a spy. The general in charge of her case is, naturally, von Zorn, her ex-lover. Von Zorn offers her a chance to escape execution by becoming his mistress once more. Ennobled by her recent reunion with her husband, Dolores refuses and is executed in her Red Cross uniform.[44]

The image of nursing offered in this film is unequivocal: after a woman assumes the mantle of atonement and self-sacrifice—the Red Cross uniform—there is no limit to her capacity for self-sacrifice. She willingly gives her life rather than revert to her disreputable past. Sacrificing her own life, she also allows her husband to escape recognition. Not

only is the nurse portrayed as noble and courageous—a veritable martyr to German evil—but the nursing identification assures that she dies with all her redeemed virtue. One critic of the film felt that the Germans would not have shot a confessed spy in the uniform of the Red Cross—but recognized that the uniform served an important function regarding the viewer's perception of the character's moral transformation; "if the director had shown the heroine being deprived of her insignia it would have harmed the picture . . . because it would have shown too plainly that she had disregarded conventions even as the enemy we are now fighting does most reprehensibly." In other words, the nursing identification was the heroine's proof of moral reform; she had to wear the uniform in order to achieve a martyr's death.[45]

OTHER WAR ADVENTURES OF NURSES

Adele (United Pictures, 1919), based on the autobiography *The Nurse's Story* by Adele Bleneau, was another World War I film about the adventures of a trained nurse. What makes the film notable for the image of nursing is that the heroine, Adele, had been trained as a nurse prior to the outbreak of war; so although she is a Red Cross volunteer, she is not without experience. The plot of *Adele* follows the heroine from her home in Louisiana to the battlefronts of Europe. The heroine is the daughter of a wealthy and famous Louisiana doctor; she takes great interest in his hospital work, learns a great deal about medicine, and qualifies as a nurse. After her father dies, she finds the life of luxury boring and is among the first to volunteer as a war nurse. In Wash-

ington, D.C., she meets a handsome British officer, Captain Fraser, who falls in love with her; they later find themselves on the same ship to France. Also aboard is a Captain von Schulling, who vies for Adele's affections, but with little success.[46]

Adele's nursing assignment is near the front, and some of the scenes are gruesome in that bloodied soldiers and agony are all too realistically portrayed. When Adele learns that Captain Fraser has been seriously wounded and is stranded in an area still under fire, she organizes a rescue party and brings him to safety. Shortly thereafter von Schulling is brought into the hospital, also wounded, and placed in the same room as Fraser. The evil German creeps out of bed and rips off his rival's bandages. Adele discovers him, fights him away, and tends to her beloved. The final scenes of the film find the Allies' hospital surrounded by Germans. Von Schulling suggests that Adele either help him by betraying the Allies or else witness Fraser being executed on false charges of spying. Predictably, she foils the Germans and escapes with her beloved into a happy future.

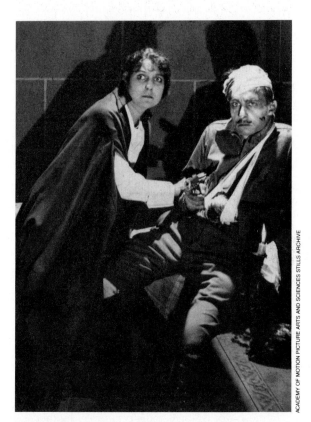

ACADEMY OF MOTION PICTURE ARTS AND SCIENCES STILLS ARCHIVE

When Adele learns that Captain Fraser has been seriously wounded and is stranded in an area still under fire, she organizes a rescue party and brings him to safety.

WAR NURSING AS A MEANS OF MORAL REGENERATION

Nursing was used mainly as a mode for moral regeneration in several war films. In *Revelation* (Metro, 1918), Nazimova plays Joline, a Paris cabaret singer and exotic dancer who also poses as a model for an American artist. The artist has placed her in poses of notorious temptresses of the past, such as Cleopatra, Salome, and others. Commissioned by a wealthy patron, the artist begins to paint Joline in the pose of the "Madonna of the Rose Bush." Therein, Joline undergoes a miraculous moral transfiguration: she abandons her lover, the artist, and her life of gaiety in exchange for a life of service to others—as a Red Cross nurse. The artist enlists in the army, and eventually the two are reunited after Joline nurses him back to health. Although the not-so-subtle hand of God effects her transformation, the concrete expression of Joline's new character is her voluntary service as a Red Cross nurse.[47]

Perhaps the most famous vamp of the silent film era was Theda Bara. In one of the earliest and most successful examples of Hollywood's ability to fashion legend from thin air, young Theodosia Goodman from Cincinnati, Ohio, became the most exotic, most

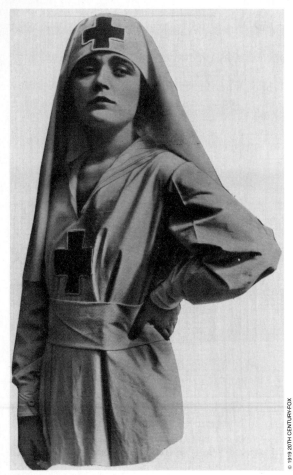

© 1919 20TH CENTURY-FOX

In The Light *(1918), Theda Bara plays Blanchette Dumonde, the "wickedest woman" in Paris. Interest from an artist who wants to use her as a model for a Madonna statue prompts Blanchette to reorder her life. She tries to enlist in the Red Cross to become a nurse, but her reputation has preceded her and she is refused.*

tantalizing and sensual wanton to emerge in the cinema. Mystery and sexual aura surrounded her. Her contracts included stipulations that would keep her from appearing in public or doing anything that might detract from her manufactured persona. According to the Hollywood press agents who created her, Theda Bara (an anagram for Arab Death) was born in Egypt under the shadow of the Sphinx —a long way from Cincinnati—to a French painter and an Arabian princess. The locale and parentage changed from time to time, but the overall notion of

exoticism and eroticism remained. Clothed seductively in period costumes and made up with kohl-darkened eyes and white powder, Bara typically stunned her audiences with her sexuality.

In 1918 Bara starred in *The Light* (Fox), a story very reminiscent of Nazimova's vehicle, *Revelation.* In *The Light,* Bara plays Blanchette Dumonde, the "wickedest woman" in Paris. Interest from an artist who wants to use her as a model for a Madonna statue prompts Blanchette to reorder her life. She tries to enlist in the Red Cross to become a nurse, but her reputation has preceded her and she is refused. Once again she plunges into an orgy of riotous living. As she is fleeing the wrath of one lover while in the company of a new one, she sees the artist, now a blind soldier. She abandons her lover to become the private-duty nurse to the blind sculptor. He recognizes her, and for a while the two live an idyllic existence. The first rejected lover arrives to kill the artist, but Blanchette shoots him instead. Then the second lover arrives with similar intentions but is overcome by the change he sees in Blanchette, so he leaves the artist and nurse alone, taking upon himself the blame for the first lover's death. Again, nursing, even "private-duty," is shown to be the only way for a woman to redeem herself in wartime. (Bara also starred in a similar film about a vamp reformed by nursing: *Her Double Life,* Fox, 1916).[48]

The war films reviewed here belong to the vast number of popular films made during the war. These films undoubtedly contributed to American resolve to struggle against the Germans and, as an unexpected legacy, revealed a good deal about how Americans pictured themselves as moral counterweights to European intriguers. Of the heroic Americans portrayed in these films, young females generally appeared in the role of volunteer nurses and always came from the ranks of morally pure, upper-class society. Their nursing identification provided them with a symbolic protection of their reputations, despite their wartime experiences. Foreign women often appeared as fallen women, but nursing provided them an avenue by which to return to a chaste state. Also, these reformed women were often regenerated by the love of an American; the nursing identification thus accompanied a type of Americanization of foreigners.

In these World War I media portrayals, another model of an angel of mercy with new values was depicted. The nursing identification provided an effective way to mask the novelty of female independence with traditional female values. These nurse portrayals gave the viewing public much-needed encouragement to accept an expanded sphere of female efforts. Nurse characters demonstrated, countless times, that women could provide enormous wartime support and make their own decisions, without jeopardizing the prewar social arrangements. This prefigured a transformation that was to take place for American women as a whole. Almost all the nurse characters came from sheltered, prosperous backgrounds, and the decision to become a nurse emerged consciously. Perhaps the greatest change in female standards to be observed in these portrayals was a consistent devaluation of those women providing no useful war service.

NOTES

1. Edith Wharton, *The Fruit of the Tree* (New York: Charles Scribner's Sons, 1907), p. 5.

2. Ibid., p. 555.

3. Ibid., p. 605–606.

4. Eleanor Hallowell Abbott, *The White Linen Nurse* (New York: The Century Co., 1913), p. 23.

5. Ibid., p. 45.

6. Ibid., p. 59.

7. Ibid., p. 70.

8. Ibid., pp. 3–7.

9. Ibid., p. 41.

10. Ibid., p. 70; p. 53.

11. Ibid., pp. 3–6.

12. William De Morgan, *Alice-for-Short* (New York: Henry Holt & Co., 1907).

13. J. Johnston Abraham, *The Night Nurse* (New York: E.P. Dutton & Co., 1914), p. 18.

14. F. Marion Crawford, *The White Sister* (New York: Grosset & Dunlap, 1909), p. 285.

15. Irving Harlow Hart," The One Hundred Leading Authors of Best Sellers in Fiction From 1895–1944," *Publishers Weekly* Vol. 149 (January 19, 1946): 285—287.

16. *See* Mary Roberts Rinehart, *My Story* (New York: Farrar and Rinehart, 1931).

17. Ibid., p. 95.

18. Mary Roberts Rinehart, "The Miracle," *McClure's* 39 (June 1912):139—148.

19. Ibid., p. 141.

20. Ibid., p. 147.

21. Mary Roberts Rinehart, *K* (Boston: Houghton-Mifflin, 1915).

22. Rinehart, *My Story,* p. 51.

23. Ibid., p. 53.

24. Rinehart, *K,* pp. 102–103.

25. Ibid., pp. 102–103.

26. Rinehart, *My Story,* p. 52.

27. Rinehart, *K,* p. 410.

28. Ibid., p. 313.

29. Ibid., p. 407.

30. Ibid., p. 103.

31. Ibid., p. 271.

32. Ibid., p. 57.

33. *The Promise Land* (Essanay, 1916), B & W, 3 reels.

34. *Dr. Neighbor* (Universal, 1916), B & W, 5 reels.

35. *The Nurse* (Edison, 1912), B & W, 10 min; *The Regeneration of Margaret* (Essanay, 1916), B & W, 3 reels; *When a Woman Sins* (Fox, 1918, B & W, 7 reels.

36. *Nurse at Mulberry Bend* (Kalem, 1913), B & W, 10 min.

37. *The Hand that Rocks the Cradle* (Universal, 1917), B & W, 6 reels; *Birth Control* (Message Photoplay, 1917), B & W, 5 reels.

38. Ibid.

39. *Nurse and Martyr* (Midland, 1916), B & W, 30 min.

40. *The Martyrdom of Nurse Cavell* (Australia Films, 1916), B & W, 5 reels; *The Woman the Germans Shot* (Select, 1918), B & W, 6 reels.

41. *The Great Victory* (Metro, 1919), B & W, 5 reels; *Why Germany Must Pay* (Metro, 1919), B & W, 5 reels.

42. *Heart of Humanity* (Universal, 1919), B & W, 9 reels.

43. *Vive La France!* (Paramount, 1918), B & W, 5 reels.

44. *The Splendid Sinner* (Goldwyn, 1918), B & W.

45. *The New York Times,* March 27, 1918.

46. *Adele* (United Pictures, 1919), B & W, 6 reels.

47. *Revelation* (Metro, 1918), B & W, 7 reels.

48. *The Light* (Fox, 1919), B & W, 5 reels; *Her Double Life* (Fox, 1916), B & W, 6 reels.

CHAPTER FOUR

GIRL FRIDAY: THE TWENTIES

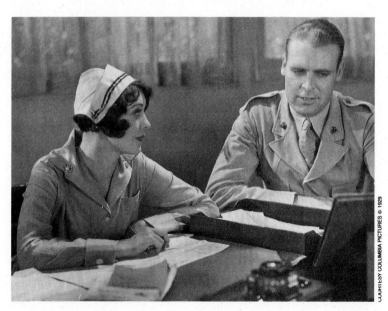

The 1920s proved to be a transitional period in the reshaping of the public image of the nurse. World War I had made it possible for women to enter new areas of activity, and 1919 brought the passage of the women's suffrage amendment in the United States. A quest for private fulfillment, motivated by the new advertising industry and national prosperity, yielded an upheaval in social mores and economic conditions.

RISING ECONOMIC AFFLUENCE

In terms of income level, material goods, and ability to consume, the American people elevated their standard of living considerably between the late-nineteenth century and the 1920s. The most reliable measure of this advancement in well-being was the rise in real income. During the period from the 1890s to 1926, in spite of a substantial increase in the cost of living, real wages more than kept pace. In 1926, some 14 million workers were earning 233 percent more in average hourly wages than they had earned in the 1890s, and 125 percent more than in 1914. After adjusting for inflation, this was equivalent to an expansion in purchasing power of 38 percent and 30 percent, respectively. Much of the rise in real full-time weekly earnings came after 1920. Thus, the 1920s were a period of prosperity in the sense that most wage earners saw their standard of living rise

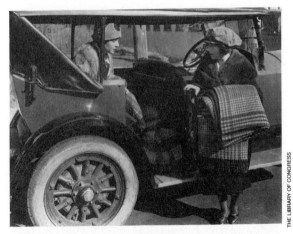

The 1920s were a period of prosperity in that most wage earn-ers saw their standard of living rise appreciably as compared to the more moderate increases of previous decades. Expensive purchases like this 1921 automobile became common.

THE LIBRARY OF CONGRESS

appreciably as compared to the more moderate increases of previous decades.

No previous generation of Americans had experienced visible advances in material well-being of such magnitude. Higher per capita income allowed people to spend a smaller portion of their income on food, clothing, and housing. They could now afford more expensive items such as meat, dairy products, and fresh fruits and vegetables; and they had more money for medical care, entertainment, and gadgets. Electric lighting, gas cooking, and new household appliances such as refrigerators, electric irons, and washing machines lightened household chores in middle-class and some working-class homes. So too did the shift to factory-made clothing, store-bought bread, and canned foods that occurred widely during the 1920s. By the late 1920s many Americans spent more on cars than on clothing. At the same time, family size was shrinking so a larger family income supported a smaller household.

More and more women, including wives and mothers, were demonstrating their capacity to hold jobs outside their homes above the level of domestic servant or file clerk. Refusing to be merely marginal or slave-wage laborers, they were beginning to compete with men as skilled typists, bookkeepers, and operators of machinery. Men as husbands and fathers might deplore this departure from female dependence, but men as employers were making the most of women as inexpensive assets in offices and factories. Even some daughters of prosperous parents were insisting on taking jobs and—even more disturbing—living independently, spending their earnings as they liked, and meeting and marrying men of their own choice.

SMALLER FAMILIES

In the early years of the twentieth century women had continued to experiment, at their own risk and illegally, with birth control techniques. The birth control clinic was at the center of a particularly controversial public health nursing crusade spearheaded by Margaret Sanger, a liberal New York nurse. Born Margaret Higgins in 1883, she was the sixth of eleven children in the family of a Corning, New York, stonecutter. Her mother, depleted from childbirth and the demands of a large family, died in her forties, while her father lived until he was eighty years old. Sanger became permanently indignant about women's lot in

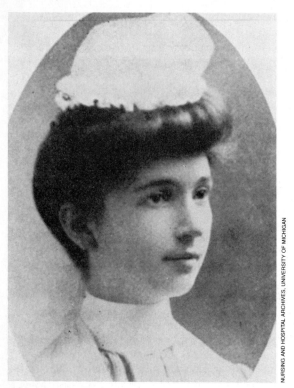

NURSING AND HOSPITAL ARCHIVES, UNIVERSITY OF MICHIGAN

The birth control clinic was at the center of a particularly controversial public health nursing crusade spearheaded by Margaret Sanger, a liberal New York nurse.

1913, when, as a nurse, she saw a law-abiding physician withhold contraceptive information from a poor woman and later learned of the woman's tragic death following an inept $5 abortion. Thus inspired, she began a crusading career that took her into court, put her in prison, and placed her before a Senate committee to plead for legislation to legalize the communication and dissemination of birth control information. Increasing publicity made her name a household word on several continents.

Although the government and the medical profession had opposed forms of birth control, the political agitation of women like Margaret Sanger had helped to educate women about their options regarding childbearing and had lessened their fears of unwanted pregnancies. By the 1920s, desire to reduce family size culminated in the establishment of a significant number of birth control clinics in the large metropolitan areas, mainly supported by middle-class women and benefactors. This was a turning point in the emergence of social options for women.

One emblem of this change was the beauty queen. In 1920 the hotel owners of Atlantic City, New Jersey, thought up a promotional scheme to lengthen the summer season at the beach. Their idea was to host a beauty contest late in September when most vacationers had gone home—a contest to select America's reigning beauty, its Miss America. They raised the beauty contest to a level of national attention and enshrined it as a typically American institution. And more than anything else, they provided the ultimate symbol of what the American woman in the 1920s was supposed to be—which was not just a wife and mother.

HEALTH AND HOSPITAL CONDITIONS

The health of the American people improved dramatically during this period. Life expectancy increased more in the first three decades of the twentieth century than in the preceding 100 years. Males born in 1900 could expect to live 48 years; by 1930 their life expectancy had reached almost 60. Infant mortality dropped sharply, especially in the 1920s. Infectious diseases such as tuberculosis, diphtheria, and pneumonia took a much lower toll. Improvements in health resulted largely from better diet, housing, and sanitation. Cities purified water supplies and enforced requirements for pasteurization of milk. But as people lived longer, the afflictions of aging, such as cancer and heart disease, became increasingly significant causes of death. And by 1930 automobile accidents joined the list of major killers.

Between the end of World War I and the beginning of the depression of the 1930s, hospital construction continued at a rapid pace. By 1928 there were 6,852 hospitals in operation—the largest number ever registered. Finding that the use of student nurses was an extremely economical method of filling nurse staffing needs, almost every hospital began its own nurse training program. This trend resulted in a tremendous lack of uniformity in the quality of nursing education programs, and consequently, nursing leaders saw a need to upgrade and standardize educational programs so that nursing could gain

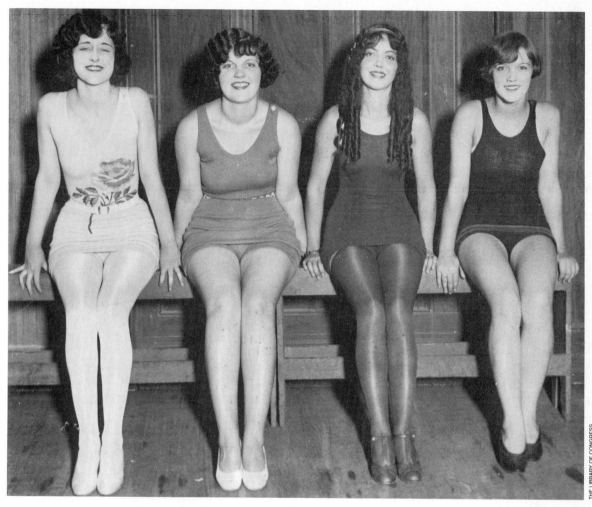

THE LIBRARY OF CONGRESS

Beauty contests more than anything else provided the ultimate symbol of what the American woman in the 1920s was supposed to be.

acceptance as a profession. By the early 1920s all states had nurse practice laws which legitimized the control of nursing through the approval of schools and the setting of nursing standards. Despite these efforts, during its first half century, nursing education developed in such a way that the nursing student worked primarily in the hospital that educated her. Over the years, the close relationship between the school, the department of nursing service, and the hospital worked against the adequate financing of nursing education.

FASHIONS OF THE TWENTIES

The transition from the Gibson Girl to the flapper as the prominent image of American womanhood represented a radical shift in feminine iconography. Both physically and philosophically, the flapper repudiated the image of the Gibson Girl. The stable, reassuring quality of the Gibson Girl had been replaced by the frenetic energy of the flapper, who threatened the traditional moral code as surely as the Gibson Girl had guarded it. Both the flapper and

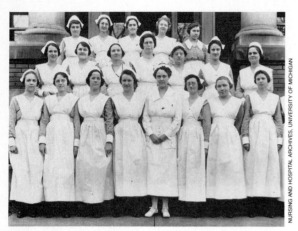

Nurse training was unique as an educational program in that it was often more dedicated to extracting service for the hospital than to educating the student. Class of 1921 at Flower Hospital in Toledo, Ohio.

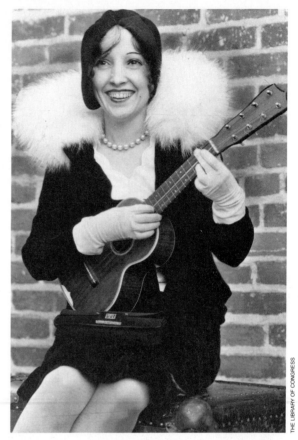

It was in the America of the 1920s that gawky, boyish flappers became the aesthetic ideal for females.

the Gibson Girl were ideal types and as such were emulated to greater or lesser degrees by many women. More important, however, both epitomized the then prevailing conception of women and their roles, and these conceptions differed radically.

The term *flapper* originated in England as a description of girls of the awkward age, the mid-teens. The awkwardness was meant literally: a girl who flapped had not yet reached mature, dignified womanhood. The flapper was supposed to need a certain type of clothing—long, straight lines to cover her awkwardness—and the stores advertised these gowns as "flapper-dresses." It was in postwar America that these gawky, boyish flappers became the aesthetic ideal.

"Turned-up nose, turned-down hose—flapper, yes sir, one of those—has anybody seen my gal?" So went a popular song of this colorful era when a girl's skirts flapped around her knees as she swung into the rumble seat of a Stutz Bearcat or danced the Charleston. It was an age of unheard-of freedom for women, hard-won in World War I. Women had proved they could take the place of men on countless fronts when the latter went off to war—that they could work beside them in the uniforms of nurses, motor corps chauffeurs, or canteen hostesses. One might almost say that the idea of equality with the men had gone to women's heads as they bobbed their hair to look like men and borrowed men's shirts, ties, and felt hats.

The flapper wore her hair short in a "Ponjola" bob, a style initiated in this country by the dancer Irene Castle in the mid-1910s but still considered radical at the end of the war. For hundreds of years women's hair—whether worn up or down, natural or wigged, powdered or oiled—had been long. After the war, bobbed hair was adopted swiftly, particularly by younger women. At first it was flaunted only by daring women. The marcel wave had been invented by a French hairdresser in 1907. Soon women were discarding curl papers and curling irons to sit under formidable electric machines that produced a permanent wave. Beauty shops sprang up after the war and became a permanent and necessary part of American culture. The henna rinse, which imparted an auburn tone, was a favorite improvement on natural hair color. Cosmetics—

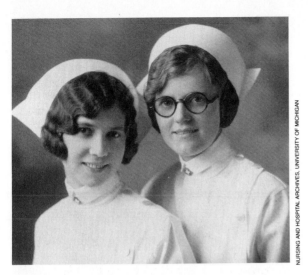

These two nurses of 1926 are wearing flapper hair styles.

rose another inch or two in 1921, went down again in 1922 and 1923 almost to the ankle, then began to rise sharply in 1924 to about ten inches off the floor. From 1925 to 1928 skirts were at knee level, just below or just above. Then in 1928 hemlines became uneven; the basic skirt line hovered about three inches below the knee. The natural waistline was almost completely lost or ignored during this period. At the beginning and end of the decade, a low, natural waistline was the model. Throughout most of the era, however, belts were worn at hip level, and draped girdle effects were placed at the same position.

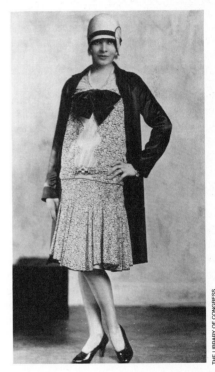

Fashions of the 1920s reflected the era: a combination of affluence and abandon. Skirts rose from a few inches above the ankle in 1919 to a daring inch above the knee.

rouge, powder, and lipstick—began to be used openly, despite the long-standing Victorian concept that no lady would paint her face.

The 1920s were a time of conspicuous makeup. The cosmetics most popular with young women emphasized artificiality and tended to draw attention to their use. Face powder was indispensable. It smoothed out an uneven surface and covered a shiny nose, giving the face a smooth, whitened finish. Rouge and lipstick then added the necessary color. Mouths were painted a brilliant red and etched in a sharp line; a full pout, known as a "cupid's bow," was the ideal shape one tried to attain. The size of the mouth was often diminished by painting "bee-sting" lips in the center and ignoring the outer corners. Eyebrows were plucked, arched, and penciled; lashes were loaded with mascara. As more women entered the business world, increased emphasis was placed on careful grooming.

Modern clothing was lighter, more flexible, and better suited for busy, athletic women. But this, too, meant a dangerous change from the Gibson Girl, who had kept herself busy only with her need to appear decorous and reputable, and who had not engaged in active sport. The 1920s featured the chemise. The silhouette was straight, slim, and simple; the effect was youthful and boyish—whether the wearer was 8, 28, or 80. A chart of the variations in hemlines through the decade would show that it started at about eight inches from the floor in 1920,

The close-fitting cloche hat, which came down over the eyebrows, was most typical of the period. Long strings of beads, dangling earrings, and multiple bracelets from wrist to elbow were in vogue. Women wore nude-colored silk or rayon stockings, which they often rolled below the knee or omitted altogether in hot weather. Shoes often had a fairly wide strap across the instep. Underneath her outer garments the flapper wore as little as possible. The corset was replaced by a girdle or nothing at all, and a brassiere-like garment was worn to minimize the breasts.

The abandonment of the traditional female aesthetic paralleled the rejection by many women of the passive sexual, social, and economic roles from which it had derived its force and relevance. Women began to breach the double standard. They smoked and drank in public; they alternately shimmied and slithered as they danced the Charleston and the tango; and they insisted on greater satisfaction in marriage as well as liberation—through birth control—from the endless cycle of child rearing. In the past women had suffered through unhappy marriages. Now couples separated more often when marriage failed to offer emotional fulfillment and companionship. While women were demanding more from marriage than in the past, many men were unable or unprepared to adjust to their new demands and attitudes. As a result the divorce rate soared. In the 1920s the United States had the highest divorce rate in the world, except possibly for the Soviet Union.

Once women became an integral part of the work force, they gained new status. As working wives they helped support the family, or they could be self-supporting though unmarried. Spending much of their time outside the home, they formed part of a previously all-male economic world. Since the 1890s middle-class single women had worked before marriage, but after marrying, they had faced either forced or voluntary unemployment and had subsided into the status of wives. By 1920 the number of working women had virtually doubled since the turn of the century, with women now representing more than one fifth of the total working population.

GIRL FRIDAY NURSES IN LITERATURE

The dominant public image of the 1920s media nurse was a transitory representation that arose out of the many changes in nursing and in society's moral climate and values. Although the older conception of the nurse as angel continued to appear well into the 1920s, the more predominant media image was a new and emerging one—the "Girl Fri-

day" portrayal. The overwhelming impression of nursing that emanated from this image was anti-professional. Nurses were seen as subordinate to physicians and, more important, placed larger emphasis on love than on their work, willingly abandoning nursing to pursue romance, marriage, or both. Their love affairs usually involved men met on the job—either doctors or patients—and the nurses stood faithfully by their lovers, helping them through thick and thin.

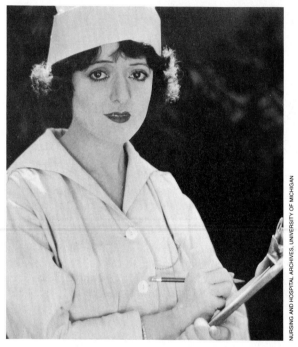

The Girl Friday nurse was the dominant mass media stereotype of the 1920s.

The Girl Friday novels can be easily divided into two separate types. The first focuses on romance, generally between the nurse and a doctor or patient, without presenting the nurse as sexually active. The second portrays the nurse pursuing romantic involvement or sexual activity—in this type, the nurse often appears as sexually adventurous to the point of promiscuity. An example of the first type is Sinclair Lewis's *Arrowsmith* (1924).

Martin Arrowsmith is a young medical student at a midwestern state university with a passion for pure science, in contrast to his classmates who "argue about whether they can make more money in a big city or town, and is it better for a young doc to play the good fellow and lodge game, or join the church and look earnest . . . get an office on a northeast corner, near a trolley car junction." Martin confides to the admiring "co-ed," Madeline Fox, that he thinks he will be a ship's doctor because at least he would not have to spend his time "trying to drag patients away from some rival doc that has an office on another deck." His friend, Angus Duer, already sees himself as "a brilliant young surgeon," and does not hesitate to say that he is out to make money. Fortunately for Martin there is one old German professor of bacteriology, Max Bottlieb—dedicated to patient, accurate, scientific investigation—who becomes his friend and scientific conscience.[1]

At the Zenith Hospital a chance encounter introduces Martin to a nurse named Leora. His initial meeting with her gives some indication of his feeling of superiority toward nurses.

> He passes several nurses rapidly, half nodding to them in the manner (or what he conceived to be the manner) of a brilliant young surgeon who is about to operate. He was so absorbed in looking like a brilliant young surgeon that he was completely lost. . . . Like all males, he hated to confess ignorance by asking directions, but grudgingly he stopped at the door of a bedroom in which a probationer nurse was scrubbing.

When the nurse answers impudently, Martin huffily retorts, "I am Dr. Arrowsmith, and I've been informed that even probationers learn that the first duty of a nurse is to stand when addressing doctors!"[2]

Martin later marries Leora, and life broadens for both as he is lured to the esteemed McGurk Institute in New York, where Martin soon isolates a germ killer that he names Phage. The publicity-conscious institute prepares a publicity campaign to promote this new drug to world fame, but Martin objects on the grounds that his findings have not been fully verified. While he works to verify them, a Frenchman also discovers Phage.

Angered at Martin, the institute nonetheless gives him a second chance, allowing him to lead a medical team fighting bubonic plague in the West Indies. Again he hesitates to use Phage, thus antagonizing both the institute and the native government. Leora dies of the plague, and as Martin reels from this

shock, the publicity-hungry institute issues a report that greatly exaggerates his accomplishments. Such events prove thoroughly unnerving to a man whose true habitat is the laboratory. In a rather unconvincing plot turn, Martin next marries a wealthy woman who tries to turn him into a fashionable scientist. But she fails and divorces him. Dr. Martin Arrowsmith then retreats to a laboratory in the Vermont woods, determined to pursue research on his own terms.

In *Arrowsmith,* Lewis makes Leora a nurse chiefly so that she can conveniently meet her future husband. However, even though we see her as a nurse for only a short time, Lewis does send us subtle messages about nursing. That she willingly leaves her career and devotes herself to helping her new husband develop his—as a conscientious Girl Friday would do—suggests that a physician's work is more important than a nurse's. It also implies that nursing is to be taken up by young, single women as a means of catching a male—then dropped as soon as that goal is accomplished.

Harry Leon Wilson's 1923 novel *Oh, Doctor!* similarly presents the nurse more as a romantic object than a professional woman. *Oh, Doctor!* is the story of a private-duty nurse, Delores Hicks, and a hypochondriac patient, Rufus Billop. Through the nurse's influence, the inactive hypochondriac is transformed into an energetic daredevil. She is initially hired by his doctor and several others who are involved in a plot to rob Rufus of a large inheritance. The doctor and his three fellow conspirators need Rufus to live for at least three more years in order for their scheme to materialize. They do not hire Delores Hicks for her expertise as a nurse but so that she can serve as a love interest for Rufus, thereby taking his mind off his imagined illnesses. She is described as an attractive young woman: they hope she will give Rufus "an interest in life, give him an aim, give him something to look at besides his tongue, give him something to talk about besides how he hurts in different spots."[3]

The nurse's concern with her profession is not the focus of this novel. Wilson concentrates instead on the development of a romance between Rufus and Delores and on how she foils the plans of the men who would rob Rufus of his inheritance. Delores's attitude toward her career seems very indifferent at times. Nursing is not the center of her life, and when she is asked how she likes her new assignment she replies, "Of course, nursing is nursing." Again the reader is left with the impression that nursing is not important as an occupation but only as a stepping-stone to romance. Delores Hicks appears not necessarily committed to her work but only to the pursuit of love.[4]

In 1929 Irwin R. Franklin published his novel *Flight, An Epic of the Air,* which was adapted from the screenplay of the same name. *Flight* is the story of a young misfit, Lefty Phelps, and the pretty marine nurse, Elinor Martin, with whom he falls in love. Again, romance is the focal point of this novel, and therefore little attention is payed to Elinor's professional life. We hardly ever see her engaging in nursing duties. Those she is shown performing seem more like secretarial tasks than nursing ones. For instance, when the reader first meets Elinor she is working as a receptionist in the offices of the senior medical officer at an aviation base in San Diego. She performs no medical activities. She merely relays messages between the senior medical officer and potential recruits waiting in his outer office. Elinor's work appears both unimportant and unattractive.[5]

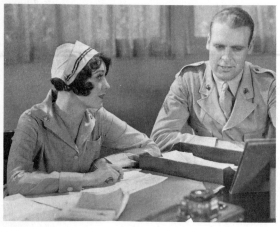

Elinor Martin (Lila Lee) and Lefty Phelps (Ralph Graves) in the motion picture version of Flight *(1929).*

COURTESY COLUMBIA PICTURES © 1929

This anti-professional portrayal of nursing continues throughout the story. When Elinor and several other nurses follow a detail of marines into a war-torn country where the marines are responsible for intervening on behalf of government forces, we might expect to see the nurses treating wounds and the like. However, the nurses are rarely depicted

doing such important work. Elinor is shown only one time applying bandages, and one time she wipes a patient's forehead to soothe him. She does, however, observe the marines at work, go on dates with Lefty, and socialize with friends. Such an anti-professional portrayal suggests that nursing is frivolous work. The message is that a woman becomes a nurse in order to pursue romance and typically leaves nursing when that pursuit ends in marriage.

One last example of a novel that concentrates on the romance of a nurse without portraying any sexual activity is *The Torch of Life* (1926), by Dr. Bertha Sher. It tells the story of Professor Geoffrey Antrobus, the superintendent of a West Coast hospital called the Pacific Philanthrophic Home. His head nurse, Julia Wentworth, is one of the book's major characters. When the novel opens, the professor and Julia have been engaged for two years. Theirs is an engagement of convenience, not of love: by marrying him, Julia hopes to increase her social standing. As for the professor, he sees the match as a convenient way to gain a director of nursing. However, the professor unexpectedly falls in love with a wealthy philanthropist, and when Julia discovers this she returns his engagement ring, resigns her post at the hospital, and leaves the nursing profession for good.[6]

Julia is initially presented as a competent head nurse—loyal, conscientious, and capable. But she is also selfishly pursuing her career as a means to catching a wealthy husband. She leaves her nursing career when she is unable to realize her goal, thus suggesting that it hardly matters that she is a nurse instead of a teacher or secretary. Nursing is used as a plot device to place her in a situation where she would be likely to meet the professor. Therefore, when the relationship between Julia and the professor ends, it makes sense for the author to have her leave the occupation to which she had no professional commitment anyway.

In general then, this first type of the Girl Friday genre does not present nursing as work that is seriously pursued out of a devotion to caring for others. Neither do these fictional nurses seem to feel any connection to their profession or any regrets as they willingly throw away years of study and work to follow romance.

The second type of the Girl Friday genre shows nurses pursuing not only romance but also sexual pleasure. This type often portrays fictional nurses engaging in premarital sex and going beyond the bounds of traditional sexual morality. In this way, it corresponds quite readily to the stereotype of the flapper with her short skirts and sexual promiscuity. One example can be found in Franz Kafka's 1925 novel, *The Trial*. This work contains a nurse character, Leni, who has an absolutely voracious sexual appetite. She works as a private-duty nurse for the lawyer, Hastler, with whom she is romantically involved. In fact, it is often difficult to remember that Leni is a nurse: one thinks of her instead as Hastler's mistress. We seldom see her performing nursing duties—she does apply liniment to her patient's chest or covers his face with a hot towel, but all her actions seem more sexual than medical. She is constantly involving herself in sexual encounters, if not with Hastler then with his clients. As Hastler himself explains, Leni finds "nearly all accused men attractive. She makes up to all of them, loves them all, and is evidently also loved in return."[7]

Conrad Aiken's short story "Bring, Bring" (1925) presents a variation on this theme. In this story the nurse, Miss Rooker, is a private-duty nurse for Mrs. Oldkirk. In the course of her stay in the Oldkirk home, she becomes physically attracted to her patient's husband, and Aiken implies that the two will become lovers. Again, the author rarely pictures the nurse performing nursing duties. Instead we are exposed to her sexual fantasies and personal memories. This nurse is nothing short of irresponsible to her patient. Although she feels sorry for Mrs. Oldkirk, she still plans to involve herself with Mr. Oldkirk. Even though Rooker is portrayed as a modern woman possessed of sexual freedom and adventurousness, her insensitivity and lack of professionalism do not suggest a very positive conception of nursing.[8]

Perhaps the best example of the second type of the Girl Friday genre is *A Farewell to Arms,* written in 1929 by Ernest Hemingway. Hemingway tells the story of a young American ambulance officer, Frederic Henry, and his romance with a British volunteer nurse, Catherine Barkley, during World War I. Catherine is a wartime nurse stationed close to the fighting, but she is seldom shown performing nursing activities. Although one would expect a wartime nurse to have little spare time to socialize and pursue recreation, we constantly see Catherine engaged in social activities. She takes walks with her lover, goes out eating and drinking with him, and goes to the horse races with him. Furthermore, when he is a patient at her hospital, she often sneaks into his room late at night and makes love with him. She does so only after seeing to all her other patients, but her actions are certainly inconsistent with the professional conduct one would hope to see associated with nurses. Hemingway's portrayal trivializes the responsibilities of a wartime nurse, suggesting that she has time to play and does not take her duties very seriously.[9]

Catherine's motivations for entering nursing reflect the emphasis on romance and adventure characteristic of many women of the 1920s. She tells Frederic that she became a nurse in order to follow her fiancé to war: "I started when he did. I remember having a silly idea he might come to the hospital where I was. With a sabre cut, I suppose, and a bandage around his head. Or shot through the shoulder. Something picturesque." Thus, nursing is, to her, merely a vehicle to place her in proximity to her love. She displays little more professional commitment to nursing when she tells Frederic that she will follow him wherever he chooses to go on an upcoming leave. When he mentions that "might be hard to manage," she assures him: "No it won't, darling. If necessary, I'll simply leave." This suggests that she has little serious devotion to her work.[10]

Leni, Miss Rooker, and Catherine Barkley all display the sexual freedom associated with the flapper, so we might expect that they would appeal to women readers of the 1920s, thereby providing nursing with a positive image. However, their conduct does not recommend nursing as a *profession* but simply as a vehicle for meeting and having sex with men.

Rupert Hughes's short story, "She Goes To War," relates the adventures of Joan Morgan, a woman who participates in the war effort in Europe during World War I. The story begins with Joan trying to figure out a way to get to Europe, where she feels all the action and adventure are and where she can be of help to the soldiers. She finally succeeds and is sent to France as one of the "Y Girls"—batallions of women sent by the YMCA to see to the soldiers' needs, selling them food and cigarettes, providing them with friendship and dance partners. The story is not about nursing, but Dorcas, a friend of Joan's, is a Red Cross nurse who makes several appearances.[11]

Red Cross nurses are presented as highly trained: Joan is told she cannot become a nurse right away, that she must first complete three years of training. Dorcas is referred to as "playing the angel to wounded allies." Red Cross nurses, in general, are described as "saints in their place" and "the Red Cross angel in snowy robes who relieved his pain and caressed his brow with her lily palm."[12]

In this story the author explicitly rejects nursing as the profession for his heroine, suggesting not only that she lacks proper training but, more important, that nursing is not an exciting enough career for the modern Joan. Accordingly, when she realizes she does not have the training to be a nurse, Joan says, "I don't think I'd care for nursing. I want to fight. I could always whip all the boys I knew, and run faster. I'm a dead shot with a pistol or a shotgun." Hughes makes it clear that this statement is not sour grapes on Joan's part, but an earnest explanation of nursing's lack of appeal to her.[13]

Thomas Mann's *The Magic Mountain,* published in 1924, does not focus on nursing, but its setting in a tuberculosis sanitarium provides exposure to several nurses. Among these is Fraulein Adriatica Von Mylendock, a minor but significant character. Von Mylendock is a nursing sister and directoress of the Berghof TB Sanitarium. A cursory glance at her responsibilities and actions might suggest a favorable image of nursing. She is in charge of the nurses at the Berghof, is often able to rely on her own judgment and initiative, and even regulates certain behaviors of the head physician, Hofrat Behrens, who has a tobacco addiction she is trying to control.

Nonetheless, the positive image suggested by Von Mylendock's autonomy is counteracted by the generally uncomplimentary view of nursing that emerges from *The Magic Mountain*. As already noted, the 1920s brought a changing ideal of womanhood, one that moved away from the angelic puritan doing good deeds to better society. The nurses at the Berghof, however, seem to have cloistered themselves in their mountain hospital unaware of the metamorphosis taking place in the world around them. They are, quite simply, women from a previous time. All are nuns and have devoted themselves to nursing out of humanitarian concern. Their understanding of their duties is couched in a religious vocabulary. For example, Von Mylendock tells a relative of one of her patients that "The Hofrat was busy, there were operations and general examinations, suffering humanity must take precedence, that was a sound Christian principle." Indeed, patients at the Berghof note the anachronistic character of Von Mylendock. One calls her "this fossil head overseer" and another, referring to her name, exclaims:

"Sounds as though she had been dead a very long time. It is positively medieval."[14]

That these nurses are nuns separates them from the flapper image in yet another way: as nuns they represent the notion of female chastity that so many women of the 1920s were rejecting. A patient, referring to Von Mylendock, notes her asexuality: "And she is distinguished from the Medici Venus by the fact that where the goddess has a bosom, she has a cross." Von Mylendock's characterization reminds us of her anti-modern nature. She is not the role model that would induce women of the 1920s to pursue nursing. While Mann's presentation of Von Mylendock may only have been intended to represent one specific nurse and not the entire profession, he does suggest a generally unfavorable view of nursing, one that clashes with the new ideal of femininity.[15]

Nurse Nancy Ashford, a major character in Lloyd Douglas's 1929 novel *Magnificent Obsession,* also has little in common with the ideal woman of the 1920s. We are told several times of her self-sacrificing devotion to the medical doctors with whom she works. Ashford shows little concern for the quality or content of her own work and is worried instead that things run smoothly for these doctors. Thus, she takes over the menial work of the hospital in order to free her idol, Dr. Hudson, to engage in the more lofty pursuit of brain surgery. "She had quickly and quietly transferred many an administrative responsibility from her chief's shoulders to her own, almost without his realizing how deftly she had eased him of an increasing volume of wearisome details." Ashford's unselfishness extends to the point of total indifference about her own career. She is unconcerned with her professional progress, but is almost obsessed with Hudson's. Accordingly, she has more in common with the angel of mercy whose last concern is her own well-being than with the flapper who seeks hedonistic autonomy. This characterization further suggests that nursing is not nearly as important as the work of the doctor. While Ashford is able to sacrifice her nursing duties to tend to administrative work, her doing so makes it possible for Hudson to delve more deeply into brain surgery—suggesting that his work, unlike hers, is too important to be forfeited.[16]

Another aspect of Ashford's character implies her connection to the Victorian imagery of the nurse. While noting Ashford's youth, Douglas presents her as a motherly figure who acts as "a general counselor at Brightwood." He explains that "many people who outranked her in years called her mother—a perfect specimen of the type that instantly invites confidences. She had become a repository for a wider diversity of confessions than come to the ear of the average priest." Ashford's charitable willingness to listen to the problems of others and Douglas's generally asexual characterization of her remind us of the attributes of a mother superior. In this way she is again more closely related to the imagery of the nurse of Victorian times.[17]

The changing image of women also resulted in some rather ambivalent portrayals of the nurse in the 1920s. Several authors tried to present nurses as both angels of mercy and modern flappers. Others developed their nurse characters with emphasis on the tension between these two competing ideologies of femininity. Isa Glenn's 1929 novel, *Transport,* introduces two nurses: one is extremely flirtatious and sexually uninhibited; the other is her exact opposite—sexually repressed, reminding one of the nunnish angels of mercy. Neither of these nurses is necessarily more likable than the other. Glenn presents an ambivalent, either/or notion of nursing— one can either follow the flapper model or the angel of mercy model—thus suggesting that there is room in the profession for both types of women.[18]

Frederick Palmer's *Invisible Wounds* (1925) put forth an equally mixed image of nursing. His nurse heroine, Irene Darcourt, certainly fits the angel of mercy characterization when seen in her capacity as a nurse in World War I. She says she has taken up her profession because nursing is a "noble" work. The role model upon which she based her occupational choice is a Nurse Stanton, whom Irene describes admiringly as making "a living by helping and healing people. . . . Irene was thinking of the triumph such as Miss Stanton had of bringing the joy of recovery to others in pain and distress." Irene is selflessly devoted to her patients and stoically represses any personal feelings when the man she loves is severely wounded and brought to her hospital for treatment. She stifles her emotions because "To help and to heal—impersonally. That was her duty." However, while Irene is shown as an angel, she also engages in a premarital love affair that results in the birth of a son out of wedlock. This is hardly consistent with Victorian morality but is instead suggestive of the newer sexual morality associated with the flapper. Irene Darcourt is the only example, in fact, of a nurse character of this period who combines serious professional conduct with a

lifestyle consonant with the sexual freedom available to modern women. As such she offered a very attractive image of nursing. She is neither prudish nor overly promiscuous, is competent, compassionate, and highly professional in her behavior. In general, however, authors of the 1920s did not combine some of the more modern attributes of the flapper with the caring and professional seriousness of nurses.[19]

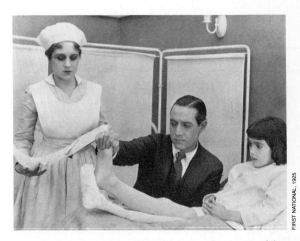

FIRST NATIONAL, 1925

In general, authors of the 1920s did not combine some of the more modern attributes of the flapper with the caring and professional seriousness of nurses.

THE IMPACT OF MOTION PICTURES

Silent films had captivated audiences since the early 1900s, and by the 1910s and 1920s there was an almost religious fervor in America focused on the epicenter of make-believe—Hollywood. Each week about 100 million Americans went to the movies, a number nearly equal to the entire population. Mass entertainment had burst upon the world. The first movie houses were built in working-class neighborhoods, but in the 1920s luxurious movie palaces were constructed in the big-city downtown districts, and impressive if less imposing theaters appeared in residential areas. By 1926 there were more than 20,000 movie theaters in all. Those in the big cities strove to rival the fantasy world that flashed across the screen: lobbies that reflected in gilt and plaster the rococo splendors of Versailles, enormous crystal chandeliers that sprayed ornate shafts of light, the thick and costly carpets favored by the most expensive hotels, fountains, lounging rooms, cathedral organs and 30-piece orchestras, and seats covered in velvet. These metropolitan wonders set the standard that, on a smaller scale, spread to countless Main Streets. A splendid new movie theater marked a town on the way up. Sinclair Lewis's character George Babbitt felt it almost a duty to visit the Chateau, the premier picture palace of his town. With exclamations of "Well, by golly!" and "You got to go some to beat this dump!" Babbitt admired it unreservedly.[20]

Movie critic and film historian Campbell MacCulloch in an article in *Theatre Arts* (October 1927) reflected on the impact of the early cinema: "No more powerful agency for the transmission of thought and custom has ever existed upon the globe than the motion picture; no greater influence toward uniting mankind has ever been developed." In their study of "Middletown" (Muncie, Indiana), Helen and Robert Lynd noted that, by the mid-1920s, among teenagers, the "sharp figures on the silver screen are always authoritatively present with their gay and confident designs for living."[21]

By the 1920s national surveys revealed that movie stars had replaced political, business, and artistic leaders as the favorite role models of American youth. During that decade, the female social role was projected on the screen by such personalities as Madge Bellamy, Clara Bow, Joan Crawford and Gloria Swanson, all vivid embodiments of the new womanhood, known to contemporaries as "the moderns." Such basic lessons were not lost on the movie audience. Studies of female moviegoers, financed by the Payne Fund and conducted between 1929 and 1933, revealed that young women paid close attention to a star's appearance and behavior. Of a Joan Crawford film, one girl said, "I watch every detail, of how she's dressed, and her make-up, and also her hair." Another surmised, "I'll bet every girl wishes she was the Greta Garbo type. I tried to imitate her walk, she walks so easy as if she had springs on her feet."[22]

Young moviegoers of the 1920s were educated in other more personal matters as well. One college girl told the Payne Fund interviewers that "movies are a liberal education in the art of making love." She went on to recount such specific benefits of this cinematic education as learning "how two screen lovers manage their arms when they are embracing; there is a definite technique; one arm over, the other

under." This young woman was grateful to the movies for providing a remedial education in a subject avoided by her straitlaced parents, while another found cinematic instructions in lovemaking "more suggestive and effective than I could possibly find in any book by say Elinor Glyn on 'How to Hold Your Man.'" The adolescent girls who flocked to the movies each week were getting their sex education through the prism of the Hollywood clinch, a training that culminated in erotic awareness if not actual necking parties. The magic of the movies brought one teenager a rich fantasy life: "Buddy Rogers and Rudy Valentino have kissed me oodles of times but they don't know it, God bless 'em!"[23]

Whatever the behavioral consequences of this education, its cultural impact cannot be denied. Movies fostered and encouraged occupation with intimate heterosexual relations. Moving pictures were clearly more effective than static literary images in detailing the active components of flapper sexuality. The employed women of the 1920s tended to congregate in a relatively new segment of the work force, deserting factories and domestic service for white-collar employment. The movie camera tended to skirt the mundane aspect of white-collar work, preferring to dwell on the glamour of a setting full of consumer goods, entertainment, and eligible men, all of which the young woman could pursue without parental interference. The demand of the economy for women's labor in this job sector, as well as women's responsiveness to this need, was nonetheless very real. By 1925, for example, 34 percent of the high school girls in Middletown aspired to be clerical workers. Fan magazines took pains to associate movie stars with these prosaic roles, pointing out that Joan Crawford was once a shop girl in Kansas City, that Janet Gaynor clerked in a shoe store, and that Frances Marion earned $25 a week as a stenographer before she became a star and screenwriter. Early films no doubt facilitated the transformation of the female work force, reflecting, endorsing, and legitimizing women's assumption of new roles.

THE GIRL FRIDAY NURSE IN THE MOVIES

Elinor Glyn, who coined the term "It" to describe the magnetism of flapper extraordinaire Clara Bow, often wrote stories featuring the modern woman. In

1925 she wrote the screenplay for and produced Metro-Goldwyn-Mayer's *Man and Maid*. In a foreword to the picture Glyn states: "Women always do one of three things to men—elevate men, degrade them, or bore them to death." The film opens during World War I, when the beautiful and blonde nurse Alathea Bulteel (Harriet Hammond) finds the body of a wounded British officer. She cares for him until help arrives, leaving before he regains consciousness. Alathea is the daughter of an impoverished English peer and must support herself after the war by working as a secretary to Sir Nicholas Thormonde (Lew Cody), a handsome and wealthy man, who appears to be the wounded officer she had found during the war. He is still convalescing and also enjoying a friendship with pretty demimondaine Suzette. However, Alathea's efficiency and hard work so impress him that he falls in love with her and kisses her. She leaves his employ, afraid that he intends to take advantage of her. Nicholas wants to marry her, but she refuses. Meanwhile, Alathea's father needs $5,000 to pay off his gambling debts, which Nicholas graciously gives him. Alathea does not know of Nicholas's unselfish generosity and offers to marry him if he will pay her father's debt. Nicholas agrees, and the two are happy until Suzette returns. Alathea believes that Nicholas is still in love with Suzette, so she leaves him. In the end, Alathea and Nicholas are reunited after learning that each married the other out of love rather than base emotions.[24]

Alathea's identification as a nurse lasts only a few scenes early in the film. Yet the rest of her story reflects some of the problems faced by veterans returning to a peacetime society, including Red Cross nurses. Before the war Alathea belonged to the leisure class, and her decision to become a volunteer nurse probably arose from the self-sacrificing instincts of members of her class. After the war Alathea cannot afford the luxury of voluntary work and is forced to take a paying job. But she does not make any use of her wartime nursing experience. It would have been very easy for the screenwriter to let Alathea work as a private nurse for the still-convalescent Nicholas; instead, she is his secretary. The implicit assumption is that nursing is not fit work for a lady *unless* there is a patriotic reason for it. Alathea's brief nursing identification served only to show the audience the truly noble nature of the leading lady and to bring her, ultimately, to her true reward—marriage with an attractive and wealthy man. Nursing

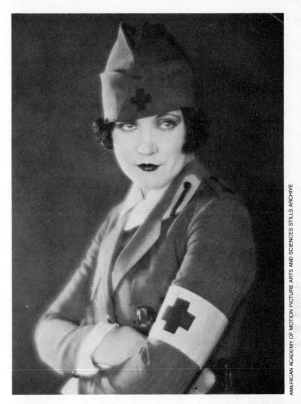

Warner Brother's Recompense *(1925) starred Marie Prevost as nurse Julie Gamelyn.*

experience itself—the practical knowledge of caring for sick and wounded—appears to be of little value.

Warner Brothers's *Recompense* (1925), which starred Marie Prevost as nurse Julie Gamelyn and Monte Blue as clergyman Peter Graham, stands as an interesting contrast to *Man and Maid* in that the nurse character continues to work as a nurse after the war. This scenario was somewhat unique in the 1920s and thus requires further explanation. The story, based on a popular novel of the same name by Robert Keable, tells of a clergyman's good works and romantic interests. Peter Graham, a clergyman and chaplain in the British Army serving in France, has fallen in love with nurse Julie Gamelyn during a stay in London. He returns to his unit, but abandons his religious work to enlist as a fighting man and serves with the same unit as Julie. The unit is transferred to South Africa, where it remains until the end of the war. Julie continues working as a nurse in a Capetown hospital while Peter works in the interior. Peter is shot by a dishonest trader, and Julie nurses him back to health. After this, Peter decides to return to London, where he opens a mission. He meets a former love, Angelica, who is pregnant, and Peter decides to marry her out of pity. Julie returns to London, too, and works in a hospital where she helps to deliver Angelica's baby. Angelica dies during delivery, and Julie and Peter finally decide to marry.[25]

The image of nursing in this film is very positive and quite realistic, given the usual melodramatic treatment of nursing. In the first place, Julie was the only film nurse character to date who was obviously a trained, professional nurse. She was not a Red Cross volunteer, but a member of the British military. She did find love during the war, but the end of the conflict did not bring about the happy conclusion of her romance. In fact, demobilization complicated her relationship with her love, because each of them had to pursue different professional or vocational callings. Julie remained a nurse in a South African hospital, while Peter fulfilled his missionary duty first in the jungle and later in London. Julie was an independent woman for her time. She may not have been a flapper, in terms of her dress or behavior, but she shared many of the traits ascribed to the liberated woman of the 1920s—self-sufficiency, spunkiness, and bravery. Even after the lovers are united for good at the end of the film, there is no indication that Julie will abandon her nursing for prosaic family life. Indeed, it might be assumed that she and Peter will work as a nurse/minister team in a hospital or mission.

In *The Child Thou Gavest Me* (First National, 1921), Barbara Castleton starred as Norma Huntley, a former World War I Red Cross nurse. While preparing to marry her fiancé, Edward, at the beginning of the film, Norma wants to tell him a sordid secret from her past, but her mother discourages her. The secret concerns an illegitimate child borne by Norma after she was raped by an unknown soldier in Belgium. Norma, who thinks the child is dead, proceeds with the wedding, only to learn shortly therafter that the child is alive and now in need of her. Her husband, Edward, agrees to adopt the child but warns Norma that he will seek out the father and kill him. Edward thinks that the father of the child is a mutual friend, Tom, and invites him to their country home. After finding Tom and Norma together in suggestive although innocent circumstances, Edward's suspi-

cions are confirmed and he shoots Tom. Norma then tells Edward the circumstances of her pregnancy, and he recognizes himself as the unknown soldier who raped her. He tries to kill himself, but Norma persuades him to live to help rear their child. Fortunately for all concerned, Tom also survives the shooting, and all are reconciled.[26]

The developments in this story are too coincidental to sustain even the mildest credibility. However, the implications of the story for the image of nursing and for the perception of the war are very clear. In this tale, nursing does not give Norma a passport of moral security. Her good works are evilly rewarded by rape and a subsequent pregnancy. (Attempted and, occasionally, actual rape by Germans was a constant threat to the nurse heroines of war films made during the war. But none of these virtuous screen heroines was made to pay the reproductive consequences of rape.) Thus, Norma's entire future is clouded by events that took place during her wartime work. The only thing Norma has to remind her of her nursing experience is a shameful secret and an unwanted child.

Forever After (First National, 1926) concerned a romance between socially distant lovers: the rich and beautiful Jennie (Mary Astor) and her handsome but poor childhood sweetheart Ted (Lloyd Hughes). Jennie and Ted have been in love for many years, but Jennie's mother intends that her daughter will marry the more socially acceptable Jack Randall. Ted hopes to earn Jennie's and her mother's acceptance by going to Harvard, at the great expense and sacrifice of his father, a none-too-successful lawyer. But when Ted's father dies, Ted has to return home to support his mother. Jennie's mother convinces Ted that he should give up his claim on her daughter because he could never adequately support her. Ted agrees and leaves town with his mother, hoping to forget Jennie. Nevertheless, Jennie refuses to marry Randall and becomes a nurse instead. During World War I, she serves in a military hospital in France and is reunited with Ted, now a wounded war hero. The film ends as she is nursing him back to health.[27]

This romance shows how the war served to reduce class differences. On the battlefield, Ted ennobles himself and earns the right to marry his sweetheart. The story ends when the war does, leaving the audience to assume that the couple will marry and live happily ever after, that Jennie will become a contented wife and mother, and that Ted will fulfill his wartime promise by entering a successful business back home. Nursing only provides Jennie with a convenient way to escape from marriage to a man she does not love and an equally convenient way to reunite her with the man she does.

A HOSPITAL ROMANCE

The portrayal of the nurse in *The Glorious Fool* (Samuel Goldwyn, 1922), though more substantial than in most other silent films of the 1920s, still associated nursing with money and marriage. This motion picture is a peculiar love story. It is set in the isolation ward of a hospital in which the heroine, known only as Nurse, is presently engaged as private-duty nurse to the young hero, Billy Grant. Billy is supposedly on his deathbed, and his compassionate nurse is deeply distraught by his condition and finds it difficult to stifle her sorrowful feelings. Billy, however, is less concerned with dying than with getting revenge on his living relatives—his cousins—who prevented his marriage by warning his fiancée's family that he was an alcoholic, which indeed he still is. To get revenge he must marry before his death in order to steer his wealth away from his cousins, and to do this he must find a readily available woman; "Nurse" is just the person for the job.[28]

Nurse, virginal and hoping for true love, is horrified by Billy's suggestion, not surprisingly, but when the minister arrives to perform the last rites for her patient, she finally submits. Her sympathy for her young patient overcomes her strong sense of propriety and her fears for her career, which may be jeopardized by marriage. After the simple wedding service, Nurse falls asleep on her knees at the foot of her husband's bed.

The next day, to Nurse's pleasure and consternation, Billy improves. Though Billy assures her that the marriage can be dissolved, he starts to fall in love with her. Not only that, but her goodness starts to rub off on him and he determines to mend his ways and give up alcohol. Meanwhile, however, the head nurse, a stern and authoritarian spinster, notes Billy's improvement and suddenly appreciates how young he is. Concerned for Nurse's reputation, she takes Billy's nurse/wife off the case and sends an older disciplinarian in her stead. Billy is, of course, quite disgusted with the new nurse and bribes the head nurse with flowers in order to get his young wife back.

Nurse returns, now fresh and beautiful after her half-day of rest, and the story ends with Billy and his nurse/wife eating breakfast together in their hospital room; clearly their marriage will stand. Their romantic tête-à-tête is observed by a curious young nurse applicant who is being shown around the hospital by the stern head nurse, who tells the new applicant what a hard, unemotional life nursing is—but the applicant, gazing at Nurse and Billy, thinks otherwise.

The most important, most strongly emphasized image of nursing in this film is that the profession demands anonymity and strict adherence to harsh regulations. To get right to the point of this story—as we are told on at least three occasions in what is a fairly short tale—"The perfect nurse is more or less of a machine. Too much sympathy is a handicap to her work and an embarrassment to her patient. A perfect, silent, reliable, fearless, emotionless machine!" This is the head nurse's maxim, often repeated to both her students and graduates.[29]

The head nurse herself is, of course, the epitome of the perfect nurse. Called Miss Smith, this middle-aged spinster is clearly the usual stereotypical supervisor who has chased all romantic sentiment from her person and embraced the sterility and joylessness of the nursing profession. Actually, she does reveal a couple of flaws in her otherwise iron-hard armor. First, she is afraid to enter the isolation ward lest she become infected. Second, she is easily swayed from hard-line rules—simply a bunch of flowers and a pleading note from Billy get him what he wants—a hint of romantic sentiment still lodges in her bosom. The only other nurse we hear about is a Miss Hart, who is also an older woman and a strict disciplinarian—another example of the spinster who is a perfect nurse. The heroine, on the other hand, is quite unable to master her machinelike role when nursing her patient, Billy. She is not a perfect nurse, but this is because she is a perfect woman.

ANOTHER WAR NURSE

The Patent Leather Kid (First National, 1927) showed how the war affected the lives of the lower classes. The film was loosely based on a short story of the same title by popular author Rupert Hughes. Hughes had a great flair for capturing the dialect and dialogue of various American regions, especially areas of New York; in addition, he appeared to be a keen

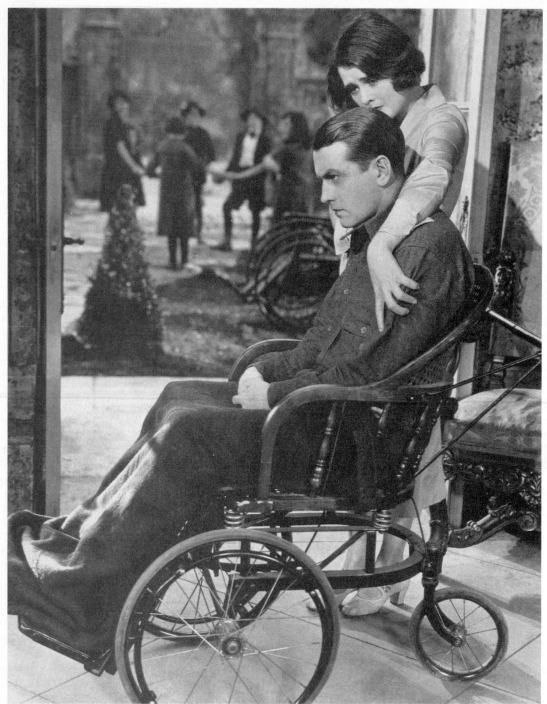

FIRST NATIONAL, 1927

In The Patent Leather Kid *(1927) Curley as a nurse lacks dignity, professional detachment, and composure. Her transformation from dance-hall girl to nurse occurs with no footage showing any training.*

and witty analyst of social mores of the 1920s. In some ways *The Patent Leather Kid* is a parody of all the romantic melodramas built around World War I. All the basic elements are there: a coward turned hero, a war nurse who saves the life of her beloved, patriotic sentiments, and a happily-ever-after ending. Yet all these stock plot elements have been modified on account of lower-class backgrounds of the leading characters.[30]

The story concerns the romance between a handsome young fighter, The Patent Leather Kid, played by screen idol Richard Barthelmess (nominated for an Academy Award for this portrayal), and a cabaret dancer named Curley Callahan, played by Molly O'Day. The Kid first meets Curley when she comes to one of his fights and taunts him and jeers at him from her ringside seat. It is love at first sight between the two; both have come from the wrong side of the tracks and understand the vulgar, tough world in which they live. Their romance is marked by passion as well as fist fights and attacks of jealousy. When America enters the war, the whole of New York, including Curley, is taken away with a rush of patriotic fervor. Army recruiters decry the Kid's refusal to enlist, and Curley thinks he ought to sign up. Curley herself heads for Europe, where she will work as a dancer and entertainer until she can learn how to be a nurse. The Kid wants nothing to do with the flag-waving crowd and steadfastly refuses to join up, even though his best friend, Puffy, volunteers. But the Selective Service catches up with the Kid, and he soon finds himself in the same unit with Puffy and on his way to France. Once in France, he makes an enemy of his superior officer, Hugo Breen, who once had been an admirer of Curley's. The Kid finds Curley dancing with Breen and starts a fist fight with the officer; he also rejects Curley's attempts to tell him that she loves him.

Soon, the unit is moved into the frontline trenches. The Kid shows no great martial talent until his friend Puffy is shot—then the Kid sees the war in more personal terms and sets out to avenge his buddy. After several feats of heroism, the Kid is buried under a pile of debris. Severely battered and wounded, he is brought to a field hospital, where a doctor, a French Red Cross nurse, and Curley, now a nurse, prepare to work on him. Curley goes slightly hysterical when she recognizes the patient; the doctor looks the Kid over and declares him a hopeless case. But Curley insists, with great histrionics, that

the doctor operate and save her man. In order to pacify the hysterical nurse, the doctor agrees, and since there is no anesthetic, the Kid suffers through the ordeal with only Curley's love to ease his pain.

Some weeks later, the Kid is in a larger hospital, suffering from complete paralysis from the neck down. Curley, who remains with him as his private nurse, assures him that all will be well, and that she'll support them when they get back to New York. But the Kid refuses to consider letting a "dame" keep him. One day, when Curley is wheeling her true love outside the hospital, they stop to watch a passing parade. As the American flag goes by, the Kid ruefully notes that when he could salute, he would not, and now that he would like to, he cannot. He asks Curley to salute for him. While she stands proudly beside him, the Kid murmurs, "Oh, God—I wanna move. I gotta move." Just then, his right hand begins to shake and slowly he brings his arm into a salute and manages to rise from the wheelchair to witness the passing of Old Glory. Thus the Kid is cured by his patriotism, and Curley is assured of a golden future with her love.[31]

The image of nursing derived from this film is mixed. Basically, Curley as a nurse lacks dignity, professional detachment, and composure. Her transformation from dance-hall girl to nurse occurs with no footage of her training. She does help to save the Kid's life, but through her hysterical outburst of emotion, not her skill. As a woman, Curley is worlds removed from the typical nurse heroine of war films. She is crude, vulgar, and poorly educated. She trades punches almost as frequently as do the prizefighters, and her language and sense of humor (she puts a wet sponge under someone about to sit down) relegate her to a low social class. She is referred to frequently as a "dame" or a "skirt," indicating that men have little respect for her. At the end of the film, she is put definitely in her true place—as an adoring sidekick and wife to the now-restored Kid.[32]

Despite these generally unflattering views of Curley as a nurse and as a woman, her character does emerge sympathetically. One might suppose that an audience could be charmed by Curley's vitality and vulgarity, as a refreshing antidote to the run of the mill, blandly proper heroines. Finally, Curley's patriotism and desire to nurse the wounded give her an opportunity to rise above her vulgar, materialistic environment, if only briefly. Curley is not transformed by her nursing work into an upper-class "lady," but she does participate in the miracle of the Kid's recovery and come to a new understanding of honor, love, and duty. And we can suppose that the Kid and Curley will settle into a less selfish domestic arrangement after the war than they appeared interested in before the war, when each sought only his or her own gratification.

FILM RECOGNITION OF THE NAVY NURSE CORPS

During the 1926 Christmas season, another film featuring wartime nursing was released: *Tell It to the Marines* turned out to be Metro-Goldwyn-Mayer's second-ranking film of the year in box office receipts. *Tell It to the Marines* relates the story of a Marine recruit's gradual transformation from an undisciplined and callow youth (played by William Haines) into a finely trained fighting man. It is also a love triangle: Private "Skeet" Burns, the recruit, and Sergeant O'Hara (Lon Chaney), his basic training superior and a weatherworn Marine, both love the same pretty Navy nurse, Norma Dale, played by Eleanor Boardman. Because the story deals with the peacetime Marine Corps of the mid-1920s, combat opportunity comes when the Marines are sent to rescue a group of Navy nurses who are tending to Chinese during an epidemic and who have been threatened by a group of Chinese bandits. Of course, Norma Dale is among these nurses, and both Burns and O'Hara go to the fight. Although the Marines are outnumbered, they still prevail. The story ends some months later, after Burns has been discharged. He and Norma, who have bought a ranch together, pay a final visit to their friend O'Hara and watch him greet a new band of recruits in the same gruff manner he used on Burns four years earlier.[33]

This film paid little attention to nursing, but it was nonetheless interesting because it featured professional military nurses who had joined the Navy in peacetime. Primarily, the main nurse character provides a romantic focus for the two male leads. There is some recognition that nurses have important work to do in peacetime, although there is no evidence of what exactly they do. The only scenes of a nurse at work feature a Miss Boardman giving a pill to the malingering Burns and later carrying a Chinese child during an evacuation. The nurses enjoy the respect and appreciation of the men at the camp: they are treated like ladies. When Skeet Burns does attempt a kiss, Norma becomes angry and marches back to the camp without him. Burns is sent to the brig for this indiscretion, but Norma later apologizes to him for having informed O'Hara of the incident. In general Norma is treated with respect. There is no hint that nursing is not a fit occupation for a lady, although it is fairly clear that Norma abandons her nursing career when she marries Burns.

Americans in the 1920s may not have known much about the real events that were taking place within the fledgling nursing profession, but they did know what the ideal woman was like—and that nurses were not like her. In a decade marked by materialism, the image of the nurse had momentarily deteriorated into a mere Girl Friday. Economic forces were fast emerging, however, that would very soon "remoralize" American values, and the status of the nurse image would soar upward even as the state of the national economy plunged downward.

NOTES

1. Sinclair Lewis, *Arrowsmith* (New York: Harcourt, Brace and World, 1924).

2. Ibid., p. 68.

3. Harry Leon Wilson, *Oh, Doctor!* (New York: Cosmopolitan Books, 1923), p. 86.

4. Ibid., p. 174.

5. Irwin R. Franklin, *Flight* (New York: Grosset and Dunlap, 1929).

6. Bertha Scher, *The Torch of Life* (New York: Gem Publishing Co., 1926).

7. Franz Kafka, *The Trial* (New York: Random House, 1925), p. 229.

8. Conrad Aiken, "Bring, Bring," in *A Treasury of Nurse Stories by World Famous Authors,* ed. Sonia Barry (New York: F. Fell, 1962).

9. Ernest Hemingway, *A Farewell to Arms* (New York: Charles Scribner's Sons, 1929), p. 19.

10. Ibid., pp. 131–132.

11. Rupert Hughes, *She Goes to War and Other Stories* (New York: Grosset and Dunlap, 1929), p. 40.

12. Ibid., p. 71.

13. Ibid., p. 134.

14. Thomas Mann, *The Magic Mountain* (New York: Alfred A. Knopf, 1924), p. 551.

15. Ibid., p. 80.

16. Lloyd C. Douglas, *Magnificent Obsession* (New York: Houghton Mifflin, 1929), p. 30.

17. Ibid., pp. 29–30.

18. Isa Glenn, *Transport* (New York: Alfred A. Knopf, 1929).

19. Frederick Palmer, *Invisible Wounds,* (New York: Dodd, Mead & Co., Inc., 1925).

20. Sinclair Lewis, *Babbit* (New York: Grosset and Dunlap, 1924).

21. Campbell MacCulloch, "Movies Are Helping America," *Theatre Arts* 11 (October 1927):23–27; Robert S. Lynd and Helen Merrell Lynd, *Middletown, A Study in Contemporary American Culture* (New York: Harcourt, Brace, 1929), p. 263.

22. Henry James Forman, *Our Movie-Made Children* (New York: The MacMillan Company, 1935), p. 18.

23. Ibid., p. 41.

24. *Man and Maid* (Metro-Goldwyn-Mayer Pictures, 1925), B & W, Silent, 53 min.

25. *Recompense* (Warner Bros., 1925), B & W, Silent, 74 min.

26. *The Child Thou Gavest Me* (Associated First National Pictures, 1921), B & W, Silent, 61 min.

27. *Forever After* (First National Pictures, 1926), B & W, Silent, 63 min.

28. *The Glorious Fool* (Goldwyn, 1922), B & W, Silent, 54 min.

29. Ibid.

30. *The Patent Leather Kid* (First National, 1927), B & W, Silent, 120 min.

31. Ibid.

32. Ibid.

33. *Tell It to the Marines* (Metro-Goldwyn-Mayer, 1926), B & W, Silent, 88 min.

CHAPTER FIVE

HEROINE:
THE THIRTIES

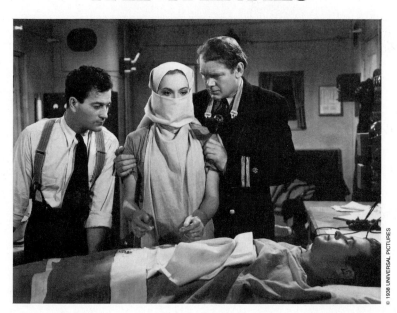

The stock market crash late in 1929 ushered in a desperate era in America that continued throughout the following decade. The collapse of the economic system created an atmosphere similar to that of war. After an unbelievable series of bank failures, bankruptcies, collapses of large corporations and small businesses, and mortgage foreclosures across the land, a black pall settled over the nation and a defeatist psychology prevailed—the exact opposite of the high spirits and optimism of the 1920s. Despite this low point in American economic history, the public image of the nurse was in the process of being elevated to an all-time high in the embodiment of the heroine representation. The mass media recognized nursing as a true profession that required education and the development of skills and knowledge for its practice. Nurses were depicted as brave, rational, dedicated, decisive, humanistic, and autonomous.

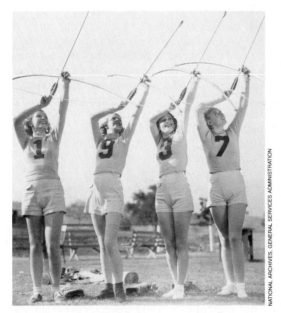

Though the 1930s was a low point in American economic history, the public image of the nurse was being elevated to an all-time high in the embodiment of the heroine.

NATIONAL ARCHIVES, GENERAL SERVICES ADMINISTRATION

THE GREAT DEPRESSION

Whether the stock market crash begot the depression or the depression begot the crash is a question that economists still argue over. What is inarguable, however, is that in the three years following the crash the whole American economy ran steadily downhill at a quickening and disastrous pace. Virtually every important industrial group suffered devastating erosion. Each responded in the only way it knew how to respond: by cutting dividends, reducing inventories, laying off workers, cutting wages and salaries, abandoning capital improvements, and operating on reduced schedules. Small and marginal businesses, even the big marginal ones, toppled like dominoes. From 1930 through 1933, a staggering total of 86,000 business enterprises failed. Farm debt increased in reverse ratio to the declining farm income, and thousands of farm families were forced off the land either by foreclosure or destitution.

But most poignant and significant were the statistics of unemployment: 4,340,000 in 1930; 8,020,000 in 1931; 12,060,000 in 1932. The 1932 figure meant that about one in every five persons in the labor force, or about one in every seven adults in the population, was out of a job. And this figure did not take into account other millions who were underemployed, that is, working only two or three days a week or one or two weeks a month. But even a full week's wages were often insufficient to take care of an average-sized family. Average weekly earnings in manufacturing, for example, slid from $24.77 in 1930 to $16.21 in 1932, a drop of approximately one-third.

The poor of that desolate winter of 1932–33 were not only the residents of the local ghetto or the down-at-heel whites from working-class neighborhoods. People were out of work not only because factories and mines and construction projects had shut down—but also banks and stores and shops and architects' offices and insurance agencies and business enterprises of every kind. The man who knocked at your door at night and asked apologetically if he could interest you in his line of brushes or encyclopedias or Christmas cards or cemetery lots might be the same fellow who a few months or a year ago had cheerfully approved your loan at the bank or written editorials in your newspaper or been the vice-president of a leading real estate company. In 1932 more than 200,000 homeowners, farmers, and businessmen lost their property because they could not keep up payments on their mortgages. Foreclosure was invariably a tragedy for the borrower, and it seldom was a bargain for the lender, since there was virtually no market for real estate, urban or rural.

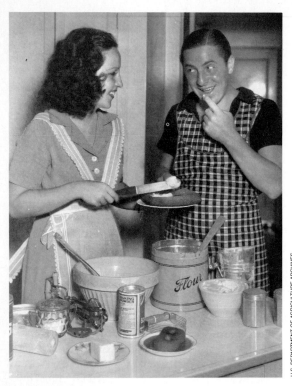

A typical middle-class family of 1935 that was not on relief consisted of two adults and 1.6 siblings living in a rented 6.4-room house or 4.5-room apartment on a gross annual income of $1,348.

U.S. DEPARTMENT OF AGRICULTURE ARCHIVES

A typical middle-class family of 1935 that was not on relief consisted of 2 adults and 1.6 siblings living in a rented, 6.4-room house or 4.5-room apartment on a gross annual income of $1,348. This is part of the U.S. Bureau of Labor Statistics profile of blue-collar and white-collar city families in which at least one member was regularly employed. Luxuries obviously played a very small part in the life of most middle-class families during the 1930s. The basic necessities—food, shelter, and clothing—absorbed at least three-quarters of the average budget, necessitating much corner-cutting, doing without, and maneuvering with one's creditors. Only about three percent of all families owned their own homes. Repairs and improvements were postponed, and tenants haggled with their landlords to fix the roof or scale down the rent. Consumption of red meat went down, and consumption of fish and poultry, which were cheaper and could often be bought from street

vendors, went up. Margarine replaced butter; Jell-O entered its golden age as the cheapest all-purpose dessert; and corn, tomatoes, and pole beans sprang up in backyards and vacant city lots. Families might use no more than a 25-watt light bulb for evening reading, for energy was seen as an expensive commodity; and home sewing was necessary to keep clothing in steady repair. About one in every two families owned an automobile. It was probably either a holdover from better days or a secondhand one bought for about $300. Somebody in the family was likely to be enough of a mechanic to grind the valves, change the oil, patch the tires, and do most of what was needed to keep it in running order.

Families that earlier would have been too proud to allow their young women to work, as much as their households needed money, were in the 1930s forced to use the services of any member of the family who could get and hold a job. In addition, women frequently had to become the breadwinners of the household because of the failure of their husbands' businesses. Indeed, by almost every measure, women's participation in work outside the home increased during the 1930s. Women's share of the labor force grew from 22 to 25 percent, while the percentage of all adult women who were in the work force rose from 24.3 to 25.4. The proportion of married women who were employed grew from 12 to 15 percent during the decade, and married women increased their share of the female labor force from 29 to 35.5 percent.[1]

FEMALE FASHIONS

The average U.S. female was 5 feet, 3 inches tall and weighed 133 pounds, according to a massive government-sponsored study that was carried out in the mid-1930s to help the garment industry set up a rational system to clothe the female form. Women from families with annual incomes of $3,000 or more were over an inch taller than those with family incomes of less than $1,000.

In reaction to the knee-high styles of the 1920s, skirts went down almost to the ankles and then remained at about ten or twelve inches above the ground during the first years of the 1930s. Gradually the hems moved upward until they stood at fifteen to seventeen inches off the floor in 1939. Early in the decade shoulders were natural and sloping; around

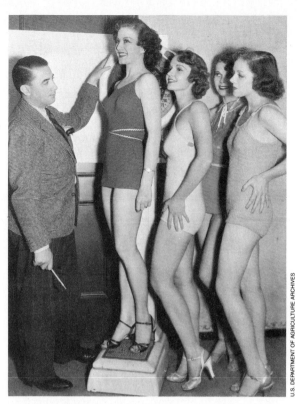

The average U.S. female of the mid 1930s was 5 feet, 3 inches tall and weighed 133 pounds, according to a massive study sponsored by the U.S. Department of Agriculture.

came into fashion. A new vogue developed for lacquering the fingernails (and toenails when they were exposed) in various shades of red.

The very short, shingled haircut and boyish bob of the 1920s was allowed to grow a bit longer in the 1930s. Coiffures were still close to the head and likely to be precisely set. The typical style early in the decade was a short bob with a definite part, neatly waved on the top of the head and done up in small curls or rolls over the ears and at the back of the neck. The all-over, often frizzy permanent wave seen in the 1920s had subsided into an end-curl. About mid-decade a pompadour style came into fashion, with the hair dressed higher over the forehead and on top of the head; clusters of curls or bangs on the forehead also appeared. A longer bob, worn rather plain around the face and with loose curls on the neck, was popularized by such movie stars as Marlene Dietrich and Carole Lombard. A long, shoulder-length pageboy bob became popular toward the end of the era, particularly with teenagers and younger women. The pageboy was worn with the ends turned under neatly in a loose roll on the shoulders; sometimes the hair was brushed back smoothly from the forehead, or it might be worn in bangs. The loose-flowing hair might be held back with a headband running behind the ears and tied on top of the head. Jean Harlow's platinum blonde hair inspired many women to bleach their own locks.

1935 sleeves became full at the shoulder, puffed or gathered, or tailored in a squared, wide style filled out with shoulder pads.

The manifestly painted face of the flapper gave way to the perfectly shaped face with its natural color heightened and brightened by makeup and with its frame of smoothly combed hair arranged flat to the head and curled behind the ears. The flapper's preference for the small "bee-sting" mouth had passed, and lips were outlined more generously. The use of rouge diminished in this decade. The pink cheek patches of the 1920s disappeared in favor of a softer tone, but often rouge was omitted. Eye shadow was used to darken the eyelids, and eyebrow pencils outlined the eyes. Eyebrows were tweezed, arched, and penciled, often to a fine line at the outer ends. During this decade, the interest in beaches and sunbathing increased the desirability of the tanned complexion, so that darker tones of face powder

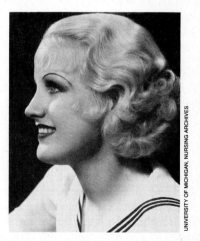

The typical female hairstyle during the early 1930s was a short bob with a definite part, neatly waved on the top of the head and done up in small curls or rolls over the ears and at the back of the neck.

THE MOVIES: THE MOST POTENT MASS MEDIUM

Eighty-five million Americans went to the movies each week, many of them as families. The average family's annual movie budget was $25.00, astonishing in light of depression admission prices. There were 17,000 theaters in the country, more than there were banks, twice as many as there were hotels, and three times as many as there were department stores. Each theater owner showed between 100 and 400 films a year. For 25¢ or less, you could enter your home-town movie theater—the Ritz, Rialto, Roxy, Castle, Tivoli, Alhambra, Stanley, or Rex—and often see two shows for the price of one. Many of the theaters were elaborate palaces, sometimes with dark blue "skies" overhead, lit by hundreds of tiny stars or complete with simulated moving clouds; some were awash with motifs taken from Chinese pagodas, Persian courts, or Egyptian temples, or were in the Art Deco style of New York's Radio City Music Hall. The larger theaters featured a Wurlizter organ that entertained movie patrons entering and exiting.

During the late-1920s and early-1930s, the motion picture industry made tremendous technical strides, which were reflected in the improved quality of films. Sound, which had been haltingly introduced in 1927, was perfected. The smooth blend of action with speed, sound effects, and music induced in the spectator a sense of reality undreamed of in the old days of pantomime. These innovations wrought a revolution not only in the movie industry but also in the popular taste for entertainment. Audiences wanted action on the screen and a coherent spoken script to go with it.

Eight companies accounted for over 75 percent of the American films released in the 1930s. They were Metro-Goldwyn-Mayer (MGM), Paramount, RKO Radio, Fox, Warner Brothers-First National (Warners), United Artists, Universal, and Columbia. Collectively they were known as the major companies, though the last two were looked upon as second-class relatives to the royal family. United Artists constituted a collection of independent producers like Samuel Goldwyn, Joseph Schenck and Mary Pickford (Miss Pickford had formed the company in 1919 along with D. W. Griffith, Douglas Fairbanks, and Charles Chaplin). Since the United Artists product was selective, that company released the fewest films, about six-teen per year. Paramount, with 50 to 60 features annually, led the majors.

The lives of movie stars were often better known than the lives of saints, and the stars' influence was infinitely more pervasive. The number of tall girls who hoped they looked like Ginger Rogers remains uncounted. Jean Harlow's platinum blonde hair set thousands of young women experimenting in the bathroom with peroxide and other bleaches. When Clark Gable stripped down in *It Happened One Night* (Columbia, 1934) to reveal himself as a no-undershirt man, the men's underwear trade was said to have suffered a slump. Most communities in the 1930s could count one or two of their progeny who had made the hopeful pilgrimage to Hollywood. If they showed up on the local screen in even a bit part, a communal chest swelled with pride.

The stars often fell into broad categories according to the types of movies in which they played. For example, there was the typical American hero played so successfully by Henry Fonda, James Stewart, and Gary Cooper; Cary Grant cornered light comedy; Charles Boyer was the unsurpassed continental lover; Spencer Tracy and Frederic March were solid and dramatic; Ronald Coleman and Leslie Howard played suave and appealing Englishmen. The predominant female image in film was affected by the grim economic reality. The carefree, dance-mad flapper of the 1920s suddenly had to go to work. Career women in films of the 1930s had intelligence and style: Claudette Colbert, Jean Arthur, Myrna Loy, Carole Lombard, Katharine Hepburn, Rosalind Russell, Kay Francis, Bette Davis, Madeleine Carroll, and Barbara Stanwyck. Women did not always have to make the choice between love and career, nor were they always objects, misused and mistreated.

Many of the women portrayed in the films of the 1930s were promoted to higher-status employment as nurses, journalists, and business executives. Rarely were women during this decade shown as only wives and mothers, unless in a sophisticated, upper-class setting. And when they were not career women, they were usually socialites, acting out fantasies about power and preferment that had been characteristic of American escape literature since at least the 1890s. But whether workers or society women, the women of 1930s films were proud and self-reliant, imperious to servants and subordinates.

The movies, particularly in periods like the 1930s when female roles were undergoing a major remodeling, constituted a powerful cultural force, shaping individual choices within the boundaries of social and economic possibilities, thus assisting in the creation of a new womanhood. The fantasies that movies wove around common female experiences contained rich meanings. The moviegoer did not merely travel through a remote fantasy land but briefly inhabited a well-contrived make-believe role that was a glamorous rendition of the social options open to women. Those vicarious lives on the screen could channel female expectations in a socially acceptable direction and then reconcile women to their lot, providing both relief and reinforcement in the guise of routine entertainment.

NURSES ON THE BIG SCREEN

In the more serious, realistic atmosphere of the 1930s, the nurse character received a great deal of positive attention. In general, nursing appeared as a worthy, important profession that enabled women to earn a respectable living. Several film genres featured nurses as frequent characters: crime and detective movies, war films, hospital and medical dramas, adventure films about aviation and ocean liners, and quite a few films about the nursing profession itself. Depression movies often featured nurses living by their wits. Films of the 1930s reflected, moreover, the recognition of nursing as a true profession requiring training, discipline, and skills.

An anonymously published, true-life account of wartime nursing entitled *War Nurse* appeared in print in 1930 and was quickly rushed into film by MGM that same year. It deals with the experiences of several nurse characters: Joy (Anita Page), a convent-educated girl who falls in love with a married man and is discharged from the hospital; "Kansas" (Helen Jerome Eddy), a small-town girl; and Babs (June Walker), the supervising nurse who falls in love with Wally (Robert Montgomery), a flier with the Lafayette Escadrille. Several of the nurse characters die before the end of the film, either from wounds incurred near the front or while giving birth to an illegitimate baby—Joy's fate. The only survivors are Babs and Wally, but their successful romance is clouded over by their war experiences and the deaths of their friends.[2]

William Wellman's *Night Nurse* (Warner Brothers, 1931) was the first civilian nursing picture of the

1930s. It raised professional issues hitherto unarticulated and also prefigured in many ways other nurse pictures of the era. A curious film, by turns exciting, grim, melodramatic, and sentimental, *Night Nurse* is about a young nurse called Lora Hart (Barbara Stanwyck) who manages to fulfill her ambitions to become a nurse despite educational shortcomings and who, after graduation, courageously fights against a corrupt establishment when she learns that two of her patients are being left to die by a crooked doctor.[3]

Although *Night Nurse* is farfetched in the way it pits an eager young idealist against the criminal world, it is no more so than many other later pictures based on a similar mold. Far more important is the film's undoubted power, due largely to Wellman's direction and to Stanwyck's entirely credible performance as Lora—and because it takes a longer, closer look at the professional nurse's lot than any film previously made.

Night Nurse breaks entirely new ground in screen history by addressing previously unmentioned questions about the profession: questions about nursing recruitment, what it means to want to be a nurse, and the suitability of certain women for the profession; and questions about the moral conflicts inherent in the profession, and how a young nurse of integrity can hope to combat corruption among her superiors. The first half of the movie chronicles how Lora gets herself accepted as a student against the will of the director of nurses and how she then copes with the ordeals of hospital life until she graduates. The remainder deals with Lora's first case as a registered nurse, when she is hired as the private nurse to the two small Richey girls, who, having left the hospital, are convalescing in their palatial family apartment under suspicious circumstances. Far from gaining in health, the girls are actually deteriorating under the medical supervision of a mysterious Dr. Ranger, while their mother drinks herself to death, encouraged by a cruel chauffeur called Nick (Clark Gable). When Lora confronts Dr. Ranger, he mentions "professional ethics" and tells her not to meddle in doctors' affairs. Undaunted, and with some assistance from a former patient who is a bootlegger, she eventually manages to save the children's lives and expose the evil Nick, who wants the children's inheritance.

A nurse who works for reform, Lora is a leader with a strong moral sense, and the bizarre context

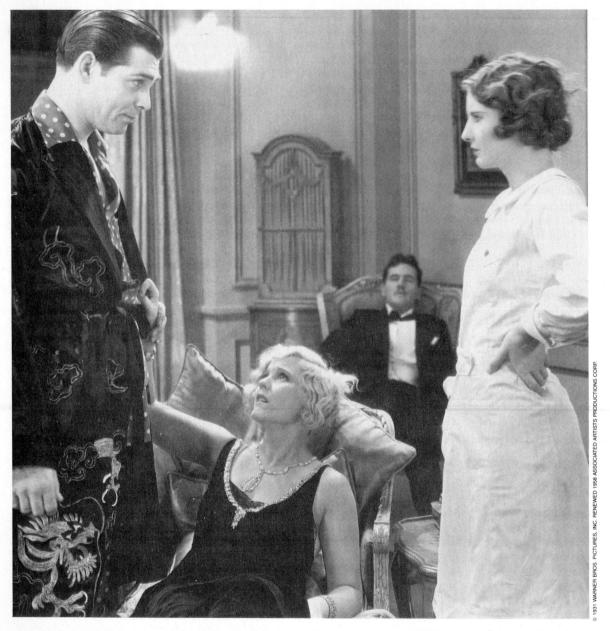

In Night Nurse *(Warner Brothers, 1931) Lora Hart (Barbara Stanwyck) manages to save two children's lives and expose the evil Nick, who wants to get his hands on the children's inheritance.*

within which she operates serves to heighten, not diminish, her character. Good and evil are melodramatically opposed in *Night Nurse,* and Lora fights for good like a latter-day avenger in this larger-than-life

drama, which constitutes a major breakthrough in the characterization of nursing. The lasting quality of this film is attested to by a recent directory of motion pictures on television, which appraises *Night*

Nurse as an "excellent, hard-bitten tale of a nurse . . . still potent today."[4]

THE WHITE PARADE

The only film entirely focused on nursing ever to be nominated for an Academy Award for Best Picture was *The White Parade* (20th Century-Fox, 1934). Although it lost out in the balloting of the Academy of Motion Picture Arts and Sciences to the smash hit *It Happened One Night, The White Parade* is an exceptional film. Based on a popular novel, it was the perfect vehicle for Fox to showcase its available female talent. Starring Loretta Young, the film explores the experiences of a group of nursing students through their 3-year training period. The film does not contain romantic complications, and the focus remains firmly on the learning of a profession.

The setting for the movie is Mitchell Reed Hospital and Nursing School in Union City, a midwestern metropolis. The Mitchell Reed School is reputed to be the finest nursing school in the country, the West Point of the nursing profession; over 10,000 young women apply to the school each year, but rigorous admission requirements allow only a limited number of them to enter. Miss Harrington (Sara Haden), the attractive, 35-year-old superintendent of the school, greets the 160 new probationers with the following speech.

> We offer the best training curriculum in America. Our department heads and instructors here are full-time workers. We are proud of that. We are also proud of the fact that, through the years, Mitchell Reed has become more like a university than a mere nurses' training school.[5]

She further enjoins the newcomers:

> In entering this profession . . . and nursing as it is practiced today is quite definitely a profession . . . you must learn to assume responsibility, and to adapt yourselves to discipline.[6]

After the brief welcoming assembly, the 160 women are divided into 10-student squads, each headed by a nursing supervisor. One of these squads, shepherded about by the gruff but kindly Miss Roberts (Jane Darwell), known as "Sailor" to her charges, is the focus of this movie. In addition to these few highlighted

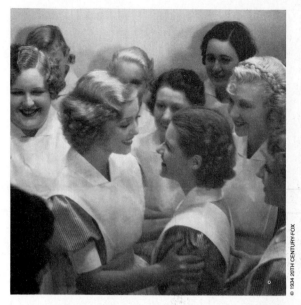

In The White Parade *(Fox, 1934) the ten young women in Sailor's squad reflect the variety of backgrounds and motivations found among the nursing students.*

characters, the film introduces scores of other students at the school who are experiencing much the same emotions and difficulties as felt by the major characters.

The ten young women in Sailor's squad reflect the variety of backgrounds and motivations found among the students. Heather Arden (Loretta Young), an attractive 17- to 18-year-old woman from a middle-class Boston family, holds romantic notions about a lot of things, but she firmly believes that a girl needs a career. She had considered being a stenographer or an actress but found the sexual pressures of her potential employers frightening, so she has entered nursing. Glenda Farley (Murial Kirkland), a 24-year-old woman from New York City, has clearly been around. Too rouged and too blonde, she holds most of the world in cynical contempt. But once, after a self-induced aborton, she landed in a hospital and met the kindest human being she had ever known—a nurse. Hoping to find satisfaction in service to others, Glenda has entered Mitchell Reed. Una Mellon (Joyce Compton), daughter of a wealthy Texas cattleman, really wanted to be an actress, but her Daddy wouldn't hear of it; Daddy suggested she attend Mitchell Reed, and she accepted the idea as the only way out of Eagle Pass, Texas.

Zita Corinna (Dorothy Wilson), a slight, pale, dark-haired girl, has always wanted to be a nurse. She found her calling in childhood when she nursed her siblings and crippled mother. Zita has little money but a great desire to succeed. Gertrude Mack (Astrid Allyn), a slightly devious young woman, wants to become a nurse because she wants to catch a doctor; her reading of novels about nurses has assured her that all nurses eventually marry "medicos." Angie Duke (Dorothea Kent), daughter of a wealthy and socially prominent Union City family, was bored with the social set; she has entered nursing because her father offered her $500,000 if she would do something useful. Lucy "Pudgy" Stebbins (June Gittelson) only shows an interest in food; a plump, lethargic, dull young woman, Lucy spends most of her time eating chocolate bars. Lucy has entered nursing school because her father said she would have to support herself, and the Mitchell Reed catalogue suggests that nursing students are well-fed. Hannah Seymour (Joan Marsh) saw a Clark Gable movie, *The White Sister,* in which the hero fell in love with a nurse; she has determined to enter nursing because it promises such romantic interludes. Mabel Wiley (Helen Lynch) left Sioux City, Iowa, for Mitchell Reed because her hometown boyfriend told her she "looked elegant in white." Hannah Fridholm (Mary Phillips), a Minnesota girl, wants to become a nurse because it promises an "honorable, profitable career of service." What seems important to the superintendent, who admits the applicants, is not so much what a young woman is, but whether or not she has the potential to become a nurse.

After receiving copies of the lengthy school of nursing rule book, the squad sorts itself out into assigned rooms, and Heather finds that tough-talking Glenda will be her roommate for 3 years. The following morning, the first day of their 5-month probationary period begins. Each of the young women struggles into her probationary uniform—flat shoes; black cotton stockings; ankle-length, striped, high-necked dress; and apron—before reporting for breakfast and assembly. Most of them grumble and complain about the uniforms and the early hour— 6 A.M. A few are sent back to their rooms to take off excess makeup, lengthen their skirts, or put on petticoats. The first order of business calls for an extensive physical examination of each new student. At the end of the first day, everyone gathers in the student lounge, exhausted and discouraged. Sailor then enters and, although it is against regulations, proceeds to chat with the girls and to establish some warmth and familiarity. The probationers learn that Sailor, a heavy and rather rough-spoken woman in her forties or fifties, received her nickname because she had been one of the few nurses in World War I assigned to duty on a battleship. She recounts a few of her more colorful adventures, such as the time when the ship was torpedoed, and manages to win the confidence and affection of most of the students.

The focal point of the entire film is the nursing school experience. At the beginning of the movie the nursing students exhibit different attitudes toward the profession. Few of them seem to have any true appreciation of nursing. Those students whose weaknesses and bad qualities outweigh their potential for improvement are quickly dropped. Angie, Lucy, Hannah Seymour, and Mabel fail the first cut at the end of the probationary period. None of these students manages to overcome her disinclination for hard work or her misconceptions about the profession; the omniscient Miss Harrington and these students' failing grades soon reveal their ineptitude.

Later, Zita is discharged from training after an attempted suicide. Despite her ardent desire to become a nurse, she cannot overcome her naiveté and inexperience. Not only does she succumb to Dr. Moore's well-known charm, but she is unable to handle the psychological consequences of her seduction. Zita had been called a natural because of her innate nursing skills and dedication; most of the young women who have entered the program have misconceptions about their chosen career and will have to be molded and trained if they are to succeed as nurses. Thus, natural qualities of self-sacrifice, compassion, or maternal instincts may enhance a young woman's nursing, but these traits alone do not qualify a woman to be a nurse. The movie emphasizes that good nurses are made, not born.

As the story develops, Heather's experiences, both romantic and professional, receive the most attention. During her first months as a probationer, Heather adjusts well and works hard at her studies; her greatest difficulty, perhaps, is her homesickness. She is popular with all the other students, except Gertrude, who resents her proper Boston accent and her sweet personality. Although Heather occasionally dates some of the interns, she shies away from serious involvement with any of them because of her "romance" with Ronald Hall III, a wealthy, polo-playing young man from Boston. In fact, her romance is entirely imaginary; Heather finds more pleasure in her daydreams of Ronald than she does with the somewhat grubby and aggressive interns. Her fantasy relationship with Ronald lasts into her senior year. Heather seems unequal to the challenge of coping with Gertrude's efforts to expose her romance as a fraud. Thus Heather turns to hardheaded and practical Glenda for help.

Most of Heather's weaknesses stem from her romantic delusions about Ronald. To her credit, Heather quickly drops her delusions after her first date with Ronald. After she witnesses his drunken and abusive behavior, she tears down her photos of him and resolves to put him out of her mind. After their subsequent reconciliation, she shows her newly won sense of independence by refusing to marry him if it means not graduating from nursing school. Apparently, her 3 years of training have wrought a significant change in her personality; she insists that getting her nursing diploma and having a profession are more important to her than being Mrs. Ronald Hall.

When Heather begins nursing school her perceptions of the profession are very limited. To her it means simply a career that will not involve running from amorous employers. By the end of her training, she realizes the significance of being a nurse. She tells Ronnie, "I'm not ashamed of being a nurse . . . I'm proud of it. . . ." Her identification with the nursing profession coincides with her maturation as a woman as well. Because she feels pride in her accomplishments she refuses to forget her training in order to become the dependent wife of a wealthy man. Even though Heather makes it clear that she does not intend to work as a nurse after her marriage, she has already succeeded in her goal—acquiring her professional credentials; as she says, "I am something." She understands that becoming a nurse is a permanent sign of her independence and self-esteem—something that no one can take away from her.[7]

FOUR GIRLS IN WHITE

The nurses' training theme was given attention again in the film *Four Girls in White* (MGM, 1939), which was dedicated to Florence Nightingale. The story traces the lives, loves, and adventures of four young women who enter a school of nursing together at a city hospital during the late-1930s. The four are Norma and Pat Page, two sisters (played by Florence Rice and Ann Rutherford), Mary Forbes (Mary Howard) and Gertie Robbins (Una Merkel). Each has chosen a nursing career for a different reason: Norma is interested in meeting and marrying a wealthy doctor or patient, Pat wishes only to follow in her sister's footsteps, Gertie appears to consider nursing as simply a job, and Mary needs a livelihood in order to support herself and her infant daughter.[8]

The film's main authority figure is Miss Tobias (Jessie Ralph), a rather elderly instructor of nursing with white hair, wrinkles, a perennial scowl, and a voice and manner reminiscent of an army drill sergeant. She is most frequently seen showing her students how to apply bandages, make beds, sterilize surgical equipment, and fill medicine bottles—tasks that her students fail to complete to her satisfaction. But Miss Tobias's gruff exterior conceals an inner warmth that, very occasionally, is permitted to break through. She cuts a refreshingly comic and outspoken figure among swarms of sweet young nurses. Above all, though, Miss Tobias has a real love of and commitment to nursing and embodies steadfastness, efficiency, and the experienced ability to instruct, guide, and discipline her students with understanding and compassion.

Norma, during the course of her three years' training, matures from an egocentric man-chaser into a heroic woman totally dedicated to her profession. The film is thematically organized to illustrate how each young woman emulates Florence Nightingale, whose presence prevails in the background throughout. In the hospital sanctuary there is a statue of Nightingale holding her lamp, and individual nurses reflect before this statue, which radiates almost religious serenity. One of the nurses, Mary, is fatally molested by an insane patient while Norma is away from assigned duty with her. Mary's name is added to the list of nurses "killed in action" inscribed on the pedestal beneath the statue; this list clearly highlights the idea of nursing as a total life commitment.[9]

After Mary is killed during Norma's unjustified absence, the other nurses shun Norma, correctly blaming her irresponsibility and selfishness for Mary's untimely death. Even Dr. Melford has only bitter words to say to this woman who is using the hospital and everyone in it for her own selfish purposes:

"And you call yourself a nurse.... Why, you don't know what the word means. You're a disgrace to the uniform you're wearing." The last scenes of the film depict Norma's initiation into the real meaning of nursing—service, symbolized by Florence Nightingale's lamp. Norma's first act of mercy is to clear Mary's name by taking the blame for what happened to her. She then resigns. During the initial call for volunteers to go to a passenger train wreck, Norma remains silent in the background. Miss Tobias tells her that in times of crisis, personal differences among the staff are forgotten. But at the site of the wreck, Norma still feels outcast. Her impulse to enter the submerged car to help those trapped inside is labeled foolishness by the other rescue workers. In the final graduation scene, however, Norma is restored to her peer group (they all receive the black-banded caps of graduate nurses) and is singled out for a special commendation. Her final action, a humble one, of transferring the medal of honor from her own cap to that of her deceased friend, Mary, dramatizes the final retribution that Norma must pay for her earlier mistake.[10]

VIGIL IN THE NIGHT

Yet another fictional melodrama centering on the nursing profession was *Vigil in the Night* (RKO Radio, 1940). This film, based on a novel by A. J. Cronin, presents a contemporary view of the nursing profession that nevertheless emphasizes the virtues of courage, self-sacrifice, dedication, and compassion. The heroine of this film, Anne Lee, played by Carole Lombard in her most impressive dramatic role, is an energetic and dedicated nurse who wants her younger sister Lucy (Anne Shirley), to be a nurse too.[11]

The movie begins in Shereham County Hospital's isolation ward. Nurse Anne Lee sits exhausted by the bed of a child seriously ill with diphtheria. It has been a night-long vigil, and now she waits anxiously for her sister to relieve her. Her sister, Lucy, is still a student and, unlike Anne, lacks dedication and diligence. She arrives late for duty, hardly sorry at all, and has not long taken over at the bedside when she leaves the boy in order to make some tea. Though she has been told to keep careful watch over her patient to ensure that the tube through which he is breathing does not become blocked, she leaves the room unattended for her break. In her absence, the tube blocks and the child dies.

After seeking Anne's help, Lucy is questioned by the doctor and matron. Another nurse, a busybody called Nurse Gregg, notices that tea has been made, which prompts Anne to claim responsibility for the tragedy. Appalled that Anne, so excellent a nurse, could act so irresponsibly, the matron reminds her that there "is nothing so bad as a bad nurse," tells her she must go, but in view of her good record allows her the privilege of resigning. Later Anne tells Lucy that she did this in order that Lucy could continue and obtain her nursing certificate, expected in a month. Although Lucy is unsure about her suitability for nursing and complains about its menial nature, Anne encourages her to go on, hopeful that they can someday work together again. Anne has no trouble finding a job in Hepperton, a neighboring town, where her professional skills soon distinguish her.[12]

On one occasion Anne observes an appendectomy on one of the most important men in town, Matt Boley, performed by the hospital's foremost physician. Anne scandalizes the matron by pointing out to the surgeon, Dr. Prescott, from the operating room gallery, that a swab still remains in the patient. Prescott admires her courage and intelligence, finding these traits unusual in a nurse.

Meanwhile Lucy obtains her nursing certificate. And on the matron's advice, Anne sets out for Shereham to bring Lucy to work with her at Hepperton. On the bus journey Anne is accompanied by the matron and by the same Nurse Gregg who knows all about Anne's past. She is now at Hepperton, too, and obviously determined to stir up trouble with her insinuating remarks. An end is put to her scandalmongering when the bus crashes down a hillside.

Anne takes command, sending for Dr. Prescott while she tends the casualties. Once again her initiative is apparent; once again her conduct impresses Dr. Prescott, who later asks Anne home for a warm drink. They discuss his desire for a properly equipped new hospital to replace the grossly inefficient one they have; the main obstacle is Matt Boley, the wealthy but miserly chairman of the hospital board, who refuses to allow the necessary monies to be spent.

Promoted to head nurse, a delighted Anne visits Boley at Prescott's request. It soon becomes clear that he wishes to show his thanks by propositioning her. When Anne realizes this, she prepares to leave, but Boley's wife enters and infers that Anne is already involved with her husband. Boley is so full of hurt pride that he readily agrees to report the nurse's behavior to the matron. The complaint of such a powerful man is sufficient to get Anne dismissed; once again her exemplary prior record is taken into consideration and she is allowed to resign.

She decides to join Lucy, who is now married to a mutual friend called Joe Shand, living in London, and nursing in a private rest home in the West End. Prescott warns Anne that he has heard that the Rolgrave Home is a disreputable establishment. When she arrives in London, Anne is shocked to find that Lucy has left Joe and is herself living at the home. The news soon breaks that a famous actress's suicide leap from a window in the Rolgrave is being blamed, in part, on the nurse in charge of her at the time—Lucy. At the inquest, however, it emerges that Lucy is blameless, but that the home itself is a highly suspect place. Instrumental in determining the truth is Prescott, who has come to London seeking financial backing for his hospital plan. Boley has again refused sufficient funds, even in the face of an outbreak of cerebrospinal fever among the children. Although Boley had been warned about the virulence of this infectious disease—"more dangerous than the worst form of tropic plague"—he had consistently refused to support Prescott's plans. Accordingly, the doctor has resigned and come in hope to London.[13]

Hearing of the matron's desperate need for volunteers to nurse the growing epidemic, Anne and Lucy return to Hepperton, where they are received with warmth and gratitude. They join a pitifully few other nurses in the unsanitary isolation ward that has been expediently fashioned from the old smallpox hospital. Courageously they enter the enclosed world of nearly a score of sick for whom they are medically able to do very little. The appalling conditions mean that even comfort is denied the patients, for Boley still resolutely refuses to allow them more linen and other such supplies. Anne takes sole charge of the isolation ward where she, Lucy, and the few others work for 12 hours at a time.

News of her return filters through to the main part of the hospital, where Anne's old friends, Nora and Glennie, decide to volunteer as well. They arrive, with a couple of other nurses, including the now regenerated Nurse Gregg, who humbly reports for duty too. Anne immediately reorganizes the isolation hospital, establishing shorter periods of duty. In addition, exasperated by Boley's obstruction, she unilaterally requisitions new linen—and decorators to provide more spacious, attractive, newly painted accommodations.

Ironically, the day Boley confronts Anne with the bills she has run up, his own little boy is brought in suffering from the illness. Dr. Prescott returns empty-handed from London and charges Boley with his share of the blame for the existing misery. With his son now affected, too, Boley's attitude changes and he recognizes the necessity for all that Anne has done.

The boy's condition deteriorates, however, and Lucy has the task of nursing him throughout the night. As she monitors his breathing, taking his ever-rising temperature regularly and placing cold compresses on his head, his strength fails him and his breathing stops. Finding the oxygen tank empty, Lucy saves the boy with mouth-to-mouth resuscitation; owing to the highly infectious nature of the illness, it is inevitable that she will contract the disease herself soon after. On her deathbed she compliments herself on saving one life to replace the other she had lost and declares that she is quite a good nurse after all. Her mind at rest, Lucy dies. Boley's gratitude for his son's recovery is expressed with extreme generosity toward the new hospital; he also buries all animosity towards Prescott and the two men become good friends. Anne returns to the main part of the hospital, ready to cope with casualties from a local pit disaster. She expresses faith in the profound good for which her profession works as the film draws to its conclusion.

Anne Lee is the central character in *Vigil in the Night,* which is the story of her self-sacrifice, courage, initiative, and strength of purpose. In contrast to her sister, Lucy, Anne is every inch a professional nurse, dedicated at all times and consistently inspired by the challenge her career offers. Neatly turned out, her hair caught at the nape of her neck in a bun, she looks splendid. The complexity of her character is profound: though beautiful, she has obviously chosen to devote herself wholeheartedly to nursing—she seems to have no private life at all. Professionally skilled and naturally gifted for her work, she still demonstrates a high degree of tolerance toward the faults of her colleagues. For despite Anne's diligence, she is never prudish or small-minded: for example, she puts up with Nora's smoking even though it is against the matron's rules.

The extent of her good nature is epitomized in the sacrifice she makes for Lucy. Taking the blame as she does could be thought unprofessional, considering

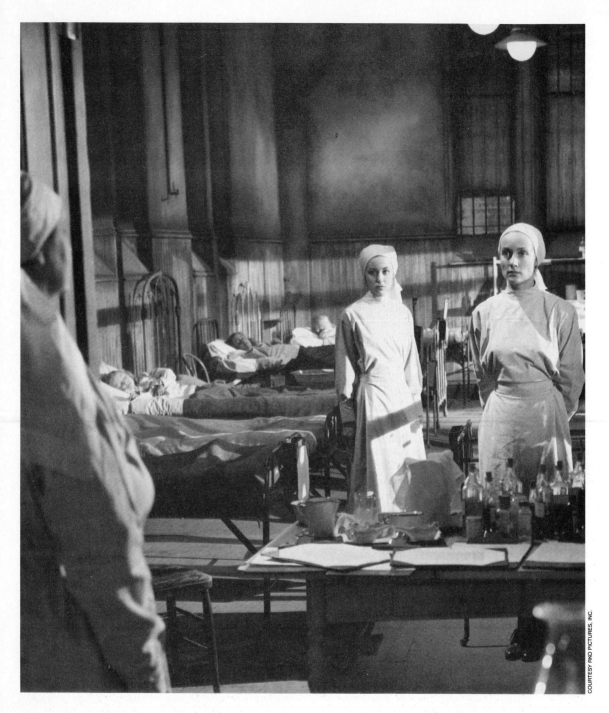

Hearing of the desperate need for volunteers to nurse children of the cerebrospinal fever epidemic, Anne and Lucy join a pitifully few other nurses in the unsanitary isolation ward.

the seriousnes of Lucy's error. Perhaps it would have been better for Lucy to have been discovered for the poor nurse she really was. Ultimately, however, Lucy's own deed of self-sacrifice exonerates Anne from any possible charge of irresponsibility.[14]

Several times during the narrative Anne speaks seriously about how important her work is to her. She *must* nurse: life without pursuing her chosen career would be unthinkable to her. Her fascination with hospital life is frequently indicated, as when she asks the matron if she may try operating room nursing because it is one of her greatest interests. Promotion to the rank of head nurse gives her "greater opportunity than [she] could have hoped for," and she wears her new uniform with an undeniable though gentle pride.

With Dr. Prescott she shares a passionate concern about replacing the existing inadequate medical facilities. Anne complains to Prescott about the skewed financial priorities—"So much for everything else; so little for the sick." This mutual interest brings doctor and nurse together, though Anne's concentration on her work precludes their getting intimate. In his quiet way, Prescott seems impressed by more than Anne's professional qualities, and he directly asks her—perhaps in desperation—if she has any other life than her work. She is adamant, however, and their relationship remains firmly based on their shared professional backgrounds.[15]

AN ESSENTIAL OPERATING ROOM NURSE

Wife, Doctor, and Nurse (20th Century-Fox), a 1937 comedy-drama about a romantic triangle, starred Warner Baxter as Dr. Judd Lewis; Virginia Bruce as nurse "Steve," or Miss Stephens; and Loretta Young as Ina, Judd's wife. As the film begins, we see the close relationship between Dr. Lewis and his pretty nurse Steve. They make a perfect surgical team: they approach their work with both humor and dedication and think nothing of spending long sessions in the operating room in order to save a patient's life. The doctor and his nurse appear perfectly relaxed in each other's company, and there is no sense of the doctor assuming a superior stance in their relationship. The extent of their dependence upon each other is revealed when Judd marries a pretty social-ite, Ina, without telling Steve about it beforehand. Ina is willing to put up with the demands of being a doctor's wife, but when she finally meets Steve and realizes that her husband's faithful surgical nurse is a beautiful young woman, she becomes a little wary. Steve, too, begins to feel some jealousy when she comes to realize that she has been in love with Judd all along. She quits her job because she realizes that she cannot handle the situation. Judd deteriorates as a husband and a doctor when he realizes how much he has depended upon Steve for support. At the end of the film, both women discover Judd in a drunken state and work together to restore him to his previous stability. The two strong and admirable young women face up to their future problems and settle down to a kind of ménage à trois.[16]

The image of nursing in this unusual romantic story remains positive throughout the film. Steve's entire characterization is based on her invaluable skills as a surgical nurse who shares the same dedication, altruism, and concern as her co-worker, Judd. That Steve and Judd work as an interdependent team becomes increasingly clear as the film progresses. We see both doctor and nurse as equally important health care providers. On the personal level, Steve is always presented in a sympathetic light. Both Steve and Ina, Judd's wife, are attractive, stylish women. The nurse character does not appear to be an unsophisticated or dowdy woman just because she works for her living. The reason for Judd's choice of Ina as a marriage partner has nothing to do with the nurse being considered a less suitable mate for a doctor. Steve's reaction to Judd's marriage is a composite of disappointment and a little jealousy; she does not exactly feel rejected because she did not recognize her own feelings for Judd before his marriage. Nevertheless, during a post-surgical period of relaxation, Steve is overcome by what she recognizes as her love for Judd. When her kiss is not reciprocated she concludes that she must get out of Judd's life for good. She is not bitter or self-pitying, and the viewer knows she is fully capable of finding another job or attracting another man. But Steve does feel that her previously warm and almost intimate relationship with Judd cannot go on. This strong depiction of a professional nurse typifies the treatment of nurses in 1930s films. Although nurse characters may become involved in happy or sad romances, they never lose their sense of professional responsibility.[17]

GREAT WOMEN OF NURSING

Film biographies, a popular Hollywood product of the 1930s, tackled two nurse heroines: *The White Angel* (Warner Brothers, 1936) and *Nurse Edith Cavell* (RKO Radio, 1939). Although the stories of Florence Nightingale and Edith Cavell had already received attention from silent-film makers, they now became the subjects of more extensive film treatment. In 1936 Kay Francis starred as Florence Nightingale in the Warner Brothers film, *The White Angel.* The film shows the terrible challenges faced by Nightingale and her band of nurses. Not only did these nurses face the accumulated filth and lack of organization in the hospital but also the overt hostility of the military doctors. The film graphically demonstrates how the nurses set about organizing and improving conditions. The scene of the nurses rhythmically sweeping out the filth captures the sense of discipline and order that characterized the Nightingale nurses. Florence became an object of veneration to the soldiers whom she helped and who appreciated what she did for them. In *The White Angel,* a woman and a nurse is portrayed as a heroic crusader who successfully defeats the forces of convention, and the nursing profession is associated with the highest level of humanitarianism.[18]

Another reverential film biography portrayed the life and death of a second great nursing heroine, *Nurse Edith Cavell,* played by Anna Neagle. The film recounts the story of the English nurse who established nursing as a profession in Belgium before World War I. When war broke out, Cavell continued her work as administrator of a Brussels hospital and nurses' training school even after the German occupation; she considered her work to be above national loyalties. She and several other Belgian women arranged for the secret transfer of Allied soldiers out of German-occupied Belgium. Cavell used her hospital as a hiding place for the soldiers and thus suffered the greatest risk. The film makes clear that Cavell helped the soldiers out of humanitarian impulses rather than patriotic ones, for she also nursed German soldiers with great compassion.

Eventually the German authorities traced the exodus of Allied soldiers to Cavell's hospital and subsequently arrested her and her suspected accomplices. Although the Germans had little solid evidence of her actions, they found her guilty of aiding the enemy and condemned her to death. In the film, the ill-fated nurse makes her final preparations with dignity and calm; her last prayers are to forgive her killers. After the war, her body is returned to England and reburied with full state honors. The film's cathedral scene, in which the casket containing Edith Cavell's body is treated to a proper funeral ceremony, is bathed in unearthly light and reverberating with angelic voices, is Nurse Cavell's only earthly reward for her martyrdom. Indeed, this true-life nursing figure is presented as a twentieth-century saint who acted decisively and eagerly in her commitment to humanity.[19]

Neither Nightingale nor Cavell concluded her labors by falling into the arms of a convenient true love; Nightingale would proceed from the Crimea to even larger tasks, and of course Cavell died. The film audience of the 1930s learned from these two films of the heroism that has occasionally marked the nursing profession as well as the contributions of strong-minded women to contemporary history. Although the 1930s and early-1940s did offer examples of nurses waylaid by romance and marriage, numerous films provided the viewer with proof that women could make a difference in the world around them and that nursing provided fertile ground for strong, altruistic, and independent women to contribute to society.

THE NURSE DETECTIVE

The largest category of 1930s films to feature nurses as major characters was detective and crime stories, in which the nurse generally contributed to the resolution of the mystery or the vindication of a falsely accused man with whom she had fallen in love. The Mary Roberts Rinehart character of "Miss Pinkerton" and Mignon Eberhart's "Sarah Keate" became popular screen characters. These nurse-detectives worked as private-duty nurses for wealthy patients and naturally became embroiled in the mysterious goings-on of the mansion's other occupants. Although these films usually ended with the nurse in the arms of her boyfriend, often a police detective, they were not primarily romantic stories. The nurse often displayed great wit, mental acuity, and courage. These nurse-detectives were worldly-wise, not easily taken in by outward appearance, and yet deep down were sympathetic and kindly women. Limited attention to actual nursing care occurred in these stories—at most the nurses administered medications, took temperatures, and delivered meals. However, by focusing attention on nurses as sleuths in complicated mysteries, Hollywood offered countless examples of nurses being appreciated for their intelligence, logic, and bravery.

MISS PINKERTON

A typical whodunit, in both its plot and its heroine, is *Miss Pinkerton* (Warner Brothers, 1932), a film taken from Mary Roberts Rinehart's mystery novel of the same name. Here the heroine's role as nurse is not the story's focus but merely a device to make her detecting more plausible. Here the crime does not arouse any great pity for the victims or moral indignation at great social problems; it is only the incident that sets in motion all the complex aspects of the puzzle that the detective must then sort out to find the culprit.[20]

Miss Pinkerton begins when old Miss Juliet Mitchell (Elizabeth Patterson) suffers nervous shock upon discovering the body of her nephew, Herbert Wynn, shot to death, apparently by his own hand. Police Inspector Patten (George Brent), believes, however, that Wynn has actually been murdered, and he requests that his friend Georgia Adams (Joan Blondell) be the one assigned to nurse old Aunt Juliet. When the nurse arrives, Patten asks her to keep alert for suspicious events in the household and secretly assist him in discovering the murderer. In recognition of her new detective role, he affectionately dubs her "Miss Pinkerton." Such an assignment keeps her busy, for everyone who inhabits or visits the house acts suspiciously. Everyone lurks behind doors and eavesdrops on the others; mysterious figures enter the house at night, shoving or strangling anyone in their way; other characters sneak about seeking, planting, or destroying clues.

Almost everyone in the story becomes suspect: Miss Juliet's longtime servants, Hugo and Mary (married); Miss Juliet's lawyer, Mr. Glen (Holmes Herbert), and her doctor (C. Henry Gordon); Paula Brent (Ruth Hall), a young society girl who, it turns out, had been secretly married to the murdered Herbert; Florence Lenz (Mary Doren), Mr. Glen's secretary and also another girlfriend of the profligate Herbert; and Charles Elliot (Donald Dilloway), a young society gentleman to whom Paula had been engaged before marrying Herbert. All of these characters

come under suspicion of murder in the course of the plot, either for motives of jealousy or because they stand to benefit from Herbert's $100,000 insurance policy. Even Miss Pinkerton herself becomes implicated when someone switches arsenic for the normal medication the nurse uses to prepare a syringe for Miss Juliet, who promptly dies.

The next night a masked, cloaked figure tries to kill Miss Pinkerton but runs away when Inspector Patten suddenly appears. The nurse never actually figures out herself who the murderer is, but her snooping supplies Inspector Patten with clues and accidently causes the culprit to be discovered and captured. It turns out to be the lawyer, who is set on eliminating everyone who stands between him and the $100,000. Georgia Adams, who initially complained about the boredom of hospital nursing, now decides she's had enough adventure and is ready to return to her normal duties. However, her personal life still promises some excitement since she and Inspector Patten have become romantically involved during their collaboration on the murder case.

The view of nursing seen in *Miss Pinkerton* was already a familiar one, and it became a standard portrayal in the nurse-detective films that followed. The patient's ailment—nervous shock in this case—rarely requires serious technical procedures or equipment; usually it needs only bed rest, comfort measures, and occasional medications. The nurse can tend to such treatments quite competently and still have plenty of time left for sleuthing. Georgia Adams, Miss Pinkerton, seems to be a vigorous, efficient, confident nurse, her humane sympathy spiced with sardonic humor. She tends Aunt Juliet carefully, straightening up her room, making her comfortable in bed, bringing meals, and preparing medications. However, since Aunt Juliet sneaks out of bed at night to conceal some incriminating evidence, Miss Pinkerton keeps an eye on her both as a suspect and as a patient.[21]

The movie studios made quite a point of advertising *Miss Pinkerton* as the first female detective in screen history, and she does supply some clues to Inspector Patten, who makes the logical deductions necessary to solve the mystery. She then returns with relief to her "boring" hospital nursing, convinced that she is not cut out for a life of sleuthing; and her continued romance with Inspector Patten seems assured. Critics recognized that the mystery was full of clichés, but the vivacious Joan Blondell gave the role of Miss Pinkerton more charm than was inherent in the character. Also, the public was drawn by the promoter's promises of "the greatest Mystery-Thriller of all time," based on the "Masterpiece by the World's Most Popular Author," that "mistress of mystery—Mary Roberts Rinehart." Again and again, posters invited the public to "Meet the screen's first sleuth in skirts."[22]

THE TRANSITION OF NURSE SARAH KEATE

This faithfulness to the original fictional character did not distinguish the movies made from Mignon Eberhart's mysteries, however—perhaps because she did not make such a good romantic heroine. In the novels, Eberhart's nurse heroine is a large, middle-aged, authoritative woman "who is stouter and crankier than she likes to admit" and who defines herself in rather stodgy terms.

> I am plain Sarah Keate, a spinster of uncertain age, unromantic tendencies, sharp eyesight, and an excellent stomach. I mention the last because it is really quite important: a good digestive apparatus and common sense walk hand in hand through life.[23]

An unsentimental, brisk woman in a starchy white uniform, she further describes herself as "a fool of an old maid," "inclined to neuralgia" and "having a white streak in my abundant reddish hair [and] lines about my eyes, which are not exactly pretty perhaps but have remarkably keen vision."[24]

Sarah defines herself primarily as a nurse, saying:

> I am not a detective, and I don't want to be a detective. Nursing is my profession. [But] there's no getting around it—there seems to have been a certain fate, a regrettable proximity, involving me and murders.[25]

Although Nurse Keate occasionally solves the murder mysteries herself, she more often just supplies clues to young, dapper detective Lance O'Leary, who makes the necessary logical deductions. In the novels, Sarah Keate is at least 15 years older than O'Leary and has no romantic interest in him at all, though she is fond of him as a friend.

Although this characterization of a redoubtable, matronly nurse-sleuth was sufficient to sell millions of novels, Hollywood felt the need for a more romantic heroine. All but one of the six films made from Mignon Eberhart novels involved Sarah in a romance, and most of them made her not only young but beautiful besides. All six films stick squarely, often unimaginatively, to Eberhart's standard whodunit formula, however, as the following brief plot synopses will demonstrate.

WHILE THE PATIENT SLEPT
(Warner Brothers, 1935)

Nurse Sarah Keate (Aline MacMahon) comes to the large gloomy home of millionaire Richard Federie (Walter Walker), who has been felled by an apoplectic stroke. Avaricious relatives and associates soon arrive, each hoping to be favorably remembered in the rich man's will. Within a few days, Federie's oldest son and his butler are murdered. The only link is that both knew that some secret was hidden in a small stone elephant Federie kept on his mantle. Sometimes endangering her own safety, Sarah vigorously pursues vital clues, which she passes on to Detective Lance O'Leary (Guy Kibble). Almost everyone is a suspect, but O'Leary soon announces that the killer is the lawyer. The elephant contained Federie's statement that the lawyer was only managing his estate for a salary, but the lawyer was planning to claim that the entire estate had been deeded over to him.

Actress Aline MacMahon plays Sarah Keate here as a youngish but very prim, austere nurse. She is intelligent, calm, brave, and compassionate; and at the end she is about to accept a marriage proposal from Lance O'Leary, here made at least 10 or 15 years older than she.[26]

THE MURDER OF DR. HARRIGAN
(Warner Brothers, 1936)

Businessman Peter Melady (Robert Strange) plans to market a new anesthetic ("Slaepan") without giving credit to the doctors who helped develop it. He comes to Melady General Hospital, which he owns, to be operated on by Dr. Harrigan (John Elderedge), one of the doctors he cheated. The nurse, here renamed Sally Keating and made young and beautiful (Kay Linaker), finds Harrigan murdered in the elevator. Melady has disappeared and is later found, also murdered. Again, almost everyone looks suspi-

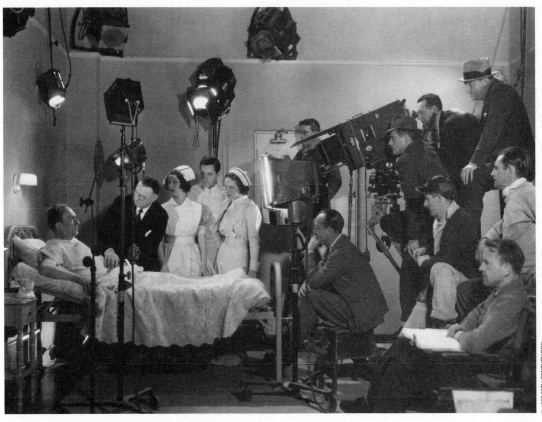

Action on the film set of The Great Hospital Mystery *(20th Century-Fox, 1937).*

© 1937 20TH CENTURY-FOX

cious to the police: Harrigan's wife, who hated him; the wife's lover; the ex-wife, who feared Harrigan would ruin her nursing career; Melady's daughter, who feared Harrigan would let her father die on the operating table. Even Sally is suspected because she brought the Slaepan formula to Melady and because she was seen sneaking Mrs. Harrigan's lover out of the hospital late one night. Sally's fiancé, intern George Lambert (Ricardo Cortez), wanting to exonerate her, pieces together enough evidence to solve the murder, though not before Sally has been attacked by the murderer (another intern who also worked on the Slaepan formula). In the last scene, Sally, fashionably dressed, announces that she has put herself into the hands of a "really *good* doctor" (George) and that she won't be returning to work.[27]

THE GREAT HOSPITAL MYSTERY
(20th Century-Fox, 1937)

Made by 20th Century-Fox instead of Warner Brothers as the others were, this is the only Eberhart film to show the nurse-sleuth as she appears in the novel—middle-aged, graying, and overweight. She is called Miss Keats here and is played by the stout, formidable Jane Darwell. The romance occurs between a young nurse, Ann Smith (Sally Blane), and a doctor (Thomas Beck) in the Samaritan Hospital. Much confusion results when Ann tries to hide her brother from murderous gangsters by asking the morgue keeper to report him dead. The morgue keeper is found murdered, as is another man, at first thought to be Ann's brother. As usual, there is much sneaking around the hospital by Miss Keats, the gangsters, and the potential victims; and the famous comedienne Joan Davis provides laughs with her slapstick rendition of Flossie, the awkward student nurse.[28]

THE PATIENT IN ROOM 18
(Warner Brothers, 1938)

Sarah Keate is once more young and beautiful (played by Ann Sheridan), and her patient at Thatcher Hospital is dapper Lance O'Leary (Patric Knowles), who has had a nervous breakdown of sorts, brought on by his failure to solve a burglary case. He lands, of course, right in the middle of another mystery. Dr. Balman (Charles Trowbridge) argues with Director Dr. Lethany (Harland Tucker) against the hospital's purchase of $100,000 worth of radium capsules for the exclusive use of Trustee Frank Warren (Edward McWade). First Warren, then Lethany, then a hospital handyman (Frank Orth) who said he witnessed the crime are all found murdered in Room 18, and the radium capsules are stolen. Again, suspects abound for one or more of the murders and the theft. Warren's nephew (John Ridgely) has just argued with him about his unpaid debts; intern Hajek (Edward Raquello) is having an affair with Lethany's wife (Jean Benedict), who tells him she'd like him better if he had more money; handyman Higgins knows from gossip how valuable the radium is; O'Leary's manservant, Bently (Eric Stanley), has a grudge against Warren, his former employer. Everyone appears in suspicious places at suspicious times, leaving clues behind. Lance O'Leary decides that the best medicine for his ailment would be to solve the mystery, which he does with Sarah's cooperation. As usual the atmosphere is made murkier by thunderstorms, an electrical blackout, and unknown assailants in the dark. O'Leary pronounces Dr. Balman the murderer, and Sarah rewards him with a long kiss.[29]

MYSTERY HOUSE
(Warner Brothers, 1938)

Banker Hubert Kingery invites the other bank officers for a weekend at his hunting lodge and then informs them that he knows one of them has been defrauding the bank through forgery and that he will reveal the name of that person later. However, before that revelation can be made, Kingery is found shot in his locked room. The death is judged suicide, but Kingery's daughter, Gwen (Anne Nagel), doesn't believe it and later invites the same party to the lodge, with the addition of detective Lance O'Leary (Dick Purcell) and her old aunt's nurse, Sarah Keate (Ann Sheridan again). Once there, they are isolated by a heavy snow storm. One bank officer's jealous wife threatens to tell "what really happened to Kingery," and she is soon found dead, another apparent suicide. Another guest admits to Gwen that he knew Kingery had proof against one of his associates; and that guest dies of a gunshot wound as he locks his bedroom door that evening, though not before leaving a note that says "the key is in my toupee." Lance O'Leary does his usual job of eliminating the false suspects (the sinister chauffeur who steals Lance's gun and knocks him out with it; the old aunt, who is not an invalid after all), and he figures out the method by which the victims were murdered alone in locked rooms. The apparently decorative guns on the walls were wired to the lock bolts so that they fired as the victims locked themselves in. Lance names the guilty associate and then settles down on the couch with Sarah to claim his "medicine"—a kiss.[30]

Despite the variety of murders in these six films featuring Sarah Keate (by whatever name), they all display a rather predictable formula of ingredients. Nearly all involved rich people, either in their gloomy mansions or as patients in private hospitals. Mignon Eberhart loved aristocrats—"thoroughbreds," as she called them—and she loved the secrets they hid. Hence, every murder investigation usually uncovers assorted adulteries and other vices along with the homicide. For all their money, the aristocrats don't have much sense, for they always seem to hide the vital piece of information or article of value in the most unsafe place. Information, formulas, jewels, radium, confessions that others would kill for are routinely hidden in vases, little stone elephants, flower pots, or toupees. Has none of these people heard of safe deposit boxes?

Nature always obliges the sense of mystery by whipping up an enormous storm, and nighttime or bad fuses provide the obligatory darkness in which Sarah can creep about in search of clues and in which she usually is mildly attacked—either by being shoved about or locked in a closet. A generous serving of comedy assures the audience that the murders are not to be considered seriously, and Sarah is usually rewarded with romance from the doctor or the detective. In the background most often is a foolish policeman who cannot solve the crime but must leave it to the amateur detectives (with or without the help of Lance O'Leary) to gather and evaluate the clues.

The image of nursing is remarkably similar in all six movies, regardless of whether Sarah is young or middle-aged, pert or austere, an independent sleuth or dependent on a man for the final deductions. Sarah (or Sally) usually looks considerably better than the minor nurse characters even though her actual nursing duties are no more impressive. On private duty, she is intelligent, compassionate, energetic, and confident. She performs her simple duties with cheerful competence and establishes good rapport with even the most difficult or crotchety patients. In the whodunits' mad atmosphere of corruption, murders, cover-ups, suspicion, and terror, Sarah is a welcome source of sanity, order, and integrity. Furthermore, she is usually the only character

developed enough for the audience to identify with at all. And since through her bravery and intelligence she gathers the information with which to either solve the mystery herself or to enable O'Leary to solve it, she is clearly meant to be a sympathetic character—in fact, the heroine.

ADVENTURES IN THE AIR

Another genre of films prevalent in the 1930s was aviation and ocean liner films. These adventure yarns routinely climaxed with characters adrift in the air or at sea and faced with the need to resolve overwhelming problems with limited resources. Since during the early days of commercial flying the airlines hired only registered nurses as stewardesses and because many sea-going vessels included a nurse among the crew, quite naturally the nurse could play an important role. Like so many other 1930s movies with nurse characters, these films portrayed the nurse as a brave, adventurous, romantic figure, a power for good and an inspiration to others.

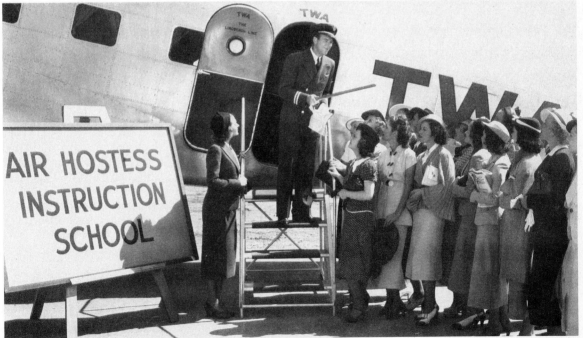

In order to make air travel appear as safe and healthful as possible, the airlines in 1930 began to hire graduate nurses to augment the regular crew of pilot and copilot.

Commercial air travel was still rather new in the 1930s, and the public was both fascinated and apprehensive, especially in the wake of a number of highly publicized crashes. In order to make air travel appear as safe and healthful as possible, the airlines in 1930 began to hire graduate nurses to augment the regular crew of pilot and copilot. Afraid that the word *nurse* might scare potential passengers away with its reminder of airsickness, the airlines instead called these women "air hostesses" or "stewardesses." Little actual nursing was needed, for even airsickness was not as common as people imagined, though it did occur in the planes' unpressurized cabins. The nurse could usually control the nausea, faintness, and/or nervousness fairly easily with an alkaline effervescent, an ammonia inhalant capsule, or a sleep-inducing amobarbital. She also carried a first aid kit for minor injuries. Primarily, however, she just kept the passengers comfortably supplied with pillows, blankets, stationery, and magazines.[31]

There were times of actual accidents when air hostesses became heroines, and some of these incidents fueled the public interest in this new and exciting field of nursing. One such case, for example, happened to Nellie Granger in April 1936. Miss Granger, who weighed only 101 pounds and stood 5 feet, 2 inches, had been a nurse-stewardess for Transcontinental and Western Air for only 6 months. When she left New York that spring morning eleven passengers were aboard her California-bound plane. The next stop was Pittsburgh. According to newspaper accounts of the events that happened, Miss Granger chatted at one time or another with all the passengers, one of whom was a woman. The flight was smooth but the sky was overcast, and just before the airplane cleared the last ridges of the Allegheny Mountains, the pilot suddenly started to "let down" through the fog. Miss Granger was sitting on her little jump seat in the rear of the plane chatting with the woman passenger, who occupied one of the last seats. Suddenly a wing of the plane sliced off a tree top. The next instant the heavy craft was cutting a wing-wide swath through a forest. At the end of 500 yards it smashed its nose against some rocks and turned over on its side. The next thing Miss Granger knew she was lying on the ground clear of the wreckage. It looked like everyone else had been killed by the terrible crash. A few wisps of smoke spiraled up from the twisted metal and a low moan issued from the jumbled mass that had been a plane.

Struggling to her feet, the nurse rushed to the wreckage and half-hauled, half-carried a large man who was dazed and injured, and the woman, whose legs were broken, some distance from the plane. By the time she had done this the wreckage had burst into flames. Administering first aid to both her charges, she covered them with blankets she had snatched from the fire and started running for help. She fought her way 4 miles through underbrush and over rocks and logs to a phone. After getting word to Pittsburgh, the little hostess, badly dazed and cut, returned with medical assistance for the two survivors. Miss Granger summed up her part in the disaster later by saying: "I just did all I could; that's all."[32]

Being a nurse-stewardess was considered a glamorous job. The number of applicants far outstripped the number of positions available. Stewardesses continued to be clearly identified as nurses for several decades until improvements in air travel (the pressurized cabins of the 1940s, for example) made the services of a nurse increasingly unnecessary. During the 1930s, at least, the air stewardess reigned as a popular film heroine and offered the public an unfailingly positive image of the nurse.

Movie reviewers occasionally praised the early air hostess films, such as *Flying Hostess* (Universal, 1936) and *Air Hostess* (Columbia, 1933), for containing situations never seen on the screen before. Nearly all the films seem to be just slightly different combinations of a few basic, recurring air hostess plot elements. There are brilliant and/or reckless pilots, almost inevitably loved by noble air hostesses. There are a variety of storms—thunder, ice, dust—to endanger the flights. There are crash landings, some of a sacrificial nature to save others. And finally there are crises that somehow disable the pilot and copilot simultaneously, leaving the plane to be brought down by the frightened but heroic hostess. These elements, stirred in with a goodly number of plugs for famous airlines and actual glimpses of planes (for the majority of people, who had never yet been in one), could be served up to the public in a variety of combinations.[33]

Without Orders (RKO Radio, 1936) is a typical nurse-stewardess film. Primarily, it is a hair-raiser, chock-full of surprises and action at every turn. The story that supports numerous cliff-hanging episodes remains true to B-movie romantic tradition. An airline owner insists that one of his most able pilots, Madison, teach the owner's cocky, devil-may-care son, Len, how to fly commercial passenger planes. Reluctantly, the pilot agrees, although his job is complicated when his student tries to steal his girlfriend, Kay, who is a stewardess for the airline company—and a registered nurse, too. Unbeknown to the pretty nurse-stewardess, the student-pilot has already had an affair with her sister and beaten her up to keep her from telling Kay about his past. The finale of the complicated story occurs when a plane full of passengers gets lost in a blizzard over the Cascade Mountains in the remote Northwest. The pilot, Len, knocks out the copilot, Madison, and jumps for safety, leaving his plane in the capable but inexperienced hands of nurse-stewardess Kay. The resultant image of the nursing profession is quite positive as Kay controls her own fears, glides the plane out of the snow-covered mountains and lands it safely.[34]

Although Kay performs no nursing or first-aid duties in the film, we recognize that the skills of a registered nurse—namely the ability to keep cool in a crisis—come in very handy in other walks of life.

The nurse-stewardess follows the radioed directions with assurance and quickness and wastes no time in pointless hysterics. Even when her plane runs out of fuel, she adopts a come-what-may attitude, doing her best to keep the plane level as it glides through the air without power. This nurse's competence and professionalism—even in fields other than nursing—are typical of many film depictions of the 1930s. The nurse characters of the 1930s frequently assumed romantic roles, yet rarely lost the respect due them as competent professionals.

HEROISM AT SEA

Only slightly less heroic were the ships' nurses in the popular sea-liner movies of the 1930s. Perhaps because the ships operated on a more leisurely schedule than the airlines, the plots of these films did not depend quite so heavily on sudden disasters or emergencies. Still, the ships' nurses had the

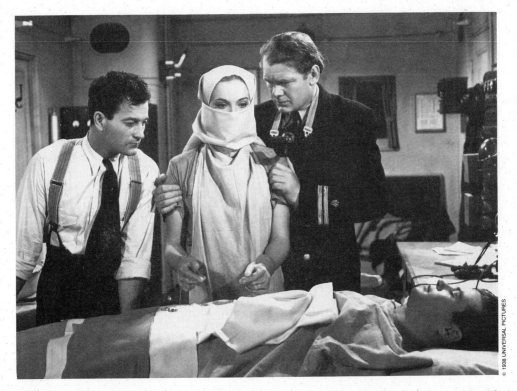

In The Storm (Universal, 1938) Nan Gray is required to perform an emergency surgery while the ship is lost at sea during a terrible storm.

chance to display the same kind of courage, resourcefulness, and romantic attractiveness that the air hostesses exhibited. Nurses often had to perform emergency surgery with only wireless instructions (*King of Alcatraz,* Paramount, 1938), assist with the birth of a baby (*Luxury Liner,* Paramount, 1933), or fight a raging cholera epidemic aboard ship (*Pacific Liner,* RKO Radio, 1939).[35]

Another example of the first act of heroism—performing emergency surgery—was seen in *The Storm* (Universal, 1938). Nan Gray played the pretty, blonde nurse, Miss Phillips, who works first on a passenger ship, where she tends to those suffering from motion sickness and hypochondria. Although clearly a bit annoyed with the passenger complaining of motion sickness before the ship is out of the harbor, the nurse maintains a cool, compassionate, and professional composure. This composure serves her in good stead when she is required to perform emergency surgery when the ship is lost at sea during a terrible storm. When the shoreside physicians in San Francisco discuss the situation after being informed via radio, the older doctor—in a remark rarely heard—tells the younger one, who is sure that no nurse is capable of performing surgery, not to place such store in the M.D. after his name. The older doctor, Striker, expresses complete confidence in the nurse's ability; and more important, the nurse herself has confidence in her ability to drain an infected appendix without instructions while the ship tosses at sea and after radio contact is broken. This film, an uninspired romantic melodrama, provides a very good example of the way 1930s directors and scenarists treated the nursing profession. The nurse remained a pretty, romantic character—the love interest in the story—but also demonstrated her ability to play an independent and courageous role in the treatment of her patients. Despite her blondeness and prettiness, the nurse appeared to be a committed and competent professional.[36]

NOTES

1. U.S. Bureau of Labor Statistics, *Handbook of Labor Statistics* (Washington D.C.: Government Printing Office, 1967).

2. *War Nurse* (Metro-Goldwyn-Mayer, 1930), B & W, 72 min.

3. *Night Nurse* (Warner Bros., 1931), B & W, 72 min.

4. Leonard Maltin, *TV Movies, 1985–86* (New York: New American Library, 1984), p. 622.

5. *The White Parade* (20th Century-Fox, 1934) B & W, 90 min.

6. Ibid.

7. Ibid.

8. *Four Girls in White* (Metro-Goldwyn-Mayer, 1939), B & W, 70 min.

9. Ibid.

10. Ibid.

11. *Vigil in the Night* (RKO Radio, 1940), B & W, 96 min.

12. Ibid.

13. Ibid.

14. Ibid.

15. Ibid.

16. *Wife, Doctor and Nurse* (20th Century-Fox, 1937), B & W, 85 min.

17. Ibid.

18. *The White Angel* (Warner Brothers, 1936), B & W, 75 min.

19. *Nurse Edith Cavell* (RKO Radio, 1939), B & W, 95 min.

20. *Miss Pinkerton* (Warner Brothers, 1932), B & W, 77 min.

21. Ibid.

22. P. Kalisch and B. Kalisch, "The Nurse-Detective in American Film," *Nursing and Health Care* 3 (March 1982):147–153.

23. Mignon G. Eberhart, *The Mystery of Hunting's End* (Garden City, New York: Doubleday, Doran & Co., 1930), p. 12.

24. Mignon G. Eberhart, *Murder by an Aristocrat* (Garden City, New York: Doubleday, Doran & Co., 1932), p. v.

25. Ibid.

26. *While the Patient Slept* (Warner Brothers, 1935), B & W, 67 min.

27. *The Murder of Dr. Harrigan* (Warner Brothers, 1936), B & W, 77 min.

28. *The Great Hospital Mystery* (20th Century-Fox, 1937), B & W, 59 min.

29. *The Patient in Room 18* (Warner Brothers, 1938), B & W, 60 min.

30. *Mystery House* (Warner Brothers, 1938), B & W, 61 min.

31. *Pittsburgh Press,* April 16, 1936.

32. Ibid.

33. *Air Hostess* (Columbia, 1933), B & W, 63 min.

34. *Without Orders* (RKO Radio, 1936), B & W, 64 min.

35. *King of Alcatraz* (Paramount, 1938), B & W, 56 min; *Luxury Liner* (Paramount, 1933), B & W, 68 min; *Pacific Liner* (RKO Radio, 1939), B & W, 76 min.

36. *The Storm* (Universal, 1938), B & W, 75 min.

CHAPTER SIX

HEROINE: WORLD WAR II

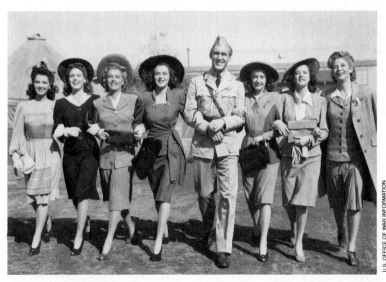

On December 7, 1941, the Japanese bombed Pearl Harbor and America mobilized for war. With the men at war, as during World War I, extensive new employment opportunities opened up to women. The lifestyles of American women were jolted considerably during World War II. As soon as it became apparent that a wartime economy could provide not only jobs for most of the unemployed men from the Depression, but also would require a large labor force to replace men in the service, women were strongly encouraged to fulfill their patriotic duty and enter male-dominated occupations.

WOMEN AT WORK

More than 16 million women, a third of the nation's working force, played a significant role in the record-breaking production of the war. Increasingly, the United States came to recognize its skilled woman-power. Women's participation in the war broke through the crust of tradition, allowing new ideas and seeds of social change to come to life. World War II largely created a new woman, somewhat different from her predecessors. Not only did this new woman tend to traditional household chores, but also she was a tool welder, a machine handler, and a factory and industrial laborer. Many people agreed with Phyllis Bottome, a distinguished British novelist, author of *Private Worlds,* who noted that there was "less and less difference in modern warfare between a man's and a woman's task." Women war workers acquired an independence that they had never known—a financial and social independence that satisfied a psychological longing. Often, while husbands, fathers, or brothers were away fighting, women became the major breadwinners and heads of households.[1]

At the beginning of the Depression the majority of nurses had been in private-duty service and therefore suffered severe unemployment as job opportunities shrank. Those who were able to find and keep jobs had low pay and long hours. The national defense and wartime periods changed the situation from one of apparently adequate supply—even surplus—to one of acute shortage. Nurses were recruited from all fields to meet the heavy needs of the armed forces, with the result that too few nurses remained to give needed care to civilians. Training programs were accelerated, and in 1943 the U.S. Cadet Nurse Corps was founded through authority of

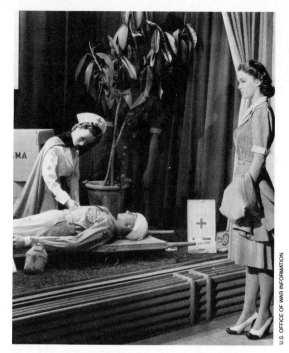

Nurses were recruited from all fields to meet the heavy needs of the armed forces, with the result that too few nurses remained to care for civilians.

U.S. OFFICE OF WAR INFORMATION

the Bolton Act. This legislation provided federal funds for the training of student nurses and for refresher and postgraduate courses. From the start of the program to its formal closing, the Corps enrolled nearly 170,000 student nurses in 1,125 of the nation's 1,300 nursing schools and graduated some 124,000.[2]

WAR FASHIONS

The styles of the 1940s were modified to accommodate the needs of a nation at war. In civilian clothing, probably the most striking aspect of the wartime silhouette was the wide, square shoulder line. Almost every garment had generous shoulder pads, not only tailored suits and coats, but even negligees, shirtwaists and blouses, cocktail dresses, and evening gowns. Women adopted mannish tailoring for suits and dresses, and the wearing of pants was more universal than in the 1930s. Slack suits and jumper suits were a favorite garb for women working in factories and on farms, driving buses, and operating elevators. Rationing of materials became necessary; woolens in particular were needed for the army. In 1942 the War Production Board issued ruling L-58, which limited the dimensions and design of garments manufactured for civilian use.

A man's double-breasted suit could not include a vest. Jackets were shortened, and vents, patch pockets, and belts were eliminated. Civilian as well as military trousers were made without cuffs. Women's dresses were reduced in yardage by some fifteen percent and were made without such extravagant items as turnover cuffs, patch pockets, balloon sleeves, matching sashes, double yokes, attached hoods, and shawls. Skirt widths were restricted to 72–80 inches, and hem and belt widths were limited to 2 inches. Some categories were exempt from these restrictions—infants' clothing, bridal gowns, maternity dresses, religious vestments, burial gowns. Throughout the war, skirts were skimpy in appearance and worn just below the knee. The tantalizing luxury of nylon hose, which had been proffered in 1939, was speedily withdrawn as nylon was channeled to parachute construction and to wardrobes of military personnel. Nylon stockings became a prized black market item, as negotiable as cigarettes in return for scarce commodities and favors. White cotton shirts and underwear for men became virtually unobtainable during these years.

Nurses in the Army Nurse Corps wore olive drab uniforms, tan shirts and scarves, brown leather bags and shoes, and olive drab visor caps. The regulation officers' overcoats were of olive drab cloth, double-breasted, worn over white uniforms, with olive drab garrison caps, white shoes, and brown wool gloves. The Army nurses' field uniform was similar to that of the Women's Army Corps. The Navy Corps nurses wore navy blue double-breasted uniforms, gilt buttons and sleeve stripes, white or navy pie caps with black ribbon headbands, white shirts, black scarves, and white skirts with white shoes or navy skirts with black shoes. Red Cross nurses wore white washable uniforms and nurses' caps; dark blue, wool, hem-length capes with dark red linings, fastened at the neck by hooks and eyes and at the chest by black frogs; and white shoes and stockings. The Red Cross nurses' aides wore French blue denim caps and jumpers, and white cotton short-sleeved shirtwaists.

Hair styles were one area where women could maintain their femininity. Most women had fairly long hair, and the flowing shoulder-length bob, which had appeared in the late 1930s, was the pre-

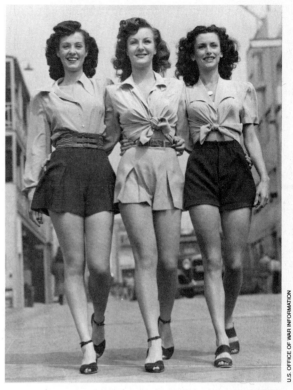

Hair styles were one area where women could maintain their femininity. Most women had fairly long hair, and the flowing shoulder-length bob, which had appeared in the late 1930s, was the prevailing mode throughout the war years.

vailing mode throughout the war years. It was worn in a variety of styles, usually softly waved and loosely curled. The pageboy bob curled under neatly in a loose roll. The hair was more often than not parted—on either side or in the middle—and combed back in a semi-pompadour to fall to the shoulders in loose curls. It might be held in place by a ribbon or band running under the hair, behind the ears, and tied on top of the head. The hair in front was frequently worn in bangs—curled, waved, or straight—or in a cluster on the forehead. A full, high pompadour effect was sometimes achieved by pushing the hair forward in a puff secured by a bow or a hair clip, or by swirling the front and side hair upward and pinning it in three or four full, spiral curls. Pinned-on bows or flower clusters were popular hair ornaments, quite often worn for daytime as well as for evening dress. When war duties required less fanciful hair treatments, the hair was pinned up on top of the head in rolls, or braided into pigtails, and the entire mop was pushed into a service or working cap. It was quite common, however, to see a Wac or a Wave with a neat service cap perched on top of a curling shoulder-length bob.

Styles in makeup called for a frankly and brightly made-up mouth, little or no rouge, and eye makeup for dress occasions. Fingernails were painted in brilliant colors, and quite often toenails were also painted. Nail polish came in such shades as Black Red, Gingerbread, Lollipop, Butterscotch, Sugar Plum, Blackberry, and Red Flannel. The advertisements said, "The lacquer-luster and color-brilliance of precious Chen Yu will turn your nails into gorgeous jewels! Choose from twenty lacquer shades— each breathtaking!"[3]

MASS MEDIA ROLE MODELS

None of the changes in women's work and fashions could have occurred without the active approval and encouragement of the principal instruments of public opinion—the mass media. Perhaps it was inevitable that, given the rash of articles, films, and books encouraging women into the war effort, Rosie the Riveter would emerge as the lauded symbol of the woman temporarily at work. On May 29, 1943, Norman Rockwell's *Saturday Evening Post* cover featuring Rosie brought the image into millions of American homes. Her ample body perched on a beam, she filled the cover with amazonian haughtiness. The image suggested a woman of middle age, competent and strong with chin held high, pausing momentarily, rivet gun in lap and goggles perched on forehead, to take a lunch break. Behind her, filling the background, was a large American flag.[4]

America entered the war in December 1941, and from then until Japan's surrender in 1945, Hollywood turned its incredible resources toward the war effort. The need for entertainment was acute, both in the armed services and on the home front. Profits came from the wartime hunger for entertainment—and from the lack of competition. Gas rationing limited the range of entertainment choices, and wartime restrictions on material eliminated competition from the nascent television industry. Meanwhile, a war-revived economy was putting dollars into the pockets of consumers—dollars that Swing-Shift Mazies and Rosie the Riveters gladly spent at the movies for a few hours' respite from their chores. Between 1941

and 1945, box-office receipts rose from $88 million to a staggering $385 million, and industry estimates claimed that 90 million people were going to the movies each week.

NURSE HEROINES ON THE SCREEN

The screen validated and encouraged nurses' military participation and civilian work. Although nursing was only one of several ways in which women could participate in the war effort, it remained the most distinctive and heroic of all possible occupations. Furthermore, the nurse characters included in films of World War II reached heights of bravery and active militancy never hinted at in the films of World War I. Several war films, many foreign-made, entered the U.S. market in the years immediately preceding U.S. entry into the war, and some featured nursing prominently. This handful did illustrate several of the conventions that would recur in later nursing-in-war films, namely the emphasis on a corps of nurses rather than individuals and the depiction of nurses suffering combat-related dangers.

For example, the Russian film, *The Girl from Leningrad* (Artkino, 1941), presented the wartime nurse as part of an organized nursing corps and as necessary to military aims. The film featured military action on the Russian-Finnish front during 1939; by the time the film reached the U.S., audiences saw it clearly as a struggle between the Russians and the Germans. The story centered on the front-line exploits of a group of nurses: Natasha (Zoya Fyodorova), Chizik (Olga Yodorina), Tamara (Maria Kapustina), Zina (Tatania Alyoshina), and Shura (Elene Melentyeva).[5]

The nurses endure the hardships of front-line conditions—worse yet, during winter—and one of their number, Natasha, is wounded when she assists a soldier in capturing an enemy post. The other nurses also take up arms when required. Although there are a few romantic interludes, the focus remains on these women as nurse-soldiers, reflective of the total war effort of the Allies in their struggle against Germany and Japan. Herein lies another significant departure from the World War I image of nursing. These nurses are shown as a cadre of women, all of whom demonstrate courage and bravery to some degree. During World War I, nurse characters appeared as individual heroines, with little relation to other nurses. In addition, the bravery and courage evinced by the Russian nurses seem to be an expected part of their role as patriotic nurses fulfilling their share of the war effort. The nurses of *The Girl from Leningrad* stand shoulder-to-shoulder with the soldiers and contribute their services in the same patriotic manner as do the men. If the nurse characters of World War II films emerged as less idealistically portrayed than counterparts in films of World War I, they also appeared to be a more integral part of the war, providing needed services rather than simple womanly tenderness.

One of the first American films to treat wartime nursing in the new conflict was *Women in War* (Republic, 1940). The film portrayed the experiences of a group of young English nurses in the Overseas Nursing Corps. It prefigured how World War II nurses would often be featured in American films: a disparate group of individuals forged into effective combat-worthy nurses in the course of their wartime experiences. The nurses undergo many ordeals, notably a bombing attack during their Channel crossing and a shelling in the French village where their hospital unit is set up. As in *The Girl from Leningrad,* these wartime nurses emerged as integral contributors to the war effort, and from them was expected a measure of courage and self-sacrifice.[6]

Atlantic Convoy (Columbia, 1942) and *Flying Tigers* (Republic, 1942) featured British nurse characters involved with Americans serving at the fringes of the war before official U.S. entry. In *Atlantic Convoy* a unit of U.S. Marines serves in Iceland, a base from which they rescue victims of German submarine warfare. On one such rescue, an English nurse (Virginia Field) and a group of children she has been escorting to America are pulled out of the sea. Most of the action centers on ferreting out the identity of a German agent who is sabotaging rescue efforts. The nurse becomes romantically involved with an American weather forecaster, who is suspected for a while of being the traitor. Again the nursing virtues emphasized in this film recall the ideals of World War I nurses—maternal love rewarded with romantic fulfillment.[7]

Another English nurse, Brooke Elliott (Ann Lee), played a maternal-romantic role in *Flying Tigers* (Republic, 1942), a story set in China before Pearl Harbor. John Wayne heads a group of American pilots working for the Chinese in the war against

Japan. Most of the plot centers on Wayne and his buddies, who risk their lives in a war that is not their own. Toward the end of the film, the U.S. declares war on Japan, and Wayne and his pilots look forward with glee to serving their own country. Brooke's primary professional duty consists of caring for children in an orphanage, but she does do some minor nursing.[8]

Universal released the 15-part serial *Don Winslow of the Navy* in 1942. Designed for juvenile audiences, the series featured Commander Don Winslow (Don Terry) of the U.S. Navy in pitched battle against the evil genius Scorpion. Based on a comic strip and successful radio serial of the same name, Don Winslow was a typical action-packed cliff-hanger. Each week, the hero was left literally at death's door—surrounded by man-eating sharks, trapped under a fallen building, engulfed in a flaming car—only to fight his way out at the beginning of the new episode. Throughout his ordeals, Don relied on his faithful buddy Lieutenant Red Pennington (Walter Sande) and to a lesser extent on two pretty young women, Misty Gaye (Anne Nagel), a secretary, and Mercedes Colby (Claire Dodd), a nurse. The presence of the two female characters served as but a nod in the direction of any girls who might be in the audience, for essentially the serial was made for boys. Without any overt signs of romance, somehow the audience was made aware that Red thought Misty to be pretty swell, and Don felt the same about

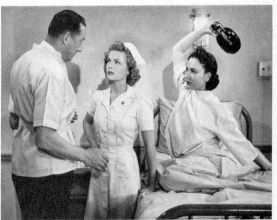

In the 15-part serial Don Winslow of the Navy *(Universal, 1942), nurse Mercedes Colby occasionally faced danger or was captured while helping out Don. Invariably she was rescued by the hero unharmed.*

Mercedes. The two male characters undertook all the initiative and suffered most of the risk. The "girls" occasionally faced danger or were captured while helping Don; invariably they were rescued by the heroes, unharmed. Once Mercedes had to nurse a captured suspected saboteur and as a result was kidnapped, to be rescued in the next episode. All in all, the "girls" were considered brave and intelligent by the two men.[9]

NURSING MOVES AHEAD IN WAR FILMS

One of the most popular films of 1942, *To the Shores of Tripoli* (20th Century-Fox), featured a nurse character in a major role and was also used in military nurse recruitment efforts. The film appealed to patriotic sentiments and served as a recruiting promotion for the Marine Corps, as the plot followed the training of a group of raw recruits and the development of esprit de corps within a headstrong young Marine.[10]

Most of the action takes place at a Marine base in the United States. Young Chris Winter (John Payne) has just enlisted in the corps to please his father. He is a devil-may-care young man, more interested in the good life than in any notions of service. The day before his enlistment begins, he has a minor run-in with Sergeant Dixie Smith (Randolph Scott), the man who will be his basic training instructor and who, because of an old friendship with Chris's father, feels responsible for making a man out of the boy. On his last night as a civilian, Chris meets a beautiful young woman in evening dress; in order to be alone with her, he tells her that her escort sent him to take his place. A little baffled at first, the young woman, Mary Carter (Maureen O'Hara) finds herself attracted to the charming, insouciant Chris, even though she suspects he may not be telling the whole truth. The evening ends in a romantic spot where Chris parks his car; a first kiss proves their mutual attraction but frightens Mary, who insists she be taken home.

The next morning, Chris reports for duty; he is the brightest, most apt man in the new platoon, but his cocky attitude spells trouble. He learns the necessary skills of basic training but refuses to accept the Marine Corps philosophy. Off duty, Chris runs into Mary Carter and discovers that she is a Navy nurse working in the dispensary. He resumes his flirtation,

but the nurse insists on being treated according to her rank as a lieutenant now that Chris is an enlisted man. The new recruit cannot believe that the Navy would commission a woman, but Sergeant Smith assures him that indeed nurses are officers. In order to get the attention he desires, Chris immediately fakes an accident. Mary assumes the management of his diagnosis and first aid. Her genuine concern for his injury quickly turns to amusing vengeance when she realizes that he is not hurt at all. To teach him a lesson, she envelops him in a mustard plaster and swaddles him in splints suspended by traction. Within hours, he is sweating, itching, and begging for release.

Back in his outfit, Chris continues to try the patience of his sergeant. Chris befriends another recruit, Johnny Dent, whose sole desire in life has been to become a fighting Marine yet whose inept-

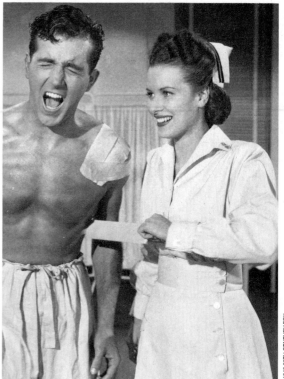

© 1942 20TH CENTURY-FOX

In To the Shores of Tripoli *(20th Century-Fox, 1942), Chris fakes an accident and Mary assumes the management of his diagnosis and first aid. Her genuine concern for his injury quickly turns to amusing vengeance when she realizes he is not hurt at all.*

ness for the job has brought on the sergeant's incessant criticism. At the end of basic training, the best of the platoon will head for training in sea duty—the coveted elite of the Marines. Chris is chosen but is incensed when he learns that Sergeant Smith has not recommended Johnny for the unit. He attacks Smith, and Mary witnesses their fist fight. Chris's expected court martial does not come about because the sergeant, out of loyalty to Chris's father, claims to have been the aggressor, and Mary confirms this story. Sergeant Dixie Smith is demoted, and the remaining members of Chris's outfit resent him for having caused the sergeant's downfall. Rather than feeling grateful to Smith, Chris is angry at being in his debt. He discharges this obligation by saving Smith's life when the former sergeant is accidentally abandoned on a target during target practice at sea. Although Chris is restored to favor among the others, his attitude toward the Marines has not changed. He intends to go through with a transfer to a desk job in Washington being arranged through the influence of a wealthy socialite who fancies herself in love with him. His attitude toward the sergeant and the corps in general has soured his chances with the nurse, Mary, and he proceeds to discard his Marine uniform for civilian clothing.

A few days after Pearl Harbor, Chris sees his unit marching toward the ship that will take them to battle. Immediately, he realizes that he does belong among the fighting men and joins them. Dixie Smith orders him out of the line, but Chris insists that his orders have not been finalized yet. His buddies close ranks around him as he tosses his civilian clothes into the crowd and dons his uniform while marching down the street. At the pier, his proud father says good-bye to him and assures him that his transfer papers will be tossed away. Aboard ship, Chris encounters Mary, who is also sailing for duty.

Mary Carter appeared to be a competent nurse. Her judgment was good enough to ascertain rather quickly that her patient was faking his injuries. However, her role in this film was to stimulate Chris Winter's moral and patriotic transformation. Whenever Mary was on screen, after the first scenes of her in evening dress, she wore a pristine nursing uniform, often with a cape, that distinguished her from other women. She contrasted especially with Helene Hunt, the thoughtless, wealthy socialite who lured Chris away from his duty with the promise of the easy life. The camera would pan from a silly Helene, arrang-

ing for someone to retrieve her errant lapdog and failing to thank the hapless savior, to a noble-looking Mary, serenely observing the spectacle. At several key moments in the film, Mary appeared in full uniform just as Chris had further damaged his chances of serving with distinction. Throughout the film, she existed as a steady beacon light, guiding Chris toward the inevitable pride he would take in being a fighting Marine. And his last-minute rejoining of his unit and the war was immediately rewarded with his return to Mary's affections.

FOCUS ON MILITARY NURSING

In 1942 Columbia Pictures produced *Parachute Nurse,* a story about a squad of trainees for the fictional National Aviation Emergency Corps—military nurses trained to parachute into remote areas to give first aid to wounded soldiers. The film opens with a group of bored civilian hospital nurses complaining about their work, which largely consists of caring for a group of hypochondriacs. A former colleague, now dressed in a military uniform, drops in to see them and explains that she is now a "paranurse." In response to this obviously exciting new field, several of the nurses declare their intention to join. Three personalities begin to emerge: Glenda White (Marguerite Chapman), a pretty, intelligent, natural leader; Dottie Morrison (Kay Harris), Glenda's cute, comical, loyal best friend; and Helen Ames (Louise Albritton), a pretty but argumentative and catty girl.[11]

Glenda, Dottie, and Helen join other nurses at the training camp, where they meet their commander, Captain Jane Morgan (played by Laurette Schimmoler, the real-life promoter of an aerial nursing corps). The nurses must endure rigorous training—calisthenics, repeated jumps from a platform to practice landing, parachute packing classes, parachute drag training with a wind machine, test drops in a parachute from a tall tower—all done to the instructors' constant litany of explanation, praise, and criticism. Between scenes of training, the nurses must learn to cooperate and live together in harmony, and romantic interests develop for some of them. Lieutenant Woods, one of the instructors, falls for Glenda, although Helen wants him for herself. Helen, who has consistently refused to get along with her fellow trainees, finally seals her fate with an act prompted by her jealousy of Glenda. She sabotages Glenda's parachute, which is to be used for a dummy drop. Woods reprimands Glenda for the careless packing, but soon everyone realizes Helen's role. Captain Morgan forces the malcontented Helen to resign. With Helen gone, the squad proceeds to its first jump.

Unfortunately, yet another member of the squad has failed to be properly assimilated into the corps. A sad-faced nurse, Gretchen Ernst, has been shunned by all but Glenda and Dottie because of her German name. Glenda watches helplessly as Gretchen makes her first jump and deliberately fails to open her parachute. Glenda's subsequent hysteria envelops her in fear and she cannot jump. Glenda decides to quit the corps and starts to pack her things, when she learns that Lieutenant Woods has crashed in an inaccessible place. Glenda begs Captain Morgan to let her replace the nurse who has volunteered to make the jump. Glenda's training comes back to her and she makes a perfect landing, only to find Woods waiting for her unharmed. His ruse to help her conquer her fear has

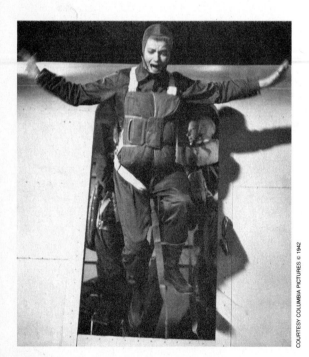

In Parachute Nurse *(Columbia, 1942), Gretchen makes her first jump and deliberately fails to open her parachute.*

been a success. The film ends with their declaration of love for each other.

The climax of this story was marked by the nurse finding romantic fulfillment through her military service, but the focus of the story remained on a group of nurses undergoing rigorous physical training to make them capable of rendering active, front-line support to the fighting men. Columbia and the cooperating Army Air Force surely intended this film to lure undecided civilian nurses into the armed forces—the early scene of bored civilian nurses may have hit home for some members of the audience. The movie emphasized the importance of nurses putting aside their individual preferences and overcoming their individual weaknesses in order to forge a strong military nursing unit. The nurses demonstrated that they were brave, compassionate, physically strong, and still feminine. The evil Helen was weeded out before she could do any real harm, and emotionally weak Gretchen took herself out of the game as well.

The film also made clear that military nurses represent the elite of the nursing profession. Captain Morgan assured Glenda that if she quit she would still be able to render valuable assistance somewhere else; but the unspoken assertion was that military nurses, and aerial nurses especially, served at the highest level possible. The portrayal of a variety of civilian nurses being forged into a courageous and competent military unit mirrored many war films of the day, which featured a squad of soldiers made up of all varieties of Americans: farmboys, ghetto roughnecks, college students, southerners, the shy and the strident—a microcosm of American diversity. Early animosities and conflicts invariably changed to strong bonds of loyalty among the men. In copying this format, *Parachute Nurse* promoted the notion that American women, just like American men, had their role to play in the war. Such "masculine" wartime traits as camaraderie, special buddies, sacrifice of self for the sake of the unit, bravery, and esprit de corps were shown as having equal applicability to women's service corps. Unlike the individual, daring, often courageous nurse characters in World War I films, nurse characters in World War II films subjected their individualism to the discipline of organized nursing corps. Instances of nurses acting with bravery occurred in the course of their nursing duties and rarely in self-determined extra missions.

COURTESY COLUMBIA PICTURES © 1942

SO PROUDLY WE HAIL

In 1943 two major motion pictures were based on the true stories of nurses at Bataan and Corregidor. These star-studded productions did much to focus attention on and increase appreciation for American military nurses. Nearly 100 American nurses were stranded with the forces on Bataan when the Japanese invasion of the Philippines began in February 1942. A handful of them managed to be evacuated before the surrender of Corregidor in May, and the stories brought home by these nurses inspired both *So Proudly We Hail* (Paramount) and *Cry Havoc!* (MGM).[12]

There is no wartime film that heralds the direct participation of women more enthusiastically than *So Proudly We Hail*. The film was voted into the Top Ten Films of the year by *Film Daily* and ranked among the year's top-grossing movies. Paramount went all out to recreate the Bataan-Corregidor tragedy, and critics cited the realism of the sets and special effects as the film's best features. The box-office success, however, depended upon its stellar cast, which included most of Paramount's leading ladies and starlets.

The film opens with a group of nurses aboard ship, heading for home. These nurses were the last evacuated from Corregidor, and one of them, Lieutenant Janet Davidson (Claudette Colbert), is practically catatonic. In order to break through her shell, the doctor asks to hear their story in hopes of finding the cause for the nurse's withdrawal. The nurses recall their first meeting aboard a ship destined for Pearl Harbor. Janet Davidson ("Davie"), the daughter

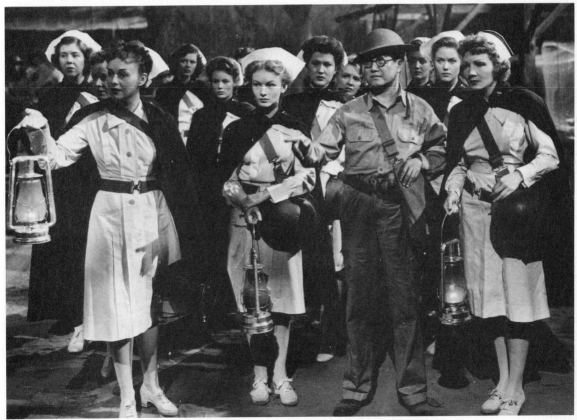

There is no wartime film that heralds the direct participation of nurses more enthusiastically than So Proudly We Hail.

of a military family and the oldest of the group, assumes the role of mother hen to the other nurses, some of whom are quite young and inexperienced. Notable among the gathered nurses are Rosemary Larson (Barbara Britton), an unsophisticated, shy girl leaving home for the first time, and Joan O'Doul (Paulette Goddard), a vivacious, pretty brunette, juggling farewells to two fiancés.

One night at sea, their ship picks up survivors of an enemy attack on another ship in the convoy. Aboard ship a temporary hospital is set up, and Janet and her nurses don their uniforms for work. One of the casualties is another nurse, Olivia D'Arcy (Veronica Lake), who is ordered to remain with Janet's group of nurses, now headed for the Philippines. Before the end of the trip, Janet becomes romantically involved with a medical technician, John Summers, and Joan finds herself strongly attracted to a former professional football player named Kansas. All the nurses get along pretty well except for Olivia, who harbors some secret hatred that makes her hard to get along with. Eventually, she breaks down and confesses that her anger stems from the death of her fiancé, shot down by the Japanese the day before their wedding. She vows to kill as many Japanese as she can.

On Bataan, Captain "Ma" McGregor, an older nurse whose bark is worse than her bite, welcomes the nurses and puts them to work at once in order to relieve other nurses who have "forgotten what the word sleep means." Unbeknown to Janet, Olivia arranges to nurse among the wounded Japanese prisoners, while Janet and Rosemary assist in surgery and Joan works in the children's ward. When Janet discovers Olivia's assignment, she rushes to the POW ward only to find Olivia sitting at her desk, unable to harm anyone. The following day the nurses change into fatigues, which they will wear throughout the remainder of the story, as laundry facilities and conditions make their whites impractical. Although the nurses submerge themselves in work, they find time to worry about their romantic interests; both Joan and Janet come to realize the depth of their feelings for Kansas and John Summers, respectively. Janet even breaks the rules and spends the night in a foxhole with John.[13]

One morning they learn that the hospital and base are to be evacuated to the jungle, and all day the nurses work to remove the patients and pack sup-

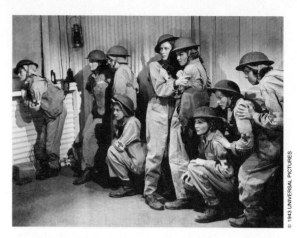

The nurses are trapped in their quarters by the Japanese and cut off from their escape vehicle with only one grenade to fend off the advancing enemy.

© 1943 UNIVERSAL PICTURES

plies. The sound of enemy gunfire accompanies them everywhere. By the day's end, only the nurses remain, but the enemy is closing in fast. Suddenly, the women are trapped in their quarters by the Japanese, cut off from their escape vehicle with only one grenade to fend off the advancing enemy. With the safety of all at stake ("I was in Nanking, I saw what happened to the women there," says one frightened nurse), Olivia steps forward and grabs the hand grenade with the words: "So long, Davie, thanks for everything . . . it's our only chance . . . it's one of us or all of us . . . good-bye." A lengthy, close shot of Olivia's face images her state of grace—the outward signs of transcendance as she prepares to die. She lets down her blonde hair and, in close-up, pulls the pin out of the grenade and inserts it in her bra before walking slowly toward the enemy soldiers. Her back to the camera, she is encircled by the sexually aroused Japanese in the moments before the detonation destroys them all.[14]

For the remaining nurses, who escape to the jungle hospital at Little Baggio, Japanese shells keep the tension high, and food and supplies run lower and lower. The nurses work themselves into exhaustion, and Joan seems especially determined to do her part without resting. Janet asks that her nurses be evacuated as they are "only going through the motions," but the commanding officer refuses, assuring Janet that the mere presence of the nurses sustains the troops' morale. An appalling air attack on the hospital paralyzes operations and prompts a decision to evacuate the nurses to the island fortress of Corregidor. Throughout the raid, Rosemary assists a surgeon with an operation, refusing to take shelter; finally, she is killed in the operating room by machine gun strafing. With the hospital buildings aflame, Janet attempts to rescue Rosemary's body only to burn her own hands in the effort. A long and dangerous evacuation to the sea is met with a lack of vessels to carry everyone across the bay to Corregidor, so Janet, with her burned hands, paddles her group of nurses into the bay to await transport.[15]

On Corregidor, thousands of men and wounded shelter in the tunnels that traverse the island; the sense of security soon palls, however, as Japanese shells batter the fortress, supplies run short, and defeat seems imminent. John Summers volunteers to join a mission to Mindanao to find quinine; Janet's protests do not shake his determination, so Janet informs Ma that she intends to marry John immediately despite Army regulations to the contrary. Ma cannot sanction the wedding officially, but arranges the impromptu affair in an empty bakery. Janet and John take their wedding gifts—peanut butter and wine—into a foxhole, where they spend the night talking before John's departure. Janet promises that she will wait for his return.

Before John's return, however, several of the nurses, including Janet and Joan, are ordered to be evacuated by submarine to Australia. Joan takes an emotional leave of Kansas, but Janet refuses to leave at all, until Ma is forced to tell her that John is presumed dead. Janet collapses and is carried aboard the evacuation vessel. Now the narrative returns to the point where the flashback began. In the final scene, the doctor pulls from his pocket a letter addressed to Janet and reads it aloud, and as the words penetrate her consciousness, Janet awakens: the letter is from John—he survived the mission. Although neither Joan nor Janet can expect to see their beloveds in the near future, the film ends on a note of hope.

Professional discipline and the sense of nursing obligations contribute to the heroic service of these nurses. Patients' welfare always outweighs the nurses' own fears; pragmatism and flexibility mark their work. When the work load becomes too heavy, the nurses discard their white uniforms for the unorthodox but practical male fatigues. The nurses set up

hospitals in the jungle and provide nursing care despite the lack of supplies and medicines. Rosemary remains in surgery despite the shelling around her; her sense of professional obligation costs her her life.

The Colbert character is used to suggest the expansion of feminine traits. Her nickname, Davie, connotes a soft boyishness, a gentle androgyny. Colbert's commanding officer, known simply as Ma, is a stern but grandmotherly presence who enforces regulations but is willing to bend the rules to allow Davie to marry John Summers just before the evacuation of Corregidor. Davie's attitudes toward her own womanhood are complex. She is the daughter of an officer now deceased, and her language is sprinkled with militarisms such as "Mind if I bunk with you?" and "Let's trench over there." When a disagreement between Joan and Olivia escalates into a fight, Davie intervenes in the tradition of all stalwart top sergeants: "Forget it and shake hands." Davie is capable of chastising her charges with a withering (and sexist) remark—"You talk like a bunch of old women"—while concurrently conveying a sense of the maternal, as when she promises to take special care of young Rosemary, whose immigrant mother's fears are thereby allayed. Davie also insists on borrowing a skirt for the brief wedding ceremony amid the bomb blasts; she clings to the vestiges of her femininity even as the American fighting forces crumble around her.[16]

Olivia's heroism benefits other women: she is an inspirational figure for her female comrades rather than for a male constituency. In the vast majority of instances in this type of drama, women are martyred or perform inspirational feats to spur the militarism of their men; in *So Proudly We Hail,* the crucial moment of self-sacrifice is by a woman for women. During the escape from Bataan, the two female leads (Goddard and Colbert) take full responsibility for their respective mates (Sonny Tufts and George Reeves). Goddard knocks out Tufts and rows him away after he decides to go down fighting, while Colbert takes the oars of another boat containing her unconscious lover. While embracing the familiar tenets of love and marriage and finally placing recuperative power in the words and spirit of the absent husband, *So Proudly We Hail* suggests seldom-seen female possibilities founded in a strength and autonomy connected to nursing.

NURSES' HEROISM IN THE PHILIPPINES COMMEMORATED AGAIN

MGM's version of the Bataan-Corregidor nursing experience, *Cry Havoc!,* did not succeed quite as spectacularly as its rival, although it too offered an all-star cast. *Cry Havoc!* offered a more introspective and less action-oriented version of the Bataan events than *So Proudly We Hail. Cry Havoc!* concerned a group of women, some nurses, most not, thrown together in the melée and disruption brought about by retreating American troops. Their varying personalities and backgrounds, not forged by strong professional and military identification, diffused the audience's perceptions and understandings of the women's nursing experiences. The film lacked the sense of movement and adventure that underlay *So Proudly We Hail.* Most events occurred in an underground dugout, and men were only seen in background sequences. In this claustrophobic environment, conflict became internalized—that is, the women concentrated on overcoming their own problems and fears.[17]

The film begins with Lieutenant Smith, or "Smitty" (Margaret Sullivan), discussing the shortage of nurses and supplies with her superior officer, Captain Marsh, or "Cap" (Fay Bainter). Cap informs Smitty that Flo (Marsha Hunt) has gone to nearby Miravelles for supplies and to pick up nine civilian women willing to work as volunteer nurses' aides in the jungle hospital. Smitty is unenthusiastic about untrained civilians but supposes that the women can do some of the menial labor, freeing the military nurses for a little rest.

The volunteers soon undergo, quite literally, a baptism of fire. Everywhere fallen trees and buildings are burning, as they carry stretchers, clean wounds, and tote buckets and supplies where they are needed. They learn that morphine is reserved only for those undergoing amputations. Weeks pass, and the women continue their work, while their hopes and fears rise and fall. One day orders arrive for the evacuation of the hospital, and the nurses and civilians are the last to depart. With the Japanese but 4 miles away, communications are cut. Soon, the shelling stops.

The nurses have been told to be ready for the trucks to take them to the sea, but back in the dugout their mood is pessimistic. Outside the women hear the sound of snipers and the rumble of tanks. Captain Marsh joins the others in the dugout but cannot answer their questions about what to expect. Suddenly, a Japanese voice demands to know who is within. Cap answers that they are eleven unarmed women. They are ordered to come out of the dugout with their arms up, and wordlessly the women comply, bravely facing imprisonment or worse.

The two nurse characters, Lieutenant Smith and Captain Marsh, stand in marked contrast to the civilian women who work as nurses' aides. Both Smitty and Cap appear disciplined, calm, and utterly in control of their emotions. Smitty, especially, demonstrates a superhuman control of herself. Not only does she work while suffering from malignant malaria, but being too proud to admit that she has secretly married against Army regulations, she keeps the knowledge of her marriage from the very people who could sympathize with her. During most of the story, Smitty is in fact abrupt and impatient with the frailties of her civilian nurses. But we understand that her icy manner stems from her rigid self-discipline—were she to relax with the women and share in their gripes or fears, she might succumb entirely to her own fears and weaknesses. Only Smitty and Cap recognize the futility of their position from the beginning; the civilians lapse in and out of hope for a rescue. Cap admits her fear to Smitty toward the end of the film, but this honest admission has never been revealed in her actions or words. For the women under her authority, Cap always maintains a calm, dignified, and patient demeanor. These two nurse characters, while sharing in the fate reserved for the other women, remain apart from them, insulated by their stronger sense of reality and their military and professional obligations.

From the beginning, the viewer realizes that the work of the civilian women cannot replace that of the professional nurses. At most, these women can take over some of the menial duties. In the course of the film, the civilian women carried stretchers, inventoried personal belongings, carried buckets and supplies, rolled bandages, operated the radio set, and offered comfort where they could to the wounded. Only Lieutenant Smith or Cap performs those nursing functions requiring specialized training. Smitty bandages the wounded and takes shrapnel out of a soldier's leg. Cap puts a cast on a fractured limb and authorizes the dispensation of morphine for an amputation. For the alert viewer, there was never confusion over who was a nurse and who was not.

NURSE WAR HEROINES IN SUPPORTING ROLES

Director John Ford, himself a former military officer, chose to make a film based on a journalist's account of America's most tragic campaign: the doomed attempt to defend the Philippines at the beginning of the war. William L. White interviewed survivors of a Navy P T boat squadron that was slowly destroyed in last-ditch attempts to impede the Japanese advance; he published these interviews in narrative form in *They Were Expendable*. The film remained very faithful to the spirit of the book, and both book and film exhibited a markedly changed tone from the gung-ho tales of Bataan and Corregidor that came out in the early months of the war. *They Were Expendable* (MGM, 1945) was about defeat and about the endurance of personal relationships in the face of disintegrating social structures. *They Were Expendable* reversed the focus of most war genre films. The conventional war film explored the bonding and fusing of individuals in support of a common goal; *They Were Expendable* chronicled the breakdown of group identity as defeat and lack of direction eroded the sense of common purpose. The heroes, fighting bravely until the end, were unable to surmount the insuperable odds against them.[18]

There is little narrative plot to the film: the action moves from the orderly, early days of the war to the chaotic improvisations that brought America to its surrender. The two main characters are Brick (Robert Montgomery), the squadron commander, and Rusty (John Wayne), a lieutenant and Brick's closest friend. It is Brick's sad duty to organize his squadron's last efforts, even though he knows that he and his men have been judged "expendable," that their fatal mission is simply to distract the Japanese as long as possible. Rusty exudes enthusiasm and actively pursues glory, but in the context of the film, this enthusiasm is pointless and more than a little sad.[19]

Almost all the main characters in the film are men, but a minor albeit important role is a young Army nurse, Sandy (Donna Reed). Sandy works in the tunnel hospital of Corregidor, where she meets Rusty during his hospitalization for a septic finger. She is a calm, professional nurse, who handles her responsibilities without complaint. All the men admire her and consider her the epitome of American womanhood. Romantic attraction flickers between Rusty and Sandy, but there is no time or opportunity for its development. Their relationship ends not on a note of hope but only of wistful wondering about what might have been. (Rusty is eventually evacuated, but Sandy is captured with the fall of Corregidor.)

Sandy serves in conditions comparable to those shown in *So Proudly We Hail*. She performs with skill in intolerable conditions, and she maintains her femininity against brutalizing events—she even manages a brief romance. Under John Ford's direction, however, this nurse and her fate become part of the cost of the war. And Sandy is not shown as a fighting nurse; her bravery and courage come in the form of emotional restraint and professional calm. Ford does not allow her any melodramatic heroics. Sandy, although totally admirable, is not used for building up morale and encouraging recruitment. In sum, the tragedy of Bataan chronicled in *So Proudly We Hail* would be vindicated by a thorough-going Allied victory; Ford's handling of the events suggests that these tragedies could never be redeemed.

Another admirable nursing image was developed in Alfred Hitchcock's problematic *Lifeboat* (20th Century-Fox, 1944), although the role and context limited the nurse's overall effectiveness. The premise of the film is very simple: a group of passengers from an American vessel sunk by a German submarine must survive in a lifeboat; their task is complicated by the presence of a German officer who manages to escape the damaged sub. The film offers no conventional patriotic sentiments; indeed it raises unsettling questions about the efficacy of cherished ideals. So troubling were the implications of the movie that the *New York Times* critic wondered if "such a picture . . . is judicious at this time."[20]

The passengers of the lifeboat include Connie Porter (Tallulah Bankhead), an effete, world-wise journalist; Gus (William Bendix), an injured seaman; Alice MacKenzie (Mary Anderson), an Army nurse; Kovak (John Hodak), a short-tempered engine room

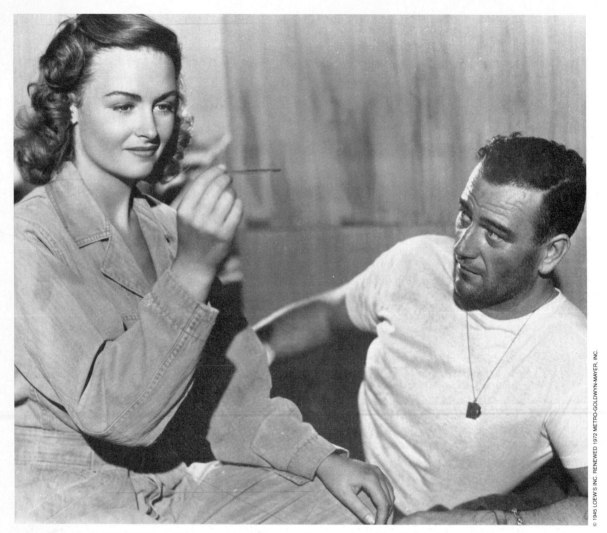

In They Were Expendable *(MGM, 1945) Sandy works in the tunnel hospital of Corregidor, where she meets Rusty during his hospitalization for a septic finger. She is a calm, professional nurse who handles her responsibilities without complaint.*

worker; Rittenhouse (Henry Hall), a millionaire businessman; Garrett (Hume Cronyn), the radio man from the ship; Mrs. Higgins (Heather Angel), a young mother whose baby died in the water; Joe (Canola Lee), the ship's black steward; and Willie (Walter Slezak), captain of the German submarine.

Kovak wants to throw the German overboard, but the rest vote to remain civilized and keep him. Gradually, the Americans grow to accept the German, especially after he performs an emergency amputation of Gus's leg. The group is disorganized, and they squabble frequently. When it becomes obvious that only the German, Willie, knows how to navigate, the others let him take charge. When they are all exhausted, Willie rows on tirelessly, singing German songs and exhorting them to cooperate to survive. Unbeknown to them, Willie has a compass and a hoarded supply of water and food for himself, and he is guiding them not toward Bermuda and safety but toward a German supply ship.

The extent of Willie's treachery becomes evident when he denies thirst-crazed Gus a drink of his water and then pushes him overboard as the others sleep. When the others find out what has happened, all but Joe turn on Willie and beat him to death. Without Willie, the passengers again begin to squabble, floating aimlessly to their doom. Connie is trying to whip them into action when a ship is suddenly sighted—the German supply ship. Again, they resign themselves—this time to visions of concentration camps. But rescue appears in the form of an American ship, which sinks the German vessel. As the group waits for the American ship to arrive, a young Nazi from the supply ship swims toward their boat. Instinctively they do the civilized thing—pull him from the water and begin to tend his wounds. When he pulls a gun on them, they quickly disarm him, and the movie ends with them all asking, "What do you do with people like that?" The answer: "You can't treat them like human beings."[21]

Lifeboat questioned the values of individualism and democracy. Discussions degenerated into pointless arguments that didn't help the survivors at all. Only the authoritarian Nazi could effect any constructive action. Yet Willie recognized no obligation beyond self-preservation. Despite their ineffectuality and their frenzied killing of Willie, the other survivors maintained the values of their civilization. At the end of the film they proffered a helping hand to another German, only to have their charity rewarded with treachery yet again. This film challenged the conventions of the American war film—namely, the assumption that Americans are not only idealistic but also brave and resourceful. If the film raised questions about the problems inherent in democracy, it did not portray the authoritarian Germans as necessarily our superiors. Perhaps none of the individual occupants of the lifeboat could compete with Willie, but together they did overcome him. For all his talents, Willie was fatally blind in one area: because he did not understand emotions beyond self-preservation, he underestimated the other occupants. His contempt for the weakness of their democratic methods led him to believe he could pursue his own ends with impunity. The squabbling representatives of democracy did unite, albeit temporarily, to avenge the killing of Gus. In all, *Lifeboat* made no absolute statements about political ideology, but it did point out the weaknesses inherent in all men and warned us to avoid the most obvious dangers.

Alice MacKenzie, the nurse character, demonstrated the best qualities found among the survivors

and, metaphorically, the best qualities of American life. She was a military officer but a pacifist at heart. Simple charity motivated her, and she, more than anyone else, initiated comfort measures and other medical necessities. She was a good nurse who, without complaint, assisted Willie (who was a surgeon before the war) with a crude amputation. Yet her goodness could not compensate for a lack of leadership, and she too allowed the German to take charge of navigation. Alice's peaceful heart did not prevent her from leading the attack on Willie—a good and peaceful person can be pushed to the limits of endurance. Significantly, she was outraged by an offense not to her national honor but to her humanitarianism. Alice reaffirmed her innate generosity when she was the first to insist on rescuing the second Nazi. She judged each German as an individual; she would probably pull yet a third German out of the sea and give him a chance, too. Of all the survivors in the lifeboat, Alice emerged as the most chari-

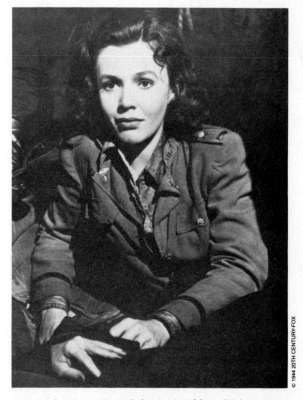

Mary Anderson as a stranded nurse in Lifeboat *(20th Century-Fox, 1944) assists a distraught mother.*

table, and it seems reasonable to assume that the strongly positive image of nurses during World War II explains why a nurse character would be chosen for this role. The nurse alone could not save the others, but she contributed more than any of them to the common welfare.

NURSING ON THE HOME FRONT

Nursing retained its distinctive and heroic allure even in stories that did not feature actual combat. Perhaps the best known of all the wartime films set at home, David O. Selznick's *Since You Went Away* (United Artists, 1944), captured how popular opinion evaluated the nursing profession. *Since You Went Away,* a long and sentimental film, chronicles daily life on the home front during the height of the war. The film unabashedly praises the sacrifices and efforts of those left behind to defend "the Unconquerable Fortress: The American Home." The center of attention is the Hilton family: Anne (Claudette Colbert), wife of Tim, who recently left to serve his country; Jane (Jennifer Jones), their older daughter, who is about 18; and Brig (Shirley Temple), an irrepressible 13-year-old. The Hilton women are devastated by Tim's absence: Anne doesn't really understand his decision to enlist, and the two girls, while very proud of their father, miss him terribly. Their comfortable, upper middle-class life also suffers. In order to economize, they must give up their faithful maid and take in a boarder, a crusty, retired Army colonel. Tony (Joseph Cotten), a handsome Naval officer and longtime family friend who is stationed in the area, stands ready to provide a masculine shoulder to lean on. Although he has long had a special regard for Anne, his sincere love of the whole Hilton family keeps his affections within the bounds of friendship. The two girls adore him, and Jane develops a painful crush on him that is only ended when she falls genuinely in love with a young soldier, Bill, the colonel's grandson.[22]

War enters the Hilton home in many ways. Aside from economizing in general, there are food rations, clothing rations, and gasoline rations to complicate their previously placid existence. They take these small problems in stride. They also handle more serious problems with courage and dignity. Not long after Tim is shipped overseas, the dreaded cablegram arrives—he is missing in action somewhere in

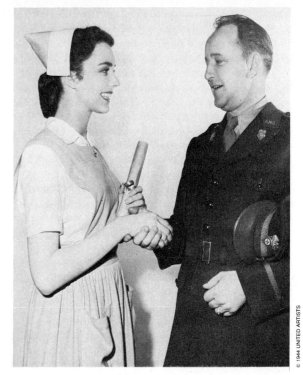

© 1944 UNITED ARTISTS

In Since You Went Away *(United Artists, 1944) Jane decides to become a nurse's aide in a local rehabilitation hospital instead of going to college as her parents expect.*

the Pacific. Anne and her daughters hold their chins high during the day, but cry themselves to sleep at night. Jane determines to become a nurse's aide in a local rehabilitation hospital rather than going to college as her parents expect. At first Anne resists Jane's plans, until she has a chance meeting with an old lady whose granddaughter was one of the nurses captured on Corregidor. Anne comes to understand that she cannot and ought not prevent her daughter from making her contribution to the war effort. Jane also becomes engaged to Bill the night before he has to leave for the front. Some weeks later another telegram arrives announcing his death in action. Again, the Hilton women close ranks and sustain each other.

The major theme of *Since You Went Away* is maturation; by the end of the story, every character has gone through some kind of trial and has been transformed by the experience. Anne, essentially a mature woman throughout the story, nevertheless finds herself capable of doing more than she ever imagined. At first she considers taking in a boarder and doing without a maid major sacrifices; by the end of the film she has become a welder. Brig loses some of her childish ways and is wearing high heels by the last scene. The crusty colonel, in perhaps the most predictable development, becomes a loving and sentimental member of his family. Even Tony is changed by the war: at the beginning of the film he views it as a great adventure; a year later, after winning the Naval Cross in combat, his devil-may-care attitude has given way to a deeper set of values. Perhaps the greatest maturation is seen in Jane. At the beginning of the war, she is pretty but basically adolescent, still given to painful crushes on older men. Her tragic love for Bill and her experiences as a nurse's aide propel her into adulthood. By the end of the story, she wears her hair pinned up and behaves with womanly restraint. She overcomes her personal loss by giving support to others; most notably, she helps a psychologically battered soldier regain his confidence.

Nursing plays an important role in facilitating Jane's transformation from girl to woman. The pride with which she wears her volunteer's uniform and recites her oath demonstrates how seriously she takes her responsibilities. Her nursing work represents her first step into the adult world, the first time she has committed herself to a role outside her family. Although her actual work is limited to menial tasks, such as passing out ice cream, transporting patients, and scrubbing bed frames, she realizes the importance of her work. When Emily Hawkins, a catty, selfish woman who hoards supplies and buys on the black market, berates Anne for letting Jane work among the riffraff of the hospital, Jane defends herself and shows the degree to which she has taken responsibility for herself and her actions. Unofficially, Jane assumes the task of helping a soldier regain his self-confidence. She provides some of the essentials of nursing, such as emotional support for a patient, and is rewarded with the patient's full recovery.

Nursing per se is a minor theme of the film, but the way Jane's role as a nurse's aide is handled emphasizes the transcendent values associated with the nursing profession. Nursing is more than patriotic service—it is also an experience that sustains even those who practice it in a modest way. After alluding to the sacrifices of those nurses on

Corregidor, the film shows how even an untrained young girl could join in the nursing effort. All the Hilton women undertake some wartime work—even Brig, who accumulates scrap materials. But among all the possible jobs being done by women, nursing still remains the most valued and admirable.

THE WAR BIRTH OF CHERRY AMES

The Cherry Ames series of adolescent novels was begun by Helen Wells in 1943 with *Cherry Ames: Student Nurse*. Written initially to inspire young women to take up nursing as a patriotic duty in World War II, the popularity of the series resulted in installments that ran until 1962. The first nine books were written by Helen Wells, then Julia Tatham assumed authorship, writing seven more. Helen Wells completed the series with nine additional titles, for a total of twenty-five. Most of these novels tend to project a positive image of nursing as an attractive, demanding, and rewarding profession. They have probably been paticularly popular, however, because each includes a gripping and often spine-chilling mystery to keep young readers captivated. The heroine of all twenty-five novels, Cherry Ames, is a young, attractive woman in her early 20s. She is an unusually sympathetic and compassionate nurse, although she can be stern with patients and other nurses if a patient's health is jeopardized. Her success with patients usually lies in her sympathetic understanding of their needs and fears. Cherry's success as a nurse also lies, however, in her strong sense of professional and moral duty, and her intelligence and quick wit.[23]

The first novel in the series, *Cherry Ames: Student Nurse,* introduces the reader to Cherry, her family, and some of her friends. More important, the book explores her decision to become a nurse and describes in an altogether positive if unrealistic way her first year as a nursing student at Spencer Hall, a hospital. Cherry meets her classmates and forms two fast friendships, one with a serious girl who wants to become an Air Force nurse (Ann Evans) and the other with a fun-loving redhead (Gwen Jones). Cherry survives her first few months as a probationer—indeed, she ranks second in her class. She makes many friends and even wins over a prospective enemy (Vivian Warren—who happens to be first in the class). She does well in the wards also, serving competently, learning how to get along with even difficult patients, and winning the devotion of a little boy whose face is almost burned away. She runs into trouble in the form of Dr. Wylie, a grouchy but highly respected surgeon, and makes friends with a friendly young intern named Dr. Jim, who likes her but is in love with Miss Baker, Cherry's first head nurse on the wards.[24]

The climax occurs when Cherry has to attend a mysterious patient of Dr. Wylie. This patient is suffering from some unknown (to Cherry) ailment, and is hidden from the rest of the hospital in what everyone else thinks is a broom closet. He is in terrible pain, and Cherry risks a reprimand to make his presence known to Dr. Jim and to recommend that his pain be relieved with an anesthetic that a hometown friend, Dr. Joe Fortune (Cherry's inspiration to enter nursing) has developed, but that the hospital is wary of using. Dr. Wylie arrives in the nick of time and approves the use of the drug; the man is saved and turns out to be a nameless but world-famous American military man, vital to the war effort (hence the secrecy over his dangerous wound).

Cherry finishes up her first year and boards the train for her hometown, Hilton. But her heart

> was in her other home, in the antiseptic-smelling corridors, in the peaceful wards ... in the cool gray stone and sterile laboratory, in the bustling clinic and the gay crowded nurses' dining room and in the hot sweet air of the operating rooms. She could not wait to see what her next years of nurse's training would bring.

The blurb below these last lines gives us some hint of what to look forward to. "Cherry has more exciting adventures in the next volume, *Cherry Ames, Senior Nurse.* Don't miss this thrilling story in which Cherry wins her cap and also solves the mystery of a stolen drug."[25]

Cherry Ames: Army Nurse, published in 1944, was the third novel in the series. In this installment, Cherry Ames, a bright, pretty, vivacious and very plucky midwesterner, has completed her training at Spencer Hospital, earned her RN, and enlisted, like many other members of her graduating class, in the Army Nurse Corps (ANC), with lieutenant's rank. The novel begins with Cherry receiving her first orders: to report for assignment, along with her old classmates, Ann Evans (the serious one), Gwen Jones (the perky redhead), and Vivian Warren (her former rival, now friend). The young officers proceed to Fort Her-

old, New Jersey, for basic training. Cherry's beau of sorts, Dr. Lex Upham, has also joined the Army and is also ordered to Ft. Herold. (The relationship between Cherry and Dr. Lex was developed in book two of the series, *Cherry Ames: Senior Nurse.* Dr. Lex has proposed to Cherry at least once before *Army Nurse* begins, and there seems to be some sort of understanding between them that they will be married, but Cherry keeps asking for more time, and their romancing never extends beyond handholding and conversation—except for Dr. Lex's obligatory proposal in the final pages of *Army Nurse.*)[26]

During basic training Cherry has great fun baiting the nurses' drill sergeant, Deake, whom she calls "lovey," and meets medical corpsman Bunce Smith, a wily, unruly, but good-hearted sprite from somewhere in rural America. Cherry has to take charge of a group of corpsmen as part of her duties in the ANC, and she and Bunce become fast friends. Her friendship with the undisciplined Bunce brings her into conflict with Captain Paul Endicott, a handsome, "regular Army" officer who serves as liaison to the military for the Spencer contingent. Endicott is a sleek, charming fellow who also turns out to be shallow and rigid. He charms Vivian Warren for a while, but Cherry, Dr. Lex, and Bunce see right through him and incur his enmity, and this precipitates the major conflicts in the novel.

Cherry takes to the military life and is happy in the ANC, but several times her humanitarian instincts clash with Army regulations, just as they had clashed with the rules and procedures at Spencer Hospital in Cherry's student days. A minor skirmish occurs between Cherry and the unbending Captain Endicott during maneuvers at Fort Herold, when Cherry is accosted by a desperate child who begs her to give first aid to her injured brother. Endicott prevents her from going, in the name of regulations, but Cherry manages to sneak off after the march to the child's rural home. She almost loses her way back to camp but fortunately runs into Bunce, who was sent out to find the missing Cherry by her frantic tentmates. It is not clear whether any punishment results from this escapade, but it foreshadows a more serious encounter with Endicott much later on, after Cherry and her friends have embarked on their first real assignment, in Panama.

While serving at the Army hospital in the Canal Zone, Cherry and Bunce discover in an abandoned house a sick old Indian who speaks an incomprehensible dialect. Cherry has a hunch that the old man is suffering from a rare form of malaria, blackwater fever, a disease for which her old friend, Dr. Joe Fortune (who has also come to Panama) has developed a miracle serum that the Army is reluctant to test. This repeats plot developments from *Cherry Ames: Student Nurse,* in which Cherry came across a famous mystery patient in need of another rare concoction of Dr. Joe's. As Student Cherry had done, Lieutenant Cherry again bends regulations for the good of a patient; rather than leaving the man in the house and reporting the case to the authorities at the U.S. Public Health Service, Cherry bravely stays by the sick Indian until the ambulance arrives. She wants to avoid the Public Health Service and force the hospital to take the patient, in the hope that the Army will finally see fit to test Dr. Joe's serum. Captain Endicott discovers this departure from regulations and convinces Dr. Wylie (Cherry's old nemesis from her student days, who has also followed her to Panama City) to put Cherry and Bunce on probation.

During the period of probation, Cherry receives her first intensive exposure to wartime nursing when several hundred injured soldiers from a torpedoed troop ship are brought into the hospital. Cherry bears up magnificently and manages to utter the book's most stirring line (to bolster a buckling Vivian Warren): "Thank God we are nurses! *Our* pity *means* something!" After several weeks of probation, Cherry learns that the information she gave the hospital regarding the old Indian has enabled the authorities to find the old man's son, who can trace the itinerary which brought the Indian to Panama City. Thus, the hospital can track down the source of the disease, which does indeed turn out to be blackwater fever, as Cherry had intuited. Vindicated, Cherry and Bunce are taken off probation. Bunce is rewarded with an assignment to the Medical Technicians' School, and Cherry is given new orders that direct her to take Dr. Joe's serum (which has, of course, proved successful) to the Pacific islands, where blackwater fever is rampant. The novel closes with Cherry being borne aloft and westward, happy in the knowledge that she has proved her mettle as an Army nurse and eager for the adventures and challenges that await her overseas. The reader is tantalized with a foretaste of these in an advertising blurb on the last pages of *Army Nurse.* "When Cherry boarded the plane for Port Janeway, she never dreamed that one of the most baffling mysteries of her career awaited her. Don't

miss *Cherry Ames, Chief Nurse,* the exciting story of Cherry's adventures as an Army nurse on an island in the Pacific."[27]

Cherry Ames, with her wholesome, all-American beauty and cheerful brightness, is a sort of idealized identification figure for the young reader. Neither beautiful nor brilliant, she is a role model for the average well-intentioned girl for whom the series was written, yet of course she represents a perfection to which the average girl could never aspire. Her small-town ordinariness allows the reader to enter into Cherry's situations, while her idealization romanticizes those situations. In the first two books of the series, Cherry enters and graduates from nursing school; in this book, the experiences of a young recruit in the Army Nurse Corps are rosily treated. *Cherry Ames: Army Nurse* deals with Cherry's first months in the ANC: her basic training, first assignment, first exposure to foreign lands, and first encounter with nursing the wounded. It gives brief expression to the natural doubts and insecurities of a young woman in Cherry's position—just as *Cherry Ames: Student Nurse* referred to Cherry's initial fears that she might not be capable of handling the challenges of nursing, while the next novel, *Chief Nurse,* takes Cherry to the war zone in the Pacific.

Army Nurse manages to settle most of Cherry's doubts about her capacity for military nursing. She is shown assuming new responsibilities in the Army. She supervises medical corpsmen and Panamanian nurses and is contrasted to people younger and weaker than herself. She is also placed in situations that demand considerable ingenuity and manages well—for example, the frightening experience with the sick old Indian in the haunted house, the depressing and discouraging period when she was placed on probation, and the draining and overwhelming exposure to multitudes of wounded men in the "Emergency" chapter. At the end of the novel, Cherry knows what we have known all along: that she will indeed make it—in fact, we can confidently predict that Cherry will *never* encounter a situation that she cannot master. Certainly the image Cherry conveys of the nurse is a highly positive one. Her hardships are mentioned but not dwelled on, and Cherry always rises above them; in addition, they are far outnumbered by her satisfactions and fun times.[28]

The novel deals in a light-hearted and reassuring way with two of the crucial problems in nursing. The first is the physical and emotional strain of the nurse's work, compounded by the frequent shortage of nurses. This matter is touched on only once, in the "Emergency" chapter, which portrays the Panamanian military hospital's response to the influx of hundreds of wounded men from a torpedoed troop ship. Even Cherry almost collapses from the strain, but she recovers enough to worry about the war-wide shortage of nurses and to make a mental plea to the girls of America to come to the aid of their country. Nothing terrible happens, and the incident ends up serving the principal purpose of allowing Cherry to prove herself to Chief Nurse Johnny Mae Cowan.

The other important nursing issue that the book raises is the conflict between a nurse's basic humanitarian impulses (which presumably lead her into nursing) and her professional discipline. In the Cherry Ames series, this conflict is a recurring theme, but one which is again and again resolved in a shallow and unconvincing way. Helen Wells always allows things to turn out in favor of Cherry's humanitarian impulses—a resolution with which the lay audience would naturally find favor. But she has it *both* ways, for in her resolutions the proper authorities (in this case, the U.S. Public Health Service) always take up the problem (in this case, the mysteriously ill Indian). In the Cherry Ames series, Cherry represents the belief that the patient's health and welfare are paramount, uncomplicated, and easily improved by applying a little intuition and common sense.

POLIO NURSES CAPTURE THE MEDIA

Meanwhile, epidemics of infantile paralysis or poliomyelitis were an annual scourge, typically appearing in the late summer and fall. The actual incidence of this disease was not high in terms of the total population. The average annual incidence during the 1930s was 7,500 cases, with a high of 16,000 cases in 1931 and a low of 2,000 cases in 1938; approximately one in ten cases was fatal. Then the number of cases soared in the 1940s from 10,000 cases in 1940 to over 40,000 cases per year in the mid-1940s. But although there were more prevalent and fatal diseases, none was more feared than polio.[29]

Polio was an elusive, faceless destroyer that medical science was all but helpless to combat. There was no prevention and no cure. It was commonly believed that the invisible virus entered the system through the respiratory tract, and consequently a variety of inoculations and nose sprays were tried without beneficial results. One such experiment permanently destroyed the sense of smell in a large group of southern school children. The safest precaution seemed to be to avoid those who might be carriers. Consequently, many people wore gauze masks whenever they stepped out of their homes during the polio season. Families who could afford to sent their children to summer camp to remove them from city crowds. Large gatherings of any kind were shunned. Public swimming pools emptied at the first hint that the infection was a community threat, and schools were closed or their openings delayed.

It was particularly distressing that polio's principal victims were children. Many children who survived were permanently paralyzed in some part of the body or condemned to metal leg braces or a wheelchair. The bulbar type of polio often led to paralysis of the circulatory and respiratory centers. For these patients, the iron lung was used—an expensive and cumbersome apparatus requiring constant professional attention. Fred Snite, a Chicago youth, achieved an unenviable fame during the 1930s by living for more than 2 years immobilized in such a mechanical cocoon.

The nurse who was to make such an impact on this disease, Elizabeth Kenny, was born in Warialda, Australia, on September 20, circa 1886. Two key events strongly influenced Elizabeth's decision to enter the Toowoomba District Hospital School of Nursing in 1906. The first happened just after the family moved north to Toowoomba, in Queensland. Elizabeth fell from a horse, fractured her wrist, and, for treatment, traveled to the home of Dr. Aeneas John McDonnell some 40 miles away and stayed there for several days. According to her autobiography, published in 1943, her acquaintance with Dr. McDonnell proved to be a pivotal event in that he "had more influence upon the subsequent course of my life than any other human being." The second decisive factor that led to her ultimate decision to become a nurse was the success of a program of physical therapy she designed for her frail younger brother, Bill. She avidly read every book she could

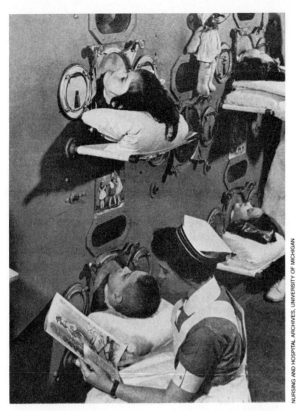

The principal victims of polio were children. The bulbar type of polio often led to paralysis of the circulatory and respiratory centers. For these patients, the iron lung was used—an expensive and cumbersome apparatus requiring constant professional attention.

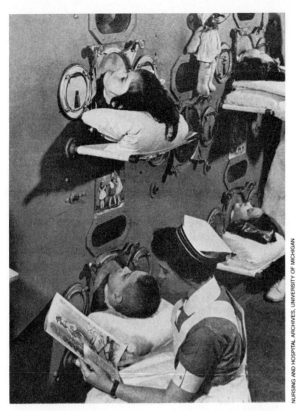NURSING AND HOSPITAL ARCHIVES, UNIVERSITY OF MICHIGAN

It was characteristic of Elizabeth Kenny's tendency to take risks and her attraction to challenge that she decided to practice nursing in the outback in Queensland. (She thought she was merely postponing a marriage, but in fact the marriage never took place.) It wasn't long before she encountered her first case of infantile paralysis, a little girl named Dorrie McIntyre. Telegraphing Dr. McDonnell for advice, she described the symptoms she observed. He replied: "Infantile paralysis. No known treatment. Do the best you can with the symptoms presenting themselves." Her first priority was to relieve the little girl's pain, which seemed to be caused by muscle spasms. Through the process of trial and error, she applied poultices of salt, then linseed meal, and finally, strips torn from a soft wool blanket, dipped in boiling water and wrung out. The child was immediately soothed and fell into a deep sleep. When she awoke, her first words were, "I want them rags that wells my legs."[32]

In the days that followed, an even more formidable problem presented itself: the child could not move her legs. Elizabeth's approach to this problem was to "re-educate" the little girl's muscles. She theorized that "incoordination" had resulted from "alienation"—in other words, that the muscles were not actually paralyzed, but that a loss of mental awareness led to the inability of the nerve impulses to convey messages to the brain to produce motion in the muscle. Using this basic approach, she treated Dorrie and five other children, totally unaware that common medical practice of the day dictated quite a different approach to therapy—complete immobilization. Yet all six patients made a total recovery.[33]

In 1913 she established a cottage hospital where she treated more victims of polio, but World War I interrupted this work. As a war nurse, she traveled to England, then to France, where she was wounded in the left leg by shrapnel; she sold her clothes at one point to help some Australian soldiers get home; and between 1915 and 1918, she made twelve round trips between Europe and Australia on ships carrying wounded men, as well as serving at land-based military hospitals. This may have been some of the hardest work of her life, dangerous as well as uncomfortable. The ships were darkened by having their portholes painted so they would not be targets of enemy attack, and they were often smitten by deadly diseases. There were large numbers of sea burials, and in October 1918, during a shipboard epidemic

procure on the muscular system, and Bill grew strong and healthy under her care.[30]

Elizabeth Kenny's leadership was evident even before she completed her basic nurse preparation program. In 1907, for example, she organized the farmers in the area, helping them to get their produce to northern markets. Thereafter, she recalled, other young people treated her as "not *nice*. A girl who knew her place looked to her male relatives to dispose of the crude details of business. It was vulgar to be healthy, ladylike to be delicate." After graduation in 1909, she was faced with several difficult choices: whether to become a bush nurse or to choose the easier life of a hospital nurse, and whether to give up nursing to marry her fiancé, since nurses were not allowed to marry.[31]

of Spanish influenza, she was one of only two nurses left to care for 500 sick and wounded soldiers. It was during the war that she attained the British and Australian supervisory nurse title, sister, which she retained for the rest of her career. When she returned from the war to work in a hospital, physicians diagnosed her as having a serious heart condition and gave her only a few months to live. Despite this grim prognosis, she regained her strength and continued her pioneering work.

After the war, Elizabeth Kenny played an important role in providing essential health care in remote areas and delightedly witnessed the development of emergency radio and ambulance plane service for the bush. One of her achievements during these years was to patent a stretcher that she described as "a rigid cot supplied with appliances for the treatment of shock while on the way to the hospital." It was characterized as having "little feet to keep patients lying on the ground up out of the mud." This invention certainly underlines Elizabeth Kenny's unusually creative ability. More important, the royalties from the stretcher patent provided the necessary resources to allow her to provide free medical care to crippled children in a clinic she opened in Townsville. Beginning with 17 patients, she was later allowed to set up a government clinic with 60. It was then, in 1933, that she met fierce opposition from the medical establishment.[34]

The common medical approach to the treatment of infantile paralysis was immobilization of affected body parts with splints and braces. Elizabeth Kenny considered immobilization, massage, and particularly abduction (separation of the legs) disastrous forms of treatment, responsible in part for deformities and loss of function. Even when it became apparent that Kenny was having considerable success in treating patients who were the victims of both polio and the ineffective conventional treatment methods, physicians turned a deaf ear to her, convinced that she was unqualified and unscientific. They especially objected to her personal terminology for the disease, including "spasm," "incoordination," "re-education," and "alienation," because it did not fit in with the concept of the disease as they understood it.

The report of the Royal Commission on the Investigation of Infantile Paralysis, issued in 1934, for example, stated that, "Her abandonment of immobilization is a grievous error and fraught with great danger. . . . " The chairman of the Commission exem-

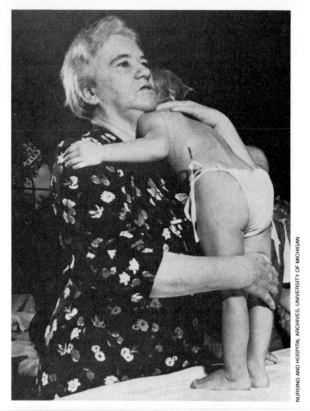

The common medical approach to the treatment of infantile paralysis was immobilization of affected body parts with splints and braces. Elizabeth Kenny considered immobilization, massage, and particularly abduction (separation of the legs) disastrous forms of treatment, responsible in part for deformities and loss of function.

plified this attitude when he explained, "Doctors are not going to be taught by a nurse." One adversary, Dr. Raphael Cilento, stooped to tactics more unscrupulous than mere ridicule, misrepresenting Miss Kenny to the press and falsifying information. He actually stole the only two existing manuscripts of her first book, but her persistent efforts to secure the return of a manuscript were rewarded by its publication in 1937. Such opponents made Elizabeth Kenny wait years for the opportunity to try her method of treatment in the acute stage of the disease, an experiment that might have provided objective evidence of its value much earlier.[35]

The weaknesses of Kenny's theoretical explanation and the physicians' need for corroboration in terms they could understand led to an impasse, and Kenny finally left Australia and the unproductive struggle of trying to reconcile two diametrically opposed forms of treatment. She did not claim to have a cure for infantile paralysis, but she did indeed have the ability to ameliorate the condition of most patients. Evidence of her growing worldwide reputation came when the desperate parents of sick children in London, Paris, and Warsaw gave her a warm welcome, and when she was invited to Buckingham Palace in June 1937.

Meanwhile, in the United States, the fact that a popular President, Franklin D. Roosevelt, was himself a polio victim occasioned public interest in and support of poliomyelitis research. The main agency for support was the National Foundation for Infantile Paralysis. This organization had grown out of a small fund-raising group that had been organized as the President's Birthday Ball Commission in 1934, the year after Roosevelt had taken office as President. The Commission was a successful enterprise, but in 1938 was phased out and replaced by the National Foundation, headed by Basil O'Connor, who had been one of Roosevelt's former law partners before he had suffered a devastating attack of paralytic poliomyelitis. O'Connor was a man of enormous energy, drive, and purpose. He succeeded to an unprecedented degree in raising huge sums of money from a willing public to support research on poliomyelitis and to provide care for all the unfortunate persons who developed the disease.

Among the supporters of the National Foundation as well as the League for Crippled Children was the popular American actress, Rosalind Russell. In 1940 she met Sister Kenny, who had just had her treatment endorsed by the National Foundation, yet who was still under attack by organized medicine in both the United States and Australia. Rosalind Russell passionately wanted to help Elizabeth Kenny in her cause by seeing that a Hollywood studio made a film biography of the nurse and her lifelong crusade. In addition, Ms. Russell fervently desired to play the role of the nurse in such a film and so began a campaign of selling the idea to Hollywood producers.

At first none of the studios were interested, but Ms. Russell was not deterred. She was solidly behind Nurse Kenny, whom she once described as looking like "an M4 tank, but her eyes were the loneliest and loveliest I've ever looked into," and wanted desperately to aid the nurse's cause. Finally, the actress told RKO studio head Charles Koerner that she would approve no other scripts until he gave serious consideration to a Kenny film. In 1945 Koerner agreed to send screenwriters Dudley Nichols and Mary McCarthy to Minneapolis, where Sister Kenny had found strong support from physicians and nurses at the University of Minnesota. A script was developed which drew heavily from Kenny's recently published 1943 autobiography, *And They Shall Walk.*[36]

SISTER KENNY REACHES THE SCREEN

Through her portrayal of this iconoclastic, richly gifted, courageous human being, Rosalind Russell imbued Sister Kenny with a stunning reality that eloquently testified to the heroine's greatness—not only in combating a dreaded disease but also in confronting the medical establishment opposed to her concepts. As the film vividly emphasizes, despite the scientific proof that the patients she nursed to recovery were living, healthy evidence of the efficacy of "The Kenny Method," the medical community was not impressed. Far from hailing Kenny's discoveries and investigating them with open minds, established orthopedic authorities waged a fierce campaign against her concepts. Fundamental to the physicians' suspicion was an inability to credit such innovative work to a nurse. Elizabeth Kenny's nursehood constituted her biggest stumbling block: not only did the specialists refuse to take her method seriously, but they generally took it as a personal affront to their profession that a nurse should so dare to challenge medical tradition. Her action was, in the eyes of many of them, a direct flouting of her nursing oath, in which she had sworn always to serve the physician.

One of the film's screenwriters, Mary McCarthy, clarified this problem in a promotional speech at a Hollywood luncheon:

> Sister Kenny didn't merely discover a new *treatment* for infantile paralysis, she scooped the entire medical profession by giving the world an entirely new concept of the disease. Her fight with the world—for the world's sake—would have been much easier if she had merely suggested a new treatment for this disease, but when she presented to the medical world the statement—now completely proven—that they had hitherto been treating a disease which didn't even exist—then the battle royal began.[37]

This adverse reaction is captured in the script of *Sister Kenny* by the character of the arrogant Dr. Brack in his relations with Elizabeth. So long as Brack's professional position is unthreatened when he meets this nurse, everything goes well. The charm disappears, however, as soon as he is expected to believe that Kenny has brought six children through polio without death or deformity by using her own kind of treatment.

Kenny's outrageously unconventional approach to treating infantile paralysis confounds Brack more because it comes from a "mere nurse" than because of its innovative nature. "Has she some degrees I don't know about?" he cynically demands. Elizabeth's friend, Dr. McDonnell, sees a tragic paradox: if Elizabeth Kenny had been a physician "she'd have used the orthodox treatments; she wouldn't have done the things she did; she wouldn't have dared!" Brack still insists that Kenny "stick to nursing and not meddle in orthopedic medicine." In Brack's view, Kenny's lack of medical qualifications discounts her opinions and her achievements. Nothing she says has any relationship to established orthopedic procedures recorded in his extensive library, so she can safely be jettisoned as a quack.[38]

The most dramatic encounter between the two antagonists, each representing his or her respective profession, occurs in a medical lecture hall.

Brack: Speak freely. Explain your theory.

Kenny: Well, Dr. Brack considers that one muscle is paralyzed and the opposing muscle is healthy. I say the opposing muscle is sick. In spa—. Well, call it a muscle condition. Now the first thing to do when you find a muscle condition like that is to apply moist heat.... The first thing to do is to keep the muscle relaxed. You put on splints, you only make the spa—, I mean, the muscle condition worse.

Brack: Yes, that would be quite reasonable if your concept were correct. Come to the convalescent stage.

Kenny: Well, after the spasm is . . .

Brack: . . . spasm!

Kenny: Yes, spasm! After the spasm is relieved, you find the muscles look perfectly normal, but they're not! They are alienated, incoordinated, and they need re-education!

Brack: There is no such thing as spasm in infantile paralysis! Incoordination! Re-education! Alienation! You'll find these words in the divorce court, not in medical science! . . . They're gibberish! You invented them!

Kenny: Yes, for a new concept! New ideas need new words.... I don't have a chance to show what I could do if I started in where you do—in the acute stage. Twenty years ago in the bush I had that chance. I had six acute cases, and they all recovered, and ever since then, over and over, I've heard the same thing, whenever a patient showed improvement, he didn't have polio!

Brack: We will never abandon immobilization! In my opinion the patient should be encased in plaster.

Kenny: To me that's terrifying.

Brack: I can show you patients whose bodies are perfectly straight as a result of using plaster.

Kenny: Yes, straight and rigid! There are thousands lying out in the graveyard that have just as much chance of recovering the use of their legs! . . . You can keep me from treating the acute cases, Dr. Brack, but not from . . . the ones you've given up. Oh . . . if you need any more braces, steel corsets or other instruments of medieval torture, I can send them to you. I've taken plenty off your patients.

Brack: . . . To become a nurse, you took an oath. Do you remember the last paragraph?

Kenny: With loyalty will I endeavor to aid the physician in his work.

Brack: Instead of aiding physicians, you have the arrogance to try to teach them their profession. In the opinion of many doctors, you are no longer a nurse.

Kenny: You can't dispose of me that way, Dr. Brack. I've given up too much for the right to wear a nurse's uniform.[39]

As this stirring scene emphasizes, Nurse Kenny challenged the highest medical authorities in the orthopedic medical field, but her challenge was always undertaken in the spirit of personal humility. When accused of intellectual arrogance and contradicting medical opinion, Kenny assured her detractors that she had nothing to say against those who held views opposite to her own. She merely wished to be allowed to describe what she had seen and done and why. Kenny was not daunted by the personal agonies or professional haggling through which she had to suffer in order to pursue her goal.

The film *Sister Kenny* celebrates the life of a very remarkable nurse who fought medical authorities throughout the world for several decades for the right to treat patients the way she found best and for the right to make her contribution to health science. The image it presents is, accordingly, largely informed by the achievements of its heroine. It makes telling statements about the physician-nurse relationship that have a more general application than the immediate context of its historical background. Elizabeth Kenny's story can in many ways be interpreted as that of every nurse who has struggled for professional credibility in a world where the physician has been considered the supreme authority.

It is fitting that this chapter should end with the story of Elizabeth Kenny, whose beauty certainly did lie in her dedication and whose attraction for an audience lay well outside a conventionally romantic context. Her contribution to health care and to the image of nursing in many ways typifies all that is best about the nursing image portrayed during the early-1940s, when the spirit engendered on Corregidor inspired so many women to unequalled acts of selflessness and bravery. While romantic conventions held sway with undiminished tenacity and the vast majority of mass media nurses got themselves involved in love affairs of some sort, the sheer heroism of the war nurses—however idealistically they were presented—cannot but demand our respect—and even awe. That nurses like those in *Cry Havoc!* and *So Proudly We Hail* have created such stirring and enduring screen images testifies to the power both of their own personalities and the filmmakers' art.

NOTES

1. *The New York Times,* May 8, 1942.

2. Beatrice J. Kalisch and Philip A. Kalisch, "The U.S. Cadet Nurse Corps and World War II," *American Journal of Nursing* LXXVI (February 1976):240–242.

3. *The New York Times,* October 6, 1943.

4. Norman Rockwell, "Cover Illustration," *Saturday Evening Post* 215 (May 29, 1943), cover.

5. *The Girl From Leningrad* (Russia; Artkino, 1941), B & W, 89 min.

6. *Women in War* (Republic, 1940), B & W, 71 min.

7. *Atlantic Convoy* (Columbia, 1942), B & W, 66 min.

8. *Flying Tigers* (Republic, 1942), B & W, 102 min.

9. *Don Winslow of the Navy* (Universal, 1942, 15-part serial), B & W, 240 min.

10. *To the Shores of Tripoli* (20th Century-Fox, 1942), B & W, 86 min.

11. *Parachute Nurse* (Columbia, 1942), B & W, 65 min.

12. *So Proudly We Hail* (Paramount, 1943), B & W, 65 min.

13. Ibid.

14. Ibid.

15. Ibid.

16. Ibid.

17. *Cry Havoc!* (Metro-Goldwyn-Mayer, 1943), B & W, 97 min.

18. *They Were Expendable* (Metro-Goldwyn-Mayer, 1945), B & W, 135 min.

19. Ibid.

20. *The New York Times,* January 13, 1944.

21. *Lifeboat* (20th Century-Fox, 1944), B & W, 96 min.

22. *Since You Went Away* (United Artists, 1944), B & W, 172 min.

23. Helen Wells, *Cherry Ames: Student Nurse* (New York: Grosset and Dunlap, 1943).

24. Ibid.

25. Ibid., p. 212.

26. Helen Wells, *Cherry Ames: Army Nurse* (New York: Grosset and Dunlap, 1944).

27. Ibid., p. 213.

28. Ibid.

29. J. R. Paul, *A History of Poliomyelitis* (New Haven: Yale University Press, 1971).

30. V. Cohn, *Sister Kenny: The Woman Who Challenged the Doctors* (Minneapolis: University of Minnesota Press, 1975), pp. 19–30.

31. E. Kenny, *And They Shall Walk: The Life Story of Sister Elizabeth Kenny* (New York: Dodd, Mead & Co., 1943).

32. Ibid., p. 11.

33. Ibid., p. 23.

34. Ibid., p. 39.

35. H. J. Levine, *I Knew Sister Kenny: A Story of a Great Lady and Little People* (Boston: Christopher Publishing House, 1954), pp. 2–4.

36. R. Russell, *Life Is a Banquet* (New York: Random House, 1977), p. 143.

37. Kenny, op cit., (3rd appendix), p. 279.

38. *Sister Kenny* (RKO, 1946), B & W, 116 min.

39. D. Nichols, A. Knox, and M. McCarthy, *Sister Kenny: A Screen Play* (Los Angeles: RKO Radio Pictures, Inc., 1945), pp. 61–64.

CHAPTER SEVEN

WIFE AND MOTHER: POSTWAR TO 1965

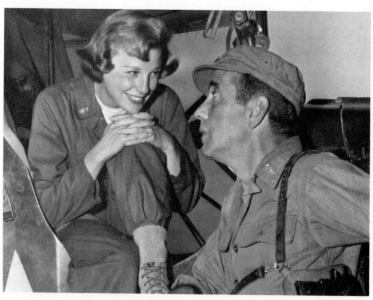

When World War II was finally over, Americans could relax and think about the good life once more after several years of austerity. A swift economic expansion began after World War II and continued throughout the 1950s. Wartime rationing and scarcities faded into memory as the Office of Price Administration restrictions on most items were lifted by the end of 1946. Factories converted from wartime production and began to produce items for the home and for individual consumption. It was again possible to purchase nylon hose, to get a pair of shoes without counting out ration stamps, to find men's white shirts on the counters, and to buy a man's suit with trouser cuffs and a vest. Streamlined household appliances were once more on the market. Laundry was easier than ever before with automatic washing machines and electric clothes dryers. In the kitchen,

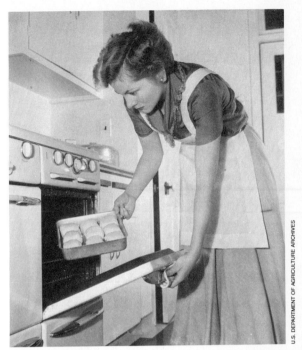

In the kitchen, time and energy could be saved with garbage disposals, freezers, dishwashers, mixers and blenders, pop-up toasters, and grills.

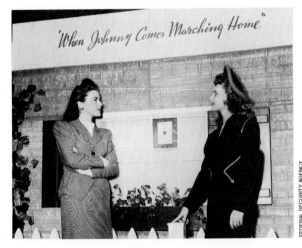

When World War II was finally over, Americans could relax and think about the good life after several years of austerity.

time and energy could be saved with electric garbage disposal units, improved stoves and refrigerators, freezers, electric dishwashers, mixers and blenders, pop-up toasters, and grills. Shortcuts to cooking were provided by frozen foods, packaged mixes, and instant coffee. Mass production, which made items of everyday living readily available at reasonable prices, also had the drawback of making every home look very much like its neighbor; and a man's suit or a woman's dress was a replica of those worn by thousands of others across the country.

SUBURBAN GROWTH

Following the war, there was a mass exodus from the cities to the suburbs, and one third of the nation's population became commuters. Large outlying shopping centers grew up to serve the suburban communities, and many cities found their downtown business districts deserted. Between 1950 and 1960, the suburbs grew five times faster than urban areas; the number of people in these areas increased from 24 percent to 35 percent of the population. Suburban houses were designed with more open spaces, often with no wall between the kitchen and the living room. Entire exterior walls were made of glass, in effect bringing the outdoors into the house. Public taste turned toward the sprawling single-story, ranch-style home or the split-level house, which combined half-stories in interesting arrangements; for example, the living room might be a few steps lower than the kitchen-dining area, with the bedrooms or recreation rooms a half-level up or down. People moved to the suburbs for their children's sake; for the grass, the air, and the space; and for prestige. Status, which became a popular sociological password in the 1950s, applied to every aspect of suburban life, from the name and location of the community, to the kind of car or cars one owned and the kind of liquor one drank.

With the migration to the suburbs came the phenomenon that David Reisman called, in his book of the same name, the "lonely crowd." He described a new breed of "outer directed" Americans, people who were primarily concerned with getting along together agreeably. They no longer consulted their inner voices for motivation or guiding principles. The new man was not an upstager or a boat rocker. He believed in team effort and pulling together and looked for his center in his "peer group." The suburbs produced coffee klatches, PTAs, Leagues of Women Voters, and Little League organizations, in all of which people cooperated with each other. Children were suddenly an organizing and socializing force. Parents' schedules revolved around dancing, skating, swimming, tennis, baton, and piano lessons. Parents met each other through their children's activities and got to know each other through their children's problems and development.[1]

To ambitious junior executives hanging their hats in Levittown and casting covetous eyes on Westchester, the right spouse was as important as a hearty chuckle and a sincere necktie. Corporations set up training programs to show company wives what they should and should not do, and *Fortune* found in interviews that the wives, especially the young ones, approved of the idea. They felt that women should become gregarious if they were shy and, if they were smarter than men, learn to hold their tongues. Several movies of the time dramatized their situation, among them *Executive Suite* and *Woman's World.* The theme in each was a corporation's search for the right man to fill a big job and how a wise mate could help her man by wearing the right dress, hiring the right interior decorator, choosing the right friends, and serving the boss his favorite menu when he came to dinner.

WOMEN IN POSTWAR AMERICA

Nothing about the late 1940s, the decade of the 1950s, and the early 1960s was more paradoxical than the role women played in it. After sharing the camaraderie of the fighting services and the hard-

ships of the war on equal terms, surely women would not go meekly back home to function solely as wives and mothers? But they did, with a fervor that would have amazed the feminists of their grandmothers' generation. During the war, the massive influx of women into the marketplace had dramatically accelerated the twentieth-century movement toward equality for American women—both in the home and in society. Women's proficiency in war jobs challenged work stereotypes, encouraging a re-evaluation of men's and women's roles in private institutions such as the home and family, as well as in the more public areas of industry, business, and government. When rearmament and the war provided new jobs for women, American society had ample reason to adjust to working women; yet a consensus had by no means been reached on the proper place of women in American society, for the postwar years witnessed renewed debate over women's roles.

When V–J Day arrived and the soldiers came home, women's independent wartime roles changed. War traditionalism was in vogue, and the patriarchal past took on a romantic hue. The deprivation of the war years made close family life attractive; women eagerly responded to the returning soldiers' desire to recreate a secure environment in the family. Ultimately, millions of women were fired from their jobs to be replaced by the returning veterans, even though many of the women had earlier expressed a desire to continue working after the war. In the two years following the termination of hostilities, the number of females in the labor force declined by about 2 million, or from 37 percent of all women in 1945 to 32 percent in 1950.

The typical age at which U.S. women married dropped from 22 to 20 and into the teens. High school marriages became an accepted practice. Children began going steady in junior high school. Girls began thinking about their weddings then or even earlier. Some social scientists and aging suffragettes worried about women's reckless haste to abandon their hard-won independence, but their voices were muffled. Unless she was a college graduate or a member of the League of Women Voters, the "ideal" woman's interest in public affairs was nil. She took pride in belonging to "the uncommitted generation." She and her husband seldom scanned a newspaper. All she expected of him was that he hold a steady job, and, as a child of the Depression, that was what he expected of himself. The name of the game was security. Both men and women believed that a woman's most important goal was to operate a home efficiently and economically. Most men thought American women spoiled. Most women thought American men didn't spend enough time with their children. *Look* magazine put out this breathtaking testimonial to the great American mother in 1956.

> The wondrous creature marries younger than ever, bears more babies and looks and acts far more feminine than the 'emancipated' girl of the Twenties or Thirties. If she makes an old-fashioned choice and lovingly tends a garden and a bumper crop of children, she rates louder Hosannas than ever before.[2]

For married women, opportunity meant *not* working in the marketplace. Since the family was credited with being the most important institution in a democratic society, women's caretaking functions were seen to demand their full attention, offering a pleasurable and important role to the wife and mother, as well as a benefit to the husband-father and an

investment to society. In the early years after the war, the baby boom carried almost all women before it. The vogue for large families—for third, fourth, even fifth and sixth babies—spread. Not since before 1914 had such large families been typical.

By the late 1950s the U.S. birth rate was approaching India's. The number of U.S. mothers who had given birth to three or more children had doubled in 20 years. The increase was most spectacular among college women; they were abandoning careers to bear four, five, and six or more children. The percentage of females in the American college population (35 percent) was lower than that in any European country and lower than the prewar figure on U.S. campuses (40 percent). Nearly two-thirds of matriculating girls dropped out before college graduation, while more than half the men stayed. Many coeds left the classroom to take menial jobs, supporting their male partners, who remained on campus; this was called the degree of "Ph.T." (Putting Husband Through). Other women quit because they had not acquired spouses. Deans' offices found that coeds were leaving at the end of the first or second year because they had found the pickings slim and wanted to try their luck elsewhere.

THE "NEW LOOK" IN WOMEN'S FASHIONS

Reinforcing the regressed role of women were the new fashions of the day. According to fashion publicists, after two decades of the "American Look," marked by slim hips, casual appearance, and short skirts, Paris couturier Christian Dior brought onto the stage what he called the "New Look"—the long skirted, hourglass fashion. By the early 1950s, these fashions reached their height in the "baby doll" look, which was characterized by a cinched-in waist, a full bosom, and long bouffant skirts. Not since the Victorian era had women's fashions been so confining.

The new styles depended on firm undergirding. Of primary importance was the waist-cincher, a tiny girdle that took inches off the waistline. Hips were frequently padded, and for the full-skirted models a bouffant petticoat was also essential. Skirts descended dramatically in 1947 from their wartime length at just below the knee to a hemline at midcalf or just above the ankles. Some skirts were very slim while others were extravagantly wide. Heels were high and slender.

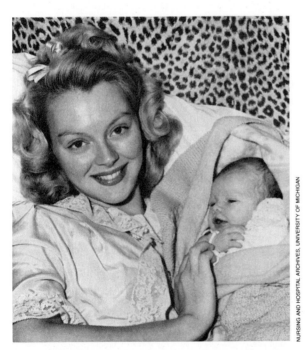

NURSING AND HOSPITAL ARCHIVES, UNIVERSITY OF MICHIGAN

The post World War II baby boom carried almost all women before it. The vogue for large families—for third, fourth, even fifth and sixth babies— spread. Not since before 1914 had such large families been typical.

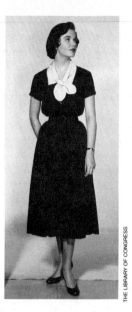

THE LIBRARY OF CONGRESS

By the early 1950s "New Look" fashions reached their height in the "baby doll" look, which was characterized by a cinched-in waist, a full bosom, and long bouffant skirts.

The shoulder-length bob of the war years gave way to a shorter cut in 1947. The preferred look in the postwar period was a neatly curled cap of hair, styled close to the head. The "poodle cut" was an all-over cap of short ringlets. The Italian, or feather, cut was longer, about 4 inches in length, and styled in loose curls often brought forward around the face. A pompadour style with wide marcel waves was popular. Soft bangs or curls on the forehead were frequently worn. Some women kept their long hair but styled it in neat rolls on the neck or in a chignon or French roll on the back of the head. Teenagers were fond of the pony tail, in which the longer hair was swept back into a single lock or flowing mane. It was held rather high on the back of the head with a rubber band or tied with a scarf and left to cascade down the back. Another short, feathered hair style featured the ducktail in back, for girls as well as boys. About 1956 a trend toward built-up and built-out hair styles started. Heads began to look larger as new bouffant and bubble coiffures appeared.

Makeup was concentrated on the eyes and lips during this era. Little rouge was worn, but eye shadow and eye liner were much used. There was a vogue for "doe eyes," a bold line drawn above the upper lashes, extended outward and curved upward to give the eyes an exotic, slightly startled look. Colors in lipstick and nail polish were softer after the hard brilliance of the wartime shades.

Metrecal, a liquid diet drink, made its appearance and found an eager mass market. So did a new Clairol slogan: "If I have only one life, let me live it as a blonde."[3] Since 1939 the average woman had shrunk three or four sizes. Instead of shopping for a dress her size, she now found one she liked and then dieted to fit into it. The bust, bosom, or cleavage became the apotheosis of erotic attention. Never, in this century at least, had so much respect been paid to mammary development. It was as though men, American men particularly, underwent a wave of nostalgia for maternal breast memories. Brassieres upholstered with foam rubber were produced as beauty aids even for the well-endowed and even for prepubescent girls. Whole careers were built on breasts. Jayne Mansfield's were insured for a million dollars.

The most important film representative of the 1950s voluptuous woman was Marilyn Monroe, who differed from the others by combining sensuality with strains of childishness reminiscent of the adolescent stars. She thereby created a powerful combination that encompassed the era. Monroe's popularity ensured the triumph of the vogue of dyed blonde hair that cosmetics companies had been promoting. Sales of hair coloring soared; platinum blondes seemed everywhere. The widespread dyeing of hair to be light blonde indicated women's acceptance of a model of looks and behavior that made them feminine, sensual, and unintellectual. Women were to seem like children, expressing their adulthood primarily through their sexuality. The "dumb blonde" who had "more fun" and whom "gentlemen preferred" now became the dominant image of beauty for American women.[4]

NURSES IN THE FEMALE WORK FORCE

In 1950 almost three quarters of all employed women fell into twenty occupational categories, of which the largest were stenographers, secretaries, teachers, and nurses. The great majority of women were employed in occupations in which they predominated. This sexual division of labor was clearly evident in the professions, even though women were only a small proportion of total professional workers. Two-thirds of all professional women were either nurses or teachers; and even in teaching there was a division between the sexes: most women taught in the primary grades, most men taught in high school. Women were notoriously underrepresented in the professions of law, medicine, engineering, and scientific research. No more than 7 percent of all professional women in 1950 were in these four categories combined. Only 6 percent of American doctors were women. In England the figure was 16 percent, and in the Soviet Union almost three-quarters of all doctors were women.

In contrast to the post-World War I era, nursing remained a high-status occupation for women after World War II. The April 1948 issue of the *Personnel and Guidance Journal* reported a study that determined the social status of 29 women's occupations. Responses to questionnaires asking what occupation was "most looked up to," which was second, and so on, were obtained from two groups of high school students and two groups of college students. The tabulated results showed that in median rank the professional nurse was second; the female physician was first and the teacher sixth.[5]

The 1951 Inventory of Nurses, conducted by the American Nurses' Association, showed about 335,000 professional registered nurses in active service and 222,000 inactive. For the United States as a whole, there were about 218 active nurses for every 100,000 persons, but the ratios varied widely among the states. The District of Columbia had 377 per 100,000 and Connecticut 361 per 100,000, while Arkansas had only 84 per 100,000. Hospitals and other institutions employed nearly half of all active professional registered nurses. The next largest group (21 percent) was engaged in private-duty service. Nearly 9 percent were reported to be in some phase of public health service. In 1953 about 101,000 students were enrolled in 1,135 state-accredited schools of nursing. The number of graduates in 1952 reached 29,000, far below the number at the peak of the war years, but somewhat higher than in 1948 or 1949.[6]

Nursing, regardless of the prestige it enjoyed among women's occupations, was low paid compared to other occupations requiring comparable training and experience. The average monthly salary of the hospital staff nurse living outside hospital quarters increased from $172 in 1946 to $205 in 1949. In 1946 public health nurses earned, on the average, $184 a month; in 1949, $238. Over the 3-year period, average monthly salaries of nurse educators rose from $207 to $256. Private-duty nurses, unlike those in other nursing fields, were usually paid by the day. In 1949 the most frequent daily rate paid in most regions of the country was $10 for 8 hours of work, a rate that did not compare favorably with earnings of other nurses, since private-duty nurses did not work on every workday of the month nor did they receive paid vacations, sick leave, or holidays. In September 1949, for example, they worked an average of less than 14 days.[7]

WIFE AND MOTHER FIGURES IN POSTWAR FILMS

The new emphasis on domesticity was everywhere apparent in mass media products, especially in films. By the end of the 1940s, most female heroines in the movies were again happy housewives. Powerful and aggressive women learned on-screen that their achievements offered them little comfort in the absence of a good man's love. Women in motion pictures were defined solely by the presence or absence of men in their lives; they were characterized as single, husband-hunting girls, housewives and mothers, spinsters, or widows and divorcées. Work was portrayed as secondary or irrelevant to a woman's fulfillment. When Rosie the Riveter was no longer needed as a recruiting symbol, she was quickly forgotten and replaced by the homemaker as the national feminine model. Marriage was the be-all and end-all. Timely plots focused on how to catch and keep a man.

In 1945 Allied victories and anticipation of a swift end to the war had led American film producers to start abandoning war pictures even before an armistice was in sight. Hollywood had, nevertheless, been exposed to strong doses of realism and social awareness, the effects of which could not readily be shaken off. Everyone's troubles did not automatically evaporate with the Japanese surrender in September 1945, and several serious, probing films confronted some major social problems.

Physical disablement formed part of the theme for William Wyler's justly acclaimed, 3-hour "tribute to the lost innocence of American Society," *The Best Years of Our Lives* (RKO Radio, 1946), in which three veterans of the war return to face the problems of readjustment. One is an air force officer (Dana Andrews) who can come to terms with neither his old job (serving in a drugstore) nor his unsuitable war bride (Virginia May); another (Frederic March) is a middle-aged ex-banker faced with having to get to know his wife (Myrna Loy) and hospital nurse daughter (Teresa Wright) all over again; the third is a sailor (Harold Russell) who has lost both hands and fears the pity of his fiancée (Cathy O'Donnell), family, and friends. Their predicaments were representative of the sufferings of many in real life (Russell, a nonprofessional, played himself in all but name) and were accurately, sincerely, and touchingly portrayed, thanks to the excellence of both the writing (screenplay by Robert Sherwood) and the acting. Four years later Fred Zinnemann dealt more specifically with the problems of paraplegic war veterans in *The Men* (United Artists, 1950), in which Marlon Brando prepared for his role with characteristic thoroughness by living for a while with actual paraplegics.[8]

Other aspects of postwar domestic disruption were explored in *Homecoming* (MGM, 1948), an attempt to deal with the sensitive subject of infidelity during wartime. Clark Gable played an Army surgeon, Ulysses Delby Johnson, who falls in love with Army nurse Lieutenant Jane "Snapshot" McCall (Lana Turner) although he has a wife (Anne Baxter) back home. Through Snapshot, nursing is presented as a commendably humanitarian and patriotic pursuit. She is an Army nurse, by her own admission fighting so that her small son can grow up in freedom. This association with the military imbues the nursing image with certain conventional notions: the woman's role is to heal the soldiers, then return them to the fray again.

As a nurse, Snapshot is impressive, not romantic. She looks tomboyish, with her dull khaki uniform and her practical, short haircut. Her main aim is to persevere in her work, in which she is able to submerge any hostile feelings she may have for the surgeon, Ulysses. Her practical skills are immediately apparent in her tireless service at the operating table. Ulysses praises her warmly and openly acknowledges his debt to her. Ultimately, her professionalism leads him to warm to her on a personal level, too. Snapshot's formidable character is apparent to Penny, Dr. Johnson's wife, even though she never meets the nurse. From the change that takes place in her husband, Penny comprehends that the influence Snapshot has had on him must be consid-

erable indeed. Only an extraordinary person could have had such a pronounced effect, teaching him to be "more understanding, wiser, more sympathetic."

Although she does not respect Ulysses initially, Snapshot assists him efficiently. As they set up the unit on their arrival in Africa, we learn from another of Ulysses's assistants that Snapshot has already ordered those items that were in short supply. She sorts and arranges instruments, preparing them for the inevitably grueling operating sessions. At these she assists with great endurance, once for over 16 hours without a break, refusing even to go to sleep when Ulysses suggests she should. "They're trying to kill the doctors—not the *nurses!*" he jokes at her. But she will not be deterred. Ulysses makes it clear that he respects and values Snapshot's personal skills very highly indeed. They exchange conversation about their patients' progress, with Snapshot consulting him about those who ought to be evacuated. "You're a very good nurse, Lieutenant," and "You're the most competent nurse I've ever had in all my experience," is how Johnson expresses his gratitude for her professional excellence. When she has to leave for another unit, Ulysses admits that he "did everything" he could to keep her with him and that he is "going to be lost" without her. They do seem to be a team of the highest order, with the surgeon aware of her unique contributions.[9]

Great importance is placed on Snapshot's power to regenerate Ulysses morally. Her influence on him changes his outlook on life profoundly, causing him to reexamine his attitudes about himself and others in a way previously unthinkable. Her humanity and compassion impress him deeply and he seeks to emulate her example; not surprisingly, he falls in love with her. Her death ironically frees him, so that he can return to his wife, Penny, as a renewed individual, ready to implement a brighter, more compassionate philosophy in their marriage and everyday life. Playing the role of surrogate wife, the nurse is thus the catalyst for the doctor's moral regeneration.

Perhaps the most thoughtful war movie of this period was *The Hasty Heart* (Warner Brothers, 1950), a melancholy portrait of an embittered Scottish corporal named Lachie (Richard Todd), who is dying in an Army hospital in Burma, and who discovers that friendship and love for a nurse (Patricia Neal) are more important than self-pity. Based on John Patrick's stage play, *The Hasty Heart* is a touching portrayal of life in the hospital just after the end

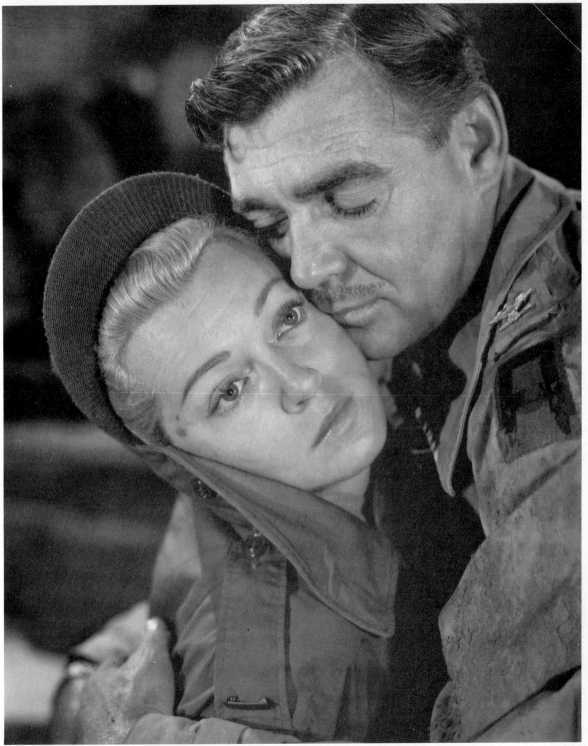

In Homecoming *(MGM, 1948) great importance is placed on Snapshot's power to regenerate Ulysses morally.*

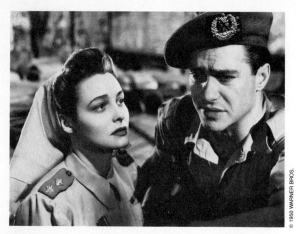

*The Hasty Heart (*Warner Brothers, 1950) *was a melancholy portrait of an embittered Scottish corporal named Lachie (Richard Todd), who is dying in an Army Hospital in Burma, and who discovers that friendship and love for a nurse (Patricia Neal) are more important than self-pity.*

of the war and concentrates on the "kindly deception" practiced by Head Nurse Parker (Neal) and the other patients on the incurably ill Lachie. In the role of Nurse Parker, Patricia Neal delivers a fine, controlled performance and does much to project a complex and convincing view of a very special military nurse.[10]

The nurse is the central organizer of the deception to make the last days of Lachie, the dying misanthrope, pleasant. Entrusted with the sensitive case by the Colonel, she urges the other men in the ward to cooperate and, even when they become discouraged by Lachie's suspicious and scowling nature, she continues to take the initiative in the kindly endeavor. She buys a Cameron Highlander's kilt and accessories for Lachie's birthday and also prepares a special tea and birthday cake for him, proving herself to be an altruistic, caring nurse with great patience and understanding. This party spurs Lachie to begin trusting other people, but the real breakthrough only comes after long sessions of trying to get him to talk about his feelings. He at first interprets her persistence as nothing but idle chatter, his narrow-minded perspective arising from his bitter view of the world. But Parker strives to free him from this view in order that he may come to love humanity.

Nurse Parker's compassion borders on unprofessional self-sacrifice. For instance, when Lachie asks

her to marry him, she agrees to do so if it is the one thing in life he wants most. And when he kisses her on the hand and then apologizes for his forwardness, she responds by kissing him full on the lips as he is lying on his bed. "Surely there's pity in every woman's love," she tells him, suggesting that her own involvement with this particular patient exceeds the bounds of normal professional concern. Once Lachie learns of his nearness to death, however, Parker can interact with him in a manner befitting her profession: she is no less compassionate, but suitably distant and objective.[11]

As the focal point of the story, Parker assumes universal qualities—as mother figure to those for whom she is responsible and as the one woman, constant and true, to remind them of the women in their own lives. As their nurse, she has their undivided attention: all her patients' emotions—anger, frustration, affection—are directed toward her, the whole and healthy one. It is not surprising, as one of the patients observes, that "everyone falls in love with his nurse; it's natural." But as he goes on to say, "just because the nurse takes good care of us and is good to us, doesn't mean she is in love with us." Even though Lachie comes very close to being deluded to the contrary, he ultimately realizes the truth, not only about his own condition, but also about the way of the world as the nurse would have him see it.[12]

GOOD AND BAD NURSES IN SOCIAL PROBLEM FILMS

One of the finest exponents of social realism in film, Elia Kazan, directed a movie for 20th Century-Fox in 1949 called *Pinky,* which told the story of a light-skinned black woman's return to her home, a rural Mississippi town, after having become a nurse in Boston and having passed as a white woman. Jeanne Crain, a very Caucasian-looking actress, played the title role; Ethel Waters played the strong grandmother, who had sent Pinky away; and Ethel Barrymore played the arrogant but honest aristocrat, whose death forces Pinky to decide between her true identity and a life of ease. Pinky has returned home because of her romantic involvement in Boston with a white physician who wants to marry her. She cannot tell him the truth about her race and yet cannot marry him without telling him—so she returns to her grandmother hoping to come to a

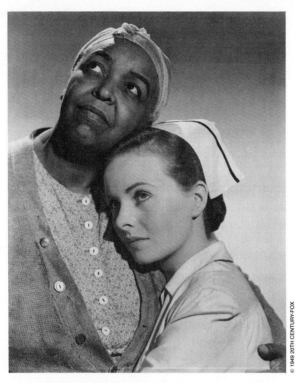

Pinky *(20th Century-Fox, 1949) told the story of a light-skinned black woman's return to her home, a rural Mississippi town, after having become a nurse in Boston and having passed as a white woman.*

decision. While home, Pinky realizes the indignities and insults faced daily by members of her race: she is arrested by crude deputies, nearly raped by drunken white men, and nearly run out of town by greedy relatives of her private-duty patient, the aristocratic Miss Em.

In deference to her grandmother's wishes, Pinky has agreed to nurse the dying Miss Em, but she and the cantankerous woman do not get along at first. Pinky defends her professional identity and resents the woman's imperious manners and expectation of menial servitude. However, Miss Em gradually comes to respect and love Pinky and gives her the best advice in the film: "Be yourself." After Miss Em dies, her will declares that Pinky has inherited her property. During the dramatic lawsuit, in which Miss Em's relatives fight to keep Pinky from having the estate, Pinky's physician suitor arrives from Boston to take her away. After he realizes Pinky's true identity, he urges her to flee with him to Denver and start a new

life. But Pinky hesitates: she loves the physician and yearns for the easier life she would have as his wife, but the trust and wisdom of Miss Em have made her realize that she must face up to her true identity. She chooses to remain in Mississippi and to use her newly inherited property to open a school for training black nurses.[13]

As the only nurse character in this often melodramatic film, Pinky is a very positive and sympathetic representative of the nursing profession. Pinky's nurse's training and her pride in her work contribute to her sense of self-respect and independence. She defends herself to Miss Em and, although she complies with the woman's orders, reminds her that in many places registered nurses are treated with respect. Pinky's professional identity has removed her from the world of her grandmother, in which members of her race submit to the established social hierarchy. Pinky fights the legal battle to retain her legacy from Miss Em and bravely faces the scorn and open hatred of the white community in which she decides to live. In addition, through her nursing skills Pinky earns the respect and approval of some of the influential white leaders of the town: Miss Em, the physician, and the judge who rules in her favor. Finally, at the end of the film, Pinky accepts Miss Em's advice to be herself: she decides to remain in the town and to use her nursing experience to help others of her race—with a free clinic and nursing school.

The identification of Pinky as a nurse is significant in its suggestion that the nursing profession offers opportunity to all. Pinky's decision to train black nurses indicates that the profession will be used to help others to overcome the handicaps of birth and poverty. Nursing is in many ways the medium through which race barriers are broken in this film. Because Pinky is a nurse she can enter the world of Miss Em and speak to her employer and the physician as an equal. The hope and promise inherent in Pinky's school for black nurses is that the coming generation of blacks in this southern town may be able to change the discriminatory patterns because of their new-found skills and education.

Nurse characters also played key roles in *The Snake Pit* (20th Century-Fox, 1948), a popular and shocking film about a state mental hospital. Based on Mary Jane Ward's best-seller, *The Snake Pit* was the third most attended and the most talked-about film of 1948. It also earned an Academy Award nomina-

© 1949 20TH CENTURY-FOX

tion for Best Actress for its star, Olivia de Havilland. Based on her own 8½ months of hospitalization in a mental institution, Ward wrote the story of Virginia Cunningham (de Havilland), who is married to Robert for just a few days when she becomes mentally ill and is diagnosed as schizophrenic. The film chronicles her experiences in a gloomy, large, overcrowded state hospital for the mentally ill.

The case history was worked out by the scriptwriters with three prominent psychiatrists, and experts claimed that it was both accurate and typical. At the hospital where Robert has her committed, Virginia comes under the care of Dr. Kik, a compassionate psychiatrist. As in the book, Juniper Hill Hospital and everyone in it, including Virginia, are seen through Virginia's eyes. The viewer is brought to experience the often degrading conditions within the hospital, from the absolute despair of ward one—from which release is possible—to the lowest depths of ward thirty-three—a true madhouse called "The Snake Pit" in reference to the crawling snake pits into which the insane were thrown centuries ago on the theory that if such an experience would drive a normal person insane, it might shock an insane person back to normality. While Virginia is still in a delusional state, she actually believes she is in prison, and indeed there seems little difference between a prison and a hospital for the mentally ill. Using electroshock therapy, hydrotherapy and narcosynthesis, Dr. Kik slowly helps Virginia to reconstruct her personality.

The nursing image found in *The Snake Pit* is multifaceted and complex. The film, being an excellent and realistic portrayal of conditions in a state psychiatric hospital in the 1940s, has several nurse characters who are accordingly distinct and individual, not at all like the melodramatic stereotypes that pervade mental hospital screen representations. For *The Snake Pit* does more than exploit a popular myth about state hospitals—that the patients are crowded together like animals and are cruelly mistreated by the staff—rather, it makes an honest effort to depict the personal conflicts that everyone—physicians, nurses, and patients—must confront and to explore how these groups go about coping with them, for good or ill.

In Miss Seiffert (Virginia Brissac), the supervising nurse who is in her 60s, we have a woman who, though seen only briefly, emerges as a professional with almost as much authority as her physician colleagues. The most striking detail of her characterization is her hearing aid (the cord for which runs down the front of her prim suit), which she has to turn on in order to hear conversations at the dinner table. It seems she prefers to enjoy her meal in peace, with the hearing aid turned off a good deal of the time, but she needs to activate it in order to confirm the report that she had told Virginia Cunningham's husband he could have his wife removed from the hospital if he moved to another state. Dr. Kik, though displeased by this, does not reprimand or criticize Miss Seiffert, who obviously has a say in such administrative decisions; we later see another doctor ask her to investigate the matter of Mrs. Cunningham's release in greater detail.

The middle-aged Miss Vance (Esther Somers) is a different kind of nurse, whose hefty figure is a useful help in her job in the severely disturbed ward. She walks about the mumbling, dancing, frantic figures, lifting a weeping patient off the floor and offering a few words of encouragement to a frightened woman, but although her work is extremely taxing, she has the endurance and dedication to do it well.

Miss Somerville (Jacqueline de Wit), former head nurse on ward one, becomes a patient herself and is a truly pathetic figure: what *Time*'s reviewer described as "the nurse whose own mind has worked loose in the buffeting, jarring atmosphere of the asylum and who now wanders through the ward, keeping imaginary records." As she walks about the ward, Miss Somerville maintains her former professional manner, wearing what appears to be a uniform—even though it is wrinkled—and solicitously taking temperatures with an emery board. She even mouths pertinent comments about overcrowding: "Bet they'll send us more than one [to take Virginia's place], they always do. And we're so crowded already I don't know where it's all going to end." This characterization, of a nurse who is so sensitive to her environment that she loses her sanity, is the most stereotypical image in *The Snake Pit,* being part of the popular misconception that those who work in mental institutions are themselves either insane, sadistic, or especially prone to mental collapse.[14]

Helen Craig's excellent performance as Miss Davis is the only unmistakably negative portrayal in the film. Plagued by crowded conditions and a strenuous workload, many of the other nurses are understandably insensitive at times. Only Miss Davis projects an intrinsically and intentionally icy attitude, which causes her staff to obey her unquestioningly and her patients to submit out of sheer terror. Miss Davis was promoted from staff nurse to head nurse in ward one, the best ward. When Virginia Cunningham is first brought there, she is met by the talkative young nurse's aide, Miss Bixby (June Storey), who warns Virginia not to sit on the bed because she might mess it up, which would irritate Miss Davis; she also tells Virginia to obey Miss Davis in everything in order to remain on her good side.

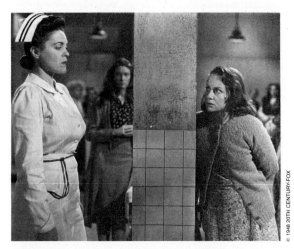

In The Snake Pit *(20th Century-Fox, 1948) when Miss Davis sees Virginia on her ward for the first time, she emphasizes that her ward is "quite pleasant—for those who are willing to cooperate."*

When Miss Davis actually sees Virginia on her ward for the first time she emphasizes that her ward is "quite pleasant—for those who are willing to cooperate." Cooperation is intended to be all on the side of the patients, however: they should obey the letter of the law with no exceptions. Miss Davis' obsession with rules is another expression of her militaristic personality. Her very appearance, standing tall and straight with her large chest pushed forward, her black hair pulled off her face to reveal thick, dark eyebrows, set lips, and a jutting jaw, is militaristic, too. Being quite tall, when looking at her patients—particularly Virginia—Miss Davis looks down on them, both literally and figuratively. But the most fascinating detail of her militaristic manner is the sound she makes when she walks; hearing her

footsteps in the corridor, coming toward us, they are distinctly loud and controlled as if she were wearing a pair of combat boots. Also, she habitually crosses her hands in front of her in an "at ease" position, as in an Army formation, in contrast to Miss Hart, who places her hands very frequently on her patients' shoulders to comfort them.[15]

The most perplexing aspect of Miss Davis is her sexuality, the source of many of her own psychological problems. Virginia's observation that Miss Davis hates her because she is jealous of the attention she receives from Dr. Kik—in other words, that Miss Davis is infatuated with the doctor—is probably true, especially if we consider Miss Davis' malicious response to the accusation—cornering Virginia and putting her into a straight jacket. In order to exercise control, Miss Davis has to deny her femininity by adopting increasingly masculine attributes, like the military posture, and by exerting power over helpless, weak, and emotionally vulnerable people. The conflict between her and Virginia arises when Virginia makes it plain that, unlike the other "ladies," she really does consider herself a writer, and thereby threatens Miss Davis's notion that she is the only woman who is productive. Virginia has the boldness to answer Miss Davis's biting comments with, "Do I tell you how to be a nurse?" This gets the unprofessional response, "All right lady, I've tried to be patient with you, but you haven't any spirit of cooperation. All you have is an exalted idea of your own importance. Let me tell you something, if it weren't for Dr. Kik, you'd never be here [ward one]."[16]

Virginia discerns the nurse's jealousy and shocks the frigid woman when she declares, "I know now why you hate me so. It's because you're in love with Dr. Kik." Miss Davis walks out of the room without saying a word; even sarcasm cannot serve her now. Virginia runs after her, pleading not to be punished or sent away for what she has said, but the nurse is not softened by the woman's supplications. Virginia locks herself in Miss Davis's bathroom for hours before the nurses discover she is there. All the while Virginia can hear them conferring outside as they search for her all over the ward, Miss Davis herself commenting in a malicious, haughty tone, "I'll find her myself. I know all their tricks." Although Miss Davis may enjoy the power of her position as head nurse in a mental ward, it seems unlikely that she actually enjoys nursing per se, but is rather dependent upon it to sustain her own self-importance.[17]

Miss Davis's attitude is directly contrasted with that of Miss Hart on one occasion. When Dr. Kik tells Miss Hart that he is taking Virginia off shock treatment, she calmly points out that the patient has not finished the full course of treatment. He courteously reassures her that he is aware of this and wants to proceed to another stage, and she accepts his decision. Miss Davis, on the other hand, also encounters Virginia in the shock therapy room and directs her to get on the table by clapping her hands with the encouragement, "Well, what are you waiting for? You should know by now—on the table!"[18]

Until *The Snake Pit* appeared in the form of both novel and motion picture, few Americans were aware that more than half a million men, women, and children were in mental hospitals in the United States in 1948, mostly state institutions, and that another 7 million, although at large, suffered from some kind of mental illness. The state mental hospitals, desperately overcrowded and understaffed, were pictured in the film to be seriously in need of federal and state tax dollars. According to the film's producer, Darryl Zanuck, twenty-six state legislatures were prodded into passing more progressive mental health legislation after public pressure generated by *The Snake Pit*. By 1951 all states had mental health programs and were spending almost $2 for every $1 contributed by the federal government.[19]

NURSES BECOMING HOUSEWIVES

Most nurse characterizations in films of the late-1940s and 1950s featured nurses seeking romantic, marital, and domestic fulfillment. Invariably, their nursing careers terminated abruptly when they found some measure of domestic stability. *Possessed* (Warner Brothers), a popular 1946 film starring Joan Crawford, explored the world of mental illness. Miss Crawford played a private-duty nurse who forms an obsessive, romantic attraction to a man who does not return her love in equal measure. Spurned by her lover, the nurse soon marries the husband of her patient, who has committed suicide. Immediately, the nurse quits her job and enjoys the material security and comfort of her husband's position. Unfortunately, her obsession with her former lover revives when he returns and begins dating her stepdaughter. Eventually, the nurse suffers a serious breakdown and has to undergo psychiatric treatment. Although this nurse character was apparently a good, competent nurse, she clearly found no personal fulfillment in her work and spent all her emotional and mental energies in a quest for perfect love.

Not As a Stranger (United Artists, 1955) captured the essence of postwar depictions of the nursing profession. Olivia de Havilland starred as Kristina, a Swedish-American nurse who falls in love with an impecunious medical student. Kristina is a capable surgical nurse who enjoys the respect of her colleagues; her expertise is so valued that she is called away from her lunch to handle a problem. She takes an interest in a younger man, a medical student, and even helps him observe an operation. The medical student, Luke, played by Robert Mitchum, is having trouble financing his medical education and courts Kristina in an unscrupulous attempt to support himself. The nurse, who is beyond the first blush of youth, is a little skeptical of his interest at first, but soon allows herself to fall hopelessly in love with him and eagerly accepts his marriage proposal.

After graduation, they move to a new town, where he takes his first job. Kris wants to start a family, but Luke is bored by his marriage of convenience and begins to look elsewhere for romance. Meanwhile, Kris becomes pregnant but cannot find a way to tell Luke because he is so involved in his work. Once, while working with a seriously ill patient, Luke calls Kris to the hospital to help him. After they save the patient, he tells her how wonderful she is, but spoils it by indicating that he appreciates her as a nurse and not as a woman. Kris eventually makes him leave their house. Before a desperate surgical operation to save his friend and mentor, Luke learns from a colleague that Kris is pregnant. The operation fails because of his mistake, and the once proud doctor runs to Kris for safety and help—she eagerly accepts him, of course.

In this film the nurse character herself sees her nursing role as distinctly subordinate to her role as mother. Not only does she want and expect a child of her own, but her final reconciliation with her husband is that of a mother accepting her wayward son. Luke returns to his wife when he needs her comfort and support after his failure in surgery. For all her suffering, Kris is a somewhat pathetic woman, clinging to a man who has used her and forgiving him after he humiliates her. But the audience is made to see Kris's actions as noble and completely understandable. After all, even the most successful professional woman would put aside her work for home

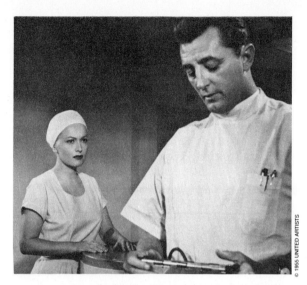

In Not As A Stranger *(United Artists, 1955) Olivia De Havilland starred as Kristina, a Swedish-American nurse who falls in love with an impecunious medical student played by Robert Mitchum.*

and children—even if her husband is one of the kids. Thus, in this postwar melodrama, the nurse is both revered for her generosity and nobility and at the same time reminded that her most important obligations concern home and family. On the medical side, there are four operations dramatically recreated in the film that are presented with admirable scientific accuracy: a laminectomy, a subtotal gastrectomy, plastic surgery on a hand, and an attempted repair of an aortal aneurysm.

In *Fear Strikes Out* (Paramount, 1957), the autobiographical account of Jimmy Piersall, famous Red Sox baseball player, the central nurse character has a contrasting role to play. Mary Teevan (Norma Moore), an attractive and fashionable young brunette, takes a leading role in winning Piersall (Anthony Perkins) for herself. Having accomplished this, she stands by him when, after a mental collapse, he is drained of all ambition: it is her drive and encouragement that invest him with the will to live. That she is a nurse is, as is so often the case, rather unimportant, particularly as we see her in uniform only once (significantly enough, when she hands in her resignation). We first see her spending an afternoon off at the Scranton minor league baseball stadium with some friends as attractive as herself. Having fallen for the shy athlete, she then proceeds to

manipulate him throughout the courtship that follows. After watching practice, for instance, she forwardly comments, "I like the way you play baseball," and then flirtingly hints for a dinner date by remarking, "Now, if only one of us could cook!" Before Piersall leaves Scranton for the winter vacation, Mary coaxes a marriage proposal out of him by forcing him to address each of the potential problems of marriage aloud in her presence.[20]

Mary's undoubted strength is her ability to offer continuing psychological support to both Piersall and others, despite emotional crises. When, for instance, the Red Sox manager suspends Piersall for starting a fight with a teammate, Mary hurries from the stands to the locker room and suggests that her husband take a period of rest and relaxation. Then, during the time of Piersall's eventual hospitalization, Mary is the only member of the Piersall family who can make rational decisions in her husband's best interest. A psychiatrist consults Mary about her husband's condition, and she agrees to the use of electroshock therapy. Furthermore, she fully understands the doctor's decision to restrict all visitors—even herself—from seeing Piersall. By contrast, the young man's father—whose psychological harassment of his son has contributed to his illness—refuses to abide by the psychiatrist's orders, secretly visits Piersall, and as a result, incites him to assault his own father. Nursing is depicted as Mary's job rather than her profession, and Mary's womanhood is as important as any other personal quality to the role she plays in *Fear Strikes Out*. In spite of this, however, that she inspires her husband and represents the unflinching face of common sense undeniably distinguishes her as one of the few entirely reasonable human beings in the picture.

At the top of the box-office ratings during the early-1960s were two films that were released in response to the success of Richard Frede's novel *The Interns*. The first, based directly on the novel, was released in 1962; the second, providing further adventures of some of the original characters and introducing several others, came out in 1964.

Set in New North Hospital, a large teaching hospital, *The Interns* (Columbia, 1962) follows the first year's experiences of four male interns—Lew Worship (James MacArthur), John Otis (Cliff Robertson), Alec Considine (Michael Callan), and Sid Lackland (Nick Adams)—and one female—Mada Bruckner (Haya Harareet), from Vienna. These doctors behave with ethical concern, with playboy enthusiasm, with callous insensitivity, and with blatant greed. Yet despite these individual traits, the world of medicine is portrayed in reverential and inspirational terms. The young men struggle with failure and success; some succumb to unethical temptations, but most last the year and prepare for the greater challenges of a hospital residency.

Nurses abound in *The Interns,* both in the background and foreground, but almost no attention is attached to the profession of nursing itself. The nurse characters are developed sketchily and then only for romantic or comic interest. In general the nurses authenticate the setting and dress up the set—they are uniformly young, pretty, and giggling. (A few older nurses do appear, occasionally in scenes of patient care, but remain incidental to the narrative.) Third-year student-nurse Gloria, played by Stephanie Powers, is elected to be Lew's girl: one of the more wolfish young doctors singles her out of a crowd of "baby nurselings" because of the "love-bite" on her neck; Lew himself is too busy studying medicine to find a girl on his own. Pretty, intelligent, and despite the "love bite," morally upright, Gloria seems to be the perfect girl for workaholic Lew, and he sets his heart on her. Toward the end of the film, Gloria announces that she wants to experience the world, to cast off her "incubator-baby" past, by working as a "tramp nurse" all over the globe. This upsets Lew, who wants to marry Gloria; of course, after the requisite painful moments for Lew, Gloria changes her mind and agrees to settle down to marriage and having babies with him.[21]

Supervising nurse Didi, played by comedienne Kay Stevens, serves as a college sorority house-mother to her nursing student charges. Didi acts as if her prime duty as nursing instructor is to arrange dates for the interns with her girls. She throws a wild new year's eve party and encourages her students to enjoy themselves in whatever way they please. The nursing supervisor summarizes the nurses' concern in her brief introductory talk about the hospital: "3000 patients in the hospital . . . means a lot of beds to make."[22]

Interestingly, the female intern of this film, Dr. Bruckner of Vienna, emerges as a very serious, sophisticated, career-minded young woman. Next to her, the young nurses appear to be callow and light-headed. To polish off the image of nursing, the new year's eve party scene reveals the true nature of repressed and shy nurse Olga: she tosses off her spectacles, lets down her hair, and dances lasciviously in her black lingerie to the fun-loving amusement of her fellow nurses and appreciative male admirers.

In the sequel, *The New Interns* (Columbia, 1964), Didi holds a baby shower that also turns into a wild party once the doctors arrive; things, therefore, are very much as they were in the original. Considine (Michael Callan) and Lew Worship (now played by Dean Jones) are again here, the former chasing a student nurse, Laura Rogers (Barbara Eden), and the latter coping with a marriage to nurse Gloria (Stefanie Powers) that is barren because of his sterility. Like its predecessor, *The New Interns* incorporates a considerable number of background nurses, who have nothing to do with the plot except to give the film hospital authenticity. Several nurses do emerge from this shadowy context, however. Didi is still head nurse and still enormous fun, a good sport of considerable talent whose skillful mounting of revues and parties takes precedence over her professional duties. Gloria is apparently an efficient children's nurse, though the audience sees only two exchanges between her and her small patients—the film instead concentrates on her handling of the infertility problem, and although a professional role is emphasized in Gloria's case more than others, her personal crisis depends for its power far more on her being a *woman* than on her being a nurse.

MILITARY NURSES PLAY HOUSEWIFE ROLES

Meanwhile, films such as *Battle Circus* (MGM, 1953), *Hellcats of the Navy* (Columbia, 1957), *South Pacific* (20th Century-Fox, 1958), and *Captain Newman, M.D.* (Universal, 1963) all featured military nurses during war who no longer make important contributions to the war effort. Instead, these pretty and sympathetic nurses concentrate their attentions on finding husbands or comforting their lovers or both.

In *Battle Circus* Humphrey Bogart played Major Webb, an Army surgeon who meets and falls in love with a young nurse, Lieutenant Ruth McCara (June Allyson), at a front-line M.A.S.H. (mobile army surgical hospital) unit. Ruth is a pretty, young, wholesome, naive, old-fashioned girl, with long blond hair, wide, wondering eyes, and full, pouting lips—

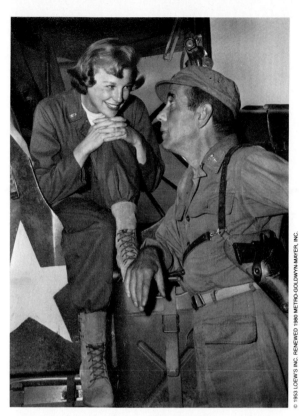

Lieutenant Ruth McCara (June Allyson) in Battle Circus *(MGM, 1953), refuses to have any relationship unless it is heading toward marriage, for she has traditional ideas about sexual morality.*

From these extracts from Ruth's conversation with Webb the morning after they have spent the night together, we can see Ruth's image of a wife is very much an extension of her nursing role. Her nursing capabilities, moreover, are shown to have their usefulness, but only within a context in which she, as wife, will play an entirely subordinate role, reminiscent of the Victorian concept of the wife as the husband's plaything or ornament.

Hellcats of the Navy tells of submarine Commander Casey Abbott (Ronald Reagan) and his efforts to chart a safe course through the Japanese mine fields in the Sea of Japan during World War II. These underwater exploits are complicated by Casey's romantic involvement with a pretty Navy Nurse, Lieutenant Helen Blair (Nancy Davis), stationed at a Navy hospital on Guam. Casey and Helen love each other, but Casey has spurned Helen because he does not want to marry until after the war. Helen, on the rebound, takes up with handsome Lieutenant Wes Barton, a frogman on Casey's submarine. When Casey is forced by the approach of a Japanese destroyer to abandon Barton in the water, crew members suspect he is trying to get rid of his rival. Helen knows that Casey has too much integrity to have left Barton to die to settle a personal grudge, and she encourages him to resume their romantic relationship. He refuses, however, to avoid confirming suspicions about his abandonment of Barton. At the end of the film, once Casey has proven himself a hero to his crew, he decides to marry Helen, who, conveniently, is waiting and waving at the dock when the submarine glides into its berth.

The main virtues of nursing in the film consist of the nurse's faith in her man, her loyalty to him, and her patience in waiting for his return. Her actual nursing duties are limited to informing Casey that he has a light concussion and sitting at a desk, ready to sign out the moment Casey appears, so that they can go out on a date. The nurse is not called upon to make any decision or to take initiative in any important situation. She is meant to be a bland prop for the heroic submarine commander. Perhaps the most telling scene of all is at the very end, when the nurse stands waving at her man returning from his adventure at sea.

An image of a World War II nurse that is indelibly stamped into American culture is presented in *Tales of the South Pacific,* by James A. Michener. The book won the 1948 Pulitzer Prize for the best work of fic-

directly in the tradition of the June Allyson heroines. Unlike the other, sexually liberated nurses in the camp, Ruth refuses to have any relationship unless it is heading toward marriage. Her sexual values, her gentle, sweet voice, and her overall femininity of manner indicate an innocent, vulnerable, and in fact exceptional young woman. Ruth's rumination about what she would like to be as a married woman is interesting, for it combines the wholesome qualities she already has with her new-found qualities as a seductress:

> I'll keep a nice house for you. . . . I'll read all the clever magazines so I'll be able to say smart things to your friends. . . . And when you're sick I'll nurse you. . . . And I'll learn to cook and bake things for you. . . . Then I'll come to see you [at work]. I'll pretend I'm a patient. Then in your private office we'll make love.[23]

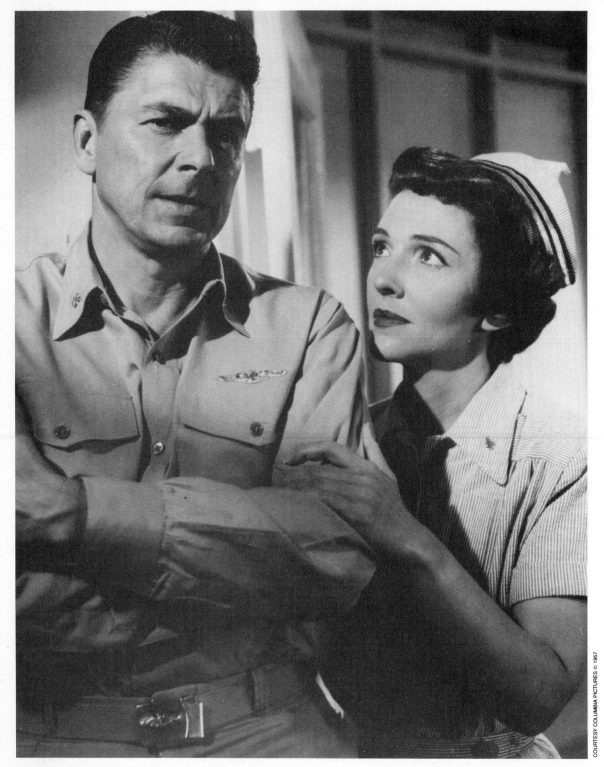

In Hellcats of the Navy *(Columbia, 1957), Lieutenant Helen Blair (Nancy Davis) is stationed at the Navy Hospital on Guam. Her nursing duties are limited to informing Casey that he has a light concussion, and sitting at a desk ready to sign out the moment Casey appears for their date.*

tion, and its adaptation as a musical play earned the 1950 Pulitzer Prize for the best American play. Twentieth Century-Fox came out with a movie version in 1958. The work, in its several mass media forms, strongly bolstered the wife and mother image of the nurse. In the book version, two of the stories involve nurses: "An Officer and a Gentleman" and "Our Heroine." "Our Heroine" served as the basis for the musical *South Pacific*. This story tells of Nellie Forbush, a young American Navy nurse stationed on a south Pacific island, who falls in love with Emile de Becque, a rich French planter. Lieutenant Joseph Cable arrives on the island with orders to conduct reconnaissance of the Japanese-held islands in the area. On the strange island of Bali Ha'i, Cable meets and falls in love with Liat—the beautiful half-caste daughter of Bloody Mary, a rambunctious native trading woman—but refuses to marry her because of her color. Then Nellie learns that de Becque has two Eurasian children by a previous marriage to a Polynesian woman. Deeply shocked, she breaks off her engagement with him, and in the mood of dejection that follows, de Becque agrees to guide Cable through the islands. Together the two men radio back to the Americans vital information about Japanese troop movements. When Nellie hears that de Becque has gone with Cable, she realizes how foolish her prejudices were. Cable is killed by the Japanese, but de Becque escapes back to the American island. At his hilltop home he finds Nellie and his two children waiting for him.

Nearly 50 nurse characters populate the cast of *South Pacific* and appear in several musical numbers and other sequences. The nurses join Nellie in her attempt to "wash that man right out of my hair" and later observe with amusement her declaration of love for Emile, "I'm in love with a wonderful guy." In addition, Nellie Forbush, who is one of the main characters, is a nurse. Despite this, nursing plays a very minimal role in the development of the narrative; the profession primarily provides a rationale for the presence of 50 young women on the island full of love-starved sailors. Nellie herself personifies the image of America womanhood—optimistic, cheerful, talented, healthy, athletic, naive, and pretty. She exhibits a provincial attitude toward the news that her true love has been married to a native woman and is the father of two Eurasian children; however, her sense of fairness and her attraction to his adorable children overcome her resistance. Lovely nurse

Nellie joyfully welcomes Emile home and into her waiting arms.[24]

Although a few critics faulted the overly artful camera work and compared the film unfavorably to the stage production, most critics and audiences found the film a warm and fully entertaining version of the tropical love story. Shot on location in Hawaii and the Fiji islands, the film combined visually enchanting scenery with a memorable musical score to make the picture a great success. Most of the songs associated with *South Pacific* have passed into musical comedy legend: "Some Enchanted Evening," "There Is Nothing Like a Dame," "Bali Ha'i," and "Gonna Wash That Man Right Out of My Hair," to name a few.

The "Nothing Like a Dame" sequence illustrates the role of nurses in the film. While the lonely sea-

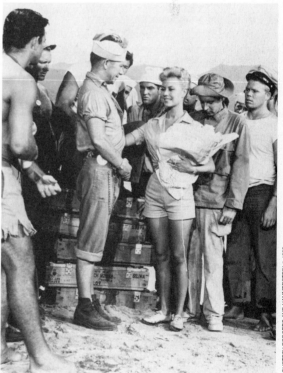

In South Pacific *(20th Century-Fox, 1958) the "Nothing Like a Dame" sequence illuminates the role of nurses in the film. While the lonely seabees recall the joys of female companionship, a group of shapely nurses jogging by diverts them. When Nellie stops for her laundry, one of the sailors notes that "She's a nice* little *girl."*

bees recall the joys of female companionship, a group of shapely nurses jogs by and diverts them momentarily. When Nellie stops for her laundry, one of the sailors notes that "she's a *nice* little girl," which just about summarizes Nellie's character and the image of the island's nurses.[25]

In *Captain Newman, M.D.* Gregory Peck plays the title role of a compassionate psychiatrist in charge of the mental ward at a stateside rehabilitation hospital during World War II. He is chronically short of staff and always looking for new nurses and orderlies. His commanding officer is under pressure to return men to duty as soon as possible, and Newman's painstaking efforts to restore his patients to health bring him some criticism. Soon into the movie, Newman manages to hoodwink a new hospital orderly, Jackson Laibowitz (Tony Curtis), into accepting a job in the psychiatric ward. However, the orderly had been meant for another ward, and a pretty nurse from that ward, Lieutenant Francie Corum (Angie Dickinson), mildly rebukes Newman for taking him. A mutual attraction develops between Newman and Francie. Francie is important for two reasons only: she is beautiful, and she is romantically involved with Captain Newman. Her role promises far more than it ultimately yields in portraying a nurse. She is an intelligent, well-trained nurse, with two years of pre-med studies at college, a full nursing course at St. Vincent's Hospital, a year and a half at Massachusetts General Hospital, and an indeterminate length of service in the Army Nurse Corps. She appears bright and understanding, discusses cases intelligently with the doctor, and is often the one Newman turns to in order to relieve his doubts. Yet despite this, Francie never does anything other than perform simple duties and stand by her patients looking sympathetic. So far as the motion picture is concerned, the qualifications with which the script imbues her are ultimately meaningless; what counts is her appearance and her passivity.

For example, when Captain Newman is trying to convince Francie to transfer into the psychiatric ward to help him, he briefly mentions all her fine qualifications but emphasizes that her physical appearance is her primary asset as a psychiatric nurse. "Francie, you're a good-looking woman. That's a good morale factor; it gives a man incentive. Take a patient cowering under the bed, for instance. He wouldn't come out for Blodgett, but one look at those legs of yours and he would come right up through the mattress."[26]

Not surprisingly, it is difficult to deduce what Francie's own attitude toward nursing is. Her impressive training indicates that she once had serious professional intentions, and indeed when she discusses patients with Newman she sounds competent and knowledgeable. Nevertheless, the minimal nursing scenes undercut that image, as does Francie's declared intention to quit nursing and have babies once the war is over. In her overly cute smile as she makes this announcement, there is the implication that making babies is what she ought to have been doing all along.

THE FLOOD OF NURSE ROMANCE NOVELS

By 1950 the paperback book industry alone was selling over a quarter of a billion books each year in drugstores and newsstands for 25¢, 35¢, and (for giants then) 50¢. Already the industry had 81,000 titles in print. During the 1950s and early-1960s, romance novels about nurses and nursing constituted the single largest occupationally linked category of mass-market paperback fiction. The major publishers of nurse romances were Dell ("Candlelight" series), Ace ("Ace Nurse Romance" series), and Harlequin; minor publishers were Arcadia House ("Valentine" series), Bantam ("Red Rose" series), New American Library (Signet Books), Pocket Books, Magnum, MacFadden, and many others. Pocket Books, which printed its first ten paperbacks in 1939, was the oldest of these mass-market publishers. The typical nurse romance adhered to a strict formula—a 200-page romance, set in an exotic locale, with a set plot and little individuality of expression. (The effectiveness of this strategy was documented by such success stories as Harlequin's growth from obscurity to the $65 million mark in a decade, and by the efforts of other mass-market houses to imitate it.) Almost 800 romantic novels about nurses were churned out as if from an assembly line. Romance situations within the context of health care institutions provided opportunities for the nurse to perform well in a number of female roles, and her future husband often witnessed her skill in nurturing surrogate husbands and children, as the nursing role was primarily equated with womanly virtues. Importantly, romance-novel nurses were portrayed as ultimately submissive women, rarely daring to question the authority of physicians, even when the physicians were wrong. Nursing was generally identified as a technical occupation rather than a profession, and education and research were deliberately de-emphasized.

The nurturing imperative that dominated these novels prescribed marriage as the ultimate goal of all romance, because with it came husband, home, and children; all other goals were subordinate. The idea that motherhood was a woman's duty and proper role meant that all other aspects of her personal and professional life were secondary. An excessively selfless devotion to the care of others resulted in the exclusion of personal interests and needs. The nurse found a mate who would materially support, protect, and love her, and any movement to a higher plane of fulfillment was short-circuited by this limited framework. Nurse romances invariably end with an engagement to marry—and an implication of "happily ever after."

The nurturing imperative also means that the maternal role is seen as the one the nurse should play in all spheres of life, not just in relation to her own children, if any, but to her patients, to physicians and other nurses, and to boyfriends, fiancé, and husband. A common theme of romance is that the nurse is so occupied with fostering others' growth that she forgets her own, but this problem takes care of itself because her competence in the nurturing role is admired by prospective husbands.

The tendency for fiancés to be physicians is significant. The doctor-nurse relationship of command and obedience supplies a highly traditional model for husband-wife relationships in many romances, as this coy scene from *Nurse on Pondre Island* demonstrates.

> "Riney, I haven't asked you if you'll marry me. Will you?"
> Primly she replied, "Now, Dr. MacDonald, when has a nurse ever defied a doctor's orders?"
> "Then I order you to." But he found a demonstration more forceful than words.[27]

The doctor's dominant role carries over into the fiancé role. "If he had held her close before, the muscular arms which had made whole again so

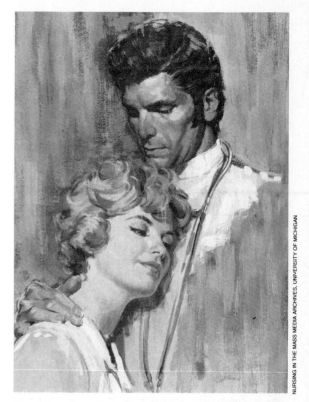

The doctor-nurse relationship of command and obedience supplies a highly traditional model for husband-wife relationships in many romances, such as Nurse on Pondre Island *(Arcadia House, 1965).*

many broken bodies, including hers, now met around Denise like a band of steel" (*Wilderness Nurse*); "So Jane had gone along meekly enough. What else could a nurse do when a doctor gave an order? Or a gal when a man was as masterful as Jeff?"[28] (*Jane Arden: Head Nurse*). The powerful embrace becomes actually forcible in *Nurse Stacey Comes Aboard.*

> Angrily, she struggled free.
> "Of all the infuriating men, you are the worst I've met, Dr. Harley! No one but you could possibly assume the right to insult a girl for days on end, and then order her to marry you! Excuse me—I must go...."
> His tall figure blocked her path....
> "Let me *go!*"
> But his arms were about her again, and this time there was no escape.[29]

The young nurse's relation to physicians is normally subservient in romance, and she is usually depicted taking orders. In *Nurses Marry Doctors,* Linda Stephens is punished unfairly for a minor infraction of rules about curfew and associating with doctors after hours. In reality, she had been returning alone from a mission of mercy when Phil (Dr. Manley) drove by and offered her a ride. Even the position of relative power that the nurse has vis-à-vis a patient is frequently infringed upon by patients, male and female, who give or refuse to accept orders; this is especially true when the patient is also the nurse's employer, as is the case with private-duty nurses (e.g., *Nurse in Acapulco, Nurse on Pondre Island*).

The future husband, whether a physician or not, also frequently makes the decision about the nurse's career: in *Nurse Into Woman,* Jim proposes that Kristine work on his ship once they are marred; in *Jane Arden: Head Nurse,* Jeff says that Jane may continue working but she "knew that if Jeff had asked her to give it up, she would have";[30] in *The Courtship of Nurse Genie Hayes,* Genie asks,

"If I marry you, may I still be Dr. Caleb's assistant?" Scott asked quietly, "Would you really like to be?"
"I would, Scott, truly, if you're sure you don't mind?"
"I don't mind anything you do, darling, so long as you do it as my wife," Scott told her gently.[31]

Even where there is no mention of the nurse's career upon engagement, other characters sometimes assume that she will leave nursing when she marries, as the Matron does in *Noonday Nurse.*[32] In *Leona Gregory, R.N.,* another nurse says,

"Will you be leaving the hospital after you're married, Leona?"
"I suppose so," Leona answered. "Bruce and I haven't discussed it. I'll do whatever he wants me to do, of course."
"Well, of course," Jane agreed as if there could not possibly be any other decision. "I suppose we'll be getting a new surgical nurse then...."[33]

A closely related theme is that nurses make better mothers. *Nurse Martin's Dilemma* and *Wilderness Nurse* come out strongly in favor of the idea that a mother should not hire another person to care for her child, and that nurse's training will help a woman be "a real wife and a real mother ... a mother who works at her job instead of shirking it."[34]

The Nurse Had a Secret incorporates a particularly rigid separation of male and female roles. The nurse is portrayed as preoccupied with trivial tasks, especially her appearance; wearing her uniform out of coquettishness and a desire to appear authoritative; doing little nursing, except setting up a routine of rest and meals for a professor and caring for him briefly after his concussion; clever only in small matters, like the social white lie; emotional and impulsive, acting on intuition and instinct rather than rationally; and blinded by love to the most significant aspects of interpersonal relationships. Men, on the other hand, are strong, calm, rational, decisive, and involved with important affairs, but they are incapable of looking after themselves, choosing clothes that go well together, or preparing their own meals.[35]

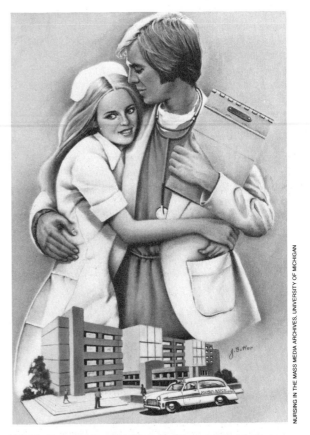

The desire to appear altruistic as well as competent in the nurturing role may motivate romance heroines to become nurses.

The desire to appear altruistic as well as competent in the nurturing role may motivate romance heroines to become nurses (*Nurse Landon's Challenge*) or volunteer for extra duties. In *Nurses Marry Doctors,* for example, Linda's rival for Julian, Evelyn, a wealthy young woman and a nurse, organizes a recreation program for orphaned and hospitalized children. "During the summer, Linda had met Evelyn Delaney one day in a tearoom, and had offered her services again. Julian had wanted her to help, and she was only trying to please him."[36]

The expectation that nurses be altruistic means they must devote themselves to the service of others even when the nature of their jobs does not require it. Thus, in *Nurse in Acapulco, A Nurse Comes Home,* and *Nurse Shelly Decides,* nurses are derided for accepting easy and luxurious positions as private-duty nurses to wealthy patients. Donna in *Nurse in Acapulco* feels a lingering sense of guilt about her do-nothing job with a rich hypochondriac, even though the decision to take a vacation was forced on her by a friend, a physician concerned about the rigors of her job as special nurse to terminally ill patients. She resolves the problem by working after hours in a charity clinic in Acapulco and by helping out during an earthquake.[37]

Nursing is viewed as offering the romantic heroine not only the training to be a good wife and mother but also the opportunity to prove her worth in this role. Devotion to duty and self-sacrifice are key elements of the altruistic imperative. For example, in *Nurse Atholl Returns,* Lyn is constantly coached by Warner, a doctor, on ignoring her own feelings and putting duty first. Each event in the novel is a lesson in doing one's duty: returning after being jilted to be a nurse at the same hospital, despite her embarrassment; leaving her friend Patsy, who is to have an emergency appendectomy because Warner insists her "duty is with tomorrow's patients—not tonight's, however personally close" to her; reassuring her former fiancé and the woman he has jilted her to marry of her good wishes despite her own pain at his betrayal.[38]

No nurse romance is more emphatically altruistic than *Nurse with Wings.* Lieutenant Shirley Andrews, an Air Force flight nurse, values patriotism, "hard work and self-sacrifice" and feels a "deep joy in service." The Nightingale, Army nurse, and flight nurse's creeds, which punctuate the text, incorporate these values. The wives of fighting men are "the real heroines of this war," the mothers of their children, the real "home-front soldiers," in Shirley's view. Like Linda in *Nurses Marry Doctors,* Shirley is compared to an angel; for the soldiers, the flight nurse is "a symbol of some beloved woman back home—a wife, a sweetheart or a mother." The mothering function is the one most often exercised by Shirley: she comforts Johnny "with an almost maternal gesture" when his fiancée breaks their engagement; she scolds young patients "with mock sternness"; she finds a place for a new mother to live and counsels the fiancée of a veteran who has lost a leg; and she plays the part of a delirious soldier's mother:

> She bent low to catch the sound, and heard him say faintly, "Hi, Mom! I'm—scared! It's dark—Mom!" The last was a whisper of childish terror. Instantly Shirley's hand closed warmly to say soothingly, "It's all right, son. It's all right! There's nothing to be afraid of!"
> . . . [with] a smile that was that of a child who comes suddenly out of a chill, lonely darkness into beloved, sheltering arms, he whispered, *"Gosh,* Mom—I was scared! . . ."
> Shirley held his head against her breast, and talked to him in a soft murmur that was unspeakably soothing to the boy's tortured nerves.[39]

This maternalistic image persisted through the 1950s and into the 1960s. In *Nurses Marry Doctors,* after working her daytime shift in the hospital, Linda sits up until 3 A.M. with a feverish child at the orphanage. In response to a doctor's criticism of her effort ("Linda, you can't look after the whole world, you know"), she says, "Nurses have an obligation to help out wherever they can." Kathie of *Noonday Nurse* thinks of all men as children, particularly her special patient, "a long, torn body who needed her as a child needs its mother," and at whom she smiled "as if he were a child."[40]

THE NURSE ROMANCE FORMULA

A choice between two or more suitors is perhaps the most frequent overall component of the romance genre, but where there is only one suitor, a triangle is still formed because the suitor (a) thinks the nurse has another suitor and is jealous of his presumed rival or rivals, (b) has another romantic involvement himself, or (c) is being pursued by another woman. Female rivalry is thus a frequent conflict.

A more serious conflict is the man's hostility toward the nurse, resulting from a general dislike or mistrust of women and misunderstandings about the nurse's character, her affections, or her social position. Like Julian of *Nurses Marry Doctors,* the man is often reluctant to become involved emotionally and afraid of marriage. He may disguise this insecurity with an outward cloak of gruffness, rudeness, or indifference, like Dr. Belmont of *Nurse Atholl Returns,* who says, "My facade of indifference was my armour against you!"[41] This misogynistic attitude may arise from an unhappy childhood, as in the case of Dr. Curt, "this brusque, dynamic, hot-tempered martinet of a surgeon," or from disappointment in love that has led to cynicism, as in the case of Rick, who tells Shirley he does not like women and fears marriage.

> "I've known women all my life, women on the stage and women 'on the outside.' And I don't seem to care a lot for any of 'em. The way they lie to each other, and chisel—the way they snag each other's men—the way they fall on each other's necks and chortle, with every evidence of undying affection, *'darling!'*—and then the minute 'darling's' back is turned, out comes a stiletto!" *(Nurse With Wings).*[42]

Dishonesty, competitiveness, hypocrisy, and affectation characterize the nurse's rival. The nurse herself sometimes resorts to subterfuge to catch the elusive male, as when Janet pursues Peter by becoming a nurse on his cruise, but such feminine wiles stop short of unscrupulousness. Romances portray a traditional kind of courtship—hence the archaic word *suitor*—in which the nurse must at least appear to be passive and allow men to do the pursuing. As Genie explains, "The poor dears go around believing it is they who do the chasing—when any girl knows that if she really wants a man, she has to run him down and brand him." *(The Courtship of Nurse Genie).*[43]

Relative independence and a spirit of adventure are usually associated with the nursing role at the beginning of the novel. Often orphaned, jilted, or relocated, the nurse is devoted to her work, concerned for her patients, wary of men, and courageous in dangerous situations. Nevertheless, this independence is partly illusory, since a physician or father figure often chooses the nurse's mission or facilitates it. For example, in *Nurse on Pondre Island,* Dr. MacDonald contrives to get Lorina away from an overly dependent mother by ensuring that she accepts a patient's offer of a new assignment.[44]

The nurse gradually loses this initial aura of independence in the ensuing series of conflicts and crises. Her vulnerability becomes increasingly evident as she is victimized to further other people's plots. The nurse's strong sense of duty, altruism, loyalty, and also her innocence make her the scapegoat in matrimonial or political schemes. A transformation from "nurse into woman" takes place, and the supposedly irrepressible feminine nature emerges from beneath the nurse's cool, calm facade.

> "When my father and mother died, I promised myself to be a nurse and help the suffering of others. You knew that. I didn't tell you I'd resolved never to marry, never to have a child—and suffer through what I loved. You say I'm a good nurse—I'll stay one! I'm not going to be a woman!"
> Her voice had risen to an almost hysterical pitch, her hands were knotted into fists. He seized them in his own, shook them. . . .
> The old nursing habit of obedience to a physician's authority held. . . .
> Tears ran down the anguished face . . . *(Nurse Into Woman).*[45]

Similarly, when Pamela gives way to tears in *The Nurse Had a Secret* because she had trusted the wrong man, she says, "I guess I'm crying, mostly, because I'm a woman. A nurse is never supposed to cry, you know."[46]

The crisis is the event that sets the heroine up to be rescued by the man she will marry, casting him in a gallant and protective role. It also provides the explanations or other evidence needed to resolve mysteries and misunderstandings about who loves whom.

Masochism may motivate the nurse to allow misunderstandings to exist when she could have clarified them earlier. This occurs where the battle between the sexes has been particularly fierce, with the result that the nurse feels helpless and thinks it hopeless to try to redeem herself. For example, in *Nurse Atholl Returns,* Dr. Belmont refuses to allow Lyn to serve temporarily as head nurse in the operating room because he thinks she has had no experience there. She had not corrected his initial misunderstanding and allows him to persist in it, and so she is humiliated in front of others.[47]

A dramatic crisis, developing a conflict between two suitors or a romantic relationship between the nurse and a suitor, is often an illness or injury of the nurse, suitor, or another character. Denise in *Wilder-*

ness Nurse sustains a serious injury to her ankle while on duty, and, facing possible amputation of her foot, has her future fiancé called in to consult. Kathie of *Noonday Nurse* faints into Dr. Fosdike's arms. In *Nurse Atholl Returns* the nurse is cared for by Dr. Fosdike after being bitten by a dog, and finally falls ill with a virus after breaking her engagement to Fosdike. The nurturing roles are momentarily reversed when her former patient, Larry, comes to claim her as his wife. Elizabeth of *A Doctor for the Nurse* breaks her wrist, re-injures it, catches a cold, and is bruised by a half-crazed suitor; each time Dr. Galland (read "Gallant") rescues her.[48]

The crisis may also be a natural disaster (an earthquake in *Nurse in Acapulco*), an act of war (the air raid in *Nurse with Wings*), an accident (the train crash in *Nurse Atholl Returns*), or any of various mysterious or dangerous situations that threaten the nurse's life, career, or love. *Navy Nurse* is a classic example of reversal: Alice is rescued by Morgan, from whom she learns that her French fiancé is a spy; she then has the opportunity to nurse Morgan through the trauma of a head wound, and he becomes her fiancé. *The Nurse Had a Secret* uses the same formula: Pamela is in love with an author who turns out to be a Communist spy and is watched over by the chauffeur, actually an FBI agent, who then becomes her fiancé.[49]

Many of these plot mechanisms—orphaning, jilting, flight from the past, victimization, misunderstanding, masochism, various kinds of crises and rescues—put the nurse in a vulnerable, dependent, and submissive role, restricting her competence to provide comfort, aid, and support. With respect to physicians, suitors, fiancé, and husband, she is the child to be commanded, rescued, protected, and nurtured (although often more in a material than in an emotional sense). In this way, nurse romances play on the fears of their readers, exploiting insecurity about the fulfillment of basic needs such as safety, love, and esteem.

Multiple engagements are often used in nurse romances in order to reinforce the marital imperative and tie up loose ends by providing mates for deserving friends, roommates, siblings, or former suitors and fiancé(s). *Lab Nurse* carries such coincidence to absurd extremes by having triplets—Faith, Hope, and Charity—all nurses in the same hospital, become engaged to three physicians. A fourth nurse, the nasty rival ironically named Felicity, is left out,

along with her scheming sister Caroline, a patient. Thus the nurse romance usually punishes the "other woman" and makes ambition seem not just selfish but evil, while the self-sacrificing, dutiful, obedient, altruistic, and loyal nurse is rewarded for not being self-seeking.[50]

Reference is rarely made to the education of the nurse, except when she is a student, and even then she is not shown attending classes or receiving instruction. In the majority of cases, it would be impossible to tell whether the nurse has graduated from a diploma program, a junior college, or a baccalaureate program. Instead, it is often assumed that the nurse was born with the capacity to give "a woman's tender care" (cover of *Nurses' Quarters*), which is seen as an intrinsic part of her feminine role. Nursing is thus depicted as a lifelong vocation by Melanie, who says: "I've wanted to be a nurse ever since I was five or six years old. . . . I entered it [nursing] because I wanted to help people, because I felt a calling. Ever since I bandaged my first doll, I've wanted to be a nurse." (*A Challenge for Nurse Melanie*). In other books, the childhood dream of becoming a nurse is fed by emulation of another person: the nurse's father in *Florida Nurse,* or an older nurse who had saved her father's life in *A Challenge for Nurse Melanie, Nurse Dawn's Discovery, Seacliff Nurse, Student Nurse,* and *The Two Faces of Nurse Roberts.*[51]

An understanding of the image of physicians in these romance novels is essential if one is to fully comprehend the roles played by nurses. The doctor is most often a surgeon, since this is the most prestigious specialty. In the romance novels' descriptions of doctors, "brilliant" comes behind only "young" and "handsome," adjectives whose prevalence is mirrored in the usual description of nurses as "young" and "beautiful" (or "lovely" or "pretty"); the formula "brilliant" (or "gifted," "talented," "promising," "intelligent") is a cliché that is, nevertheless, full of meaning. Doctors are "awesome symbols of medical authority," to quote the cover of *Doctors' Passions,* and intelligence and exceptional skill give them the right to this authority.[52]

Nurse characterizations give the overwhelming impression, on the other hand, that intelligence is not an essential quality in a nurse. Instead, good nurses are "capable," "competent," "skilled," "disciplined," "efficient," and so on. And while many doctors are described on the book jackets as "dedicated" and "hard-working," many more nurses are described as "devoted," "dedicated," "selfless," "unselfish," and "hard-working." That self-sacrifice and concern for others are viewed as essential qualities of nurses is also reflected in descriptions such as "warm," "warm-hearted," "sensitive," "sympathetic," "compassionate," and "concerned."

Traditional symbols of nursing are strongly emphasized. For example, the book covers almost invariably depict a nurse in full uniform with a cap, although nurses of this period did not generally go out of hospitals, clinics, or offices in uniform. Yet the background is frequently not the nurse's place of work, but an exotic backdrop, a gothic mansion, or some other plot-related setting. The cover nurse is most often shown with a man lurking in the background or at her side, dominating her image.

An examination of the covers of 791 paperback novels with major nurse characters revealed that (1) all of the illustrations emphasize at least one nurse character who is young and attractive, and (2) most of the illustrations (79 percent) place nurse characters in situations that are obviously romantic. Of the cover illustrations that promise a romantic story, 28 percent show a nurse in a health care setting. Of these, 25 percent show a nurse engaged in some kind of nursing activity (including holding a clipboard or a medical bag). The remaining 47 percent place the nurse in distinctly non-health care setting (for example, a field of daisies, a nautical setting, or running terrified from a dark, gothic sort of house). Of the 648 covers showing another individual or other people, 41 percent show a nurse with another character who is recognizably a doctor, 12 percent show a nurse with a doctor and at least one other character who is not a patient, and 3 percent show a nurse with a doctor and a patient; so the romantic value of physicians figures into more than half of the nurse romance cover illustrations.

NURSES ON EARLY TELEVISION

Though television had been reported as being "just around the corner" all through the 1930s, large scale production had to wait until the end of the war. The number of sets produced annually jumped from 7,500 in 1946 to 6.5 million by 1950. As of January 1, 1951, an estimated 10.5 million TV sets were in use

in 63 distinct areas served by broadcasters. Almost 40 percent of the families in these areas had sets. By the end of 1951 an estimated 15 million sets were in use. Almost 20 million, or about 46 percent, of all homes had television sets by January 1953. In 1955 there were 32 million sets, and by 1956 Americans had spent $15.6 billion on sets and repairs. In 1950 junior high school students were viewing an average of 30 hours of TV each week. By 1954 the average family watched four to five hours a day. By 1959, 44.7 million families, representing 87 percent of the nation's population, had at least one television set. The introduction of the coaxial cable that linked the east and west coasts soon effectively reduced the entire population to a single audience.

In the 1950s nurse characters largely projected either a wholesome girl-next-door profile or else, for older nurse characters, benign, motherly traits. For example, Miss Nancy Remington, the school nurse on *Mr. Peepers* (NBC, 1952–1955), lived with her parents until her marriage to the series' star, mild-mannered Robinson Peepers, a high school biology teacher. Almost no attention was given to Nancy's work as a nurse; her place in the series was determined by her status as sweetheart and later bride of Mr. Peepers. Although nursing per se received little mention, for good or ill, at least the character of Miss Remington deserved the respect of the audience— she was considered to be a fine young woman, eminently worthy of marriage to the protagonist.[53]

Janet Dean, Registered Nurse (syndicated), appearing in 1954 and starring Ella Raines, presented the life and work of an unmarried, attractive woman in her early 30s. She had been a military nurse during the war, but began practicing as a private-duty nurse for a New York agency after the war. Janet was not portrayed as a romantic figure in any of the episodes—unlike other TV nurses of the 1950s. Often she appeared as the savior and protector of the weak, in near-heroic situations. Her greatest nursing skill was her ability to identify psychological problems and handicaps that contribute to a patient's negative health status. Her efforts to help her patients often caused her to become involved in family conflicts. For example, when she nursed a small boy she discovered that part of his difficulties stemmed from over-protective parents.

The most frequent theme found Janet in a criminal or disaster-type situation calling for extraordinary bravery or solutions. For example, she agreed to enter an elevator caught between floors and hanging by a thin cable in order to treat the injured within. In another instance, she faced a bank robber determined to kill the only eyewitness to his crime, who happened to be Janet's patient. Critics noted with surprise that Janet often applied her psychological treatments "with or without the doctor's approval or help." One critic felt that Miss Dean was both "attractive and competent" but was particularly appealing in those episodes in which she was "still busy being a nurse and had not yet gotten around to the more Freudian aspects of the case." Although nursing skills infrequently received attention, the nurse character clearly emerged as a dynamic woman, a problem solver, and an individual of initiative.[54]

The 1950s also saw the first important medical drama—*Medic* (NBC, 1954–1956), a 30-minute anthology on health care themes. Although the cast of characters changed from week to week, the philosophy of the show remained the same: physicians were the priests and heroes of American society. They always demonstrated wisdom, skill, kindness, humanitarianism, and selfless dedication to the needs of others. Nurses invariably appeared as weaker, less objective, and less skilled appendages of the medical profession—admirable for their gentleness and loyalty perhaps, but definitely of limited use without a physician's supervision.

Medic was a well-written and highly realistic series that starred Richard Boone as the host-narrator, Dr. Konrad Styner. Dedicated to the profession of medicine, the series emphasized the role of the physician as "Guardian of Birth, Healer of the Sick, Comforter of the Aged." Within the series' dramatic and documentary style, the writers sought to teach and occasionally shock viewers into becoming knowledgeable about their health and safety. The profession of nursing never received much attention, with nurses generally serving as willing handmaidens to the doctors. The producers prided themselves on their accuracy and research, yet rarely explored the role of modern nursing in the hospital—although they often hired genuine registered nurses to appear in the films. The attention to realistic detail caused the downfall of the series. In a rare episode about nursing, for example, the narrative included the depiction of a cesarean delivery; network censors and the sponsors found this objectionable and unfitting for public consump-

tion and decided not to renew the series for a third season. Interestingly, episodes that included graphic scenes of surgical procedures and clinical discussions of sterility, menopause, and teenage acne passed the censors' criteria for good taste and decency.

The series paid homage to the nursing profession in an episode entitled "The Glorious Red Gallegher," the airing of which coincided with the hundredth anniversary of the birth of modern nursing. This episode, which contained the offensive scenes of a cesarean delivery, used the story of a 61-year-old nurse facing retirement to represent her profession. This nurse had dedicated her life to the treatment of the sick, especially of new mothers and their babies. She personified the virtues of motherhood, self-sacrifice, compassion, generosity, and dedication—the classic qualities associated with nursing. The show did not emphasize her judgment, intelligence, or leadership. Another episode, "Mercy Wears an Apron," departed from the standard presentation of the nurse as an appendage of the physician. In this episode, a public health nurse successfully engineered the rehabilitation of a paraplegic who was close to becoming an alcoholic. Unlike other episodes of the series, this one featured a nurse acting autonomously and actively contributing to a patient's improvement.

Perhaps the most representative episode from the series, with regard to the image of nursing, was "A Flash of Darkness," a dramatization of the events in a first-aid station in the 24 hours following a nuclear attack on the United States. Dr. Konrad Styner and his office nurse, Miss Mitchell, joined a first-aid team that included a dentist, a pharmacist, and a nurse's aide. Radio broadcasts done by Charles Collingwood reported the breakdown of public order and mounting casualties. Throughout the emergency, Miss Mitchell, replete in white uniform and cap, stood patiently at Styner's side waiting to be told what to do. Although the woman was portrayed as an experienced and trusted nurse, in this time of national disaster her dependent, traditional relationship to the physician never wavered. With the holding room filling with injured, Miss Mitchell was not even allowed to make a preliminary assessment of the patients or to treat minor wounds on her own authority. Toward the end of the episode, Styner phoned for replacement nurses. "These girls can't stay on their feet .

much longer—it's been nearly 24 hours." Of course he uttered not a word to indicate his own exhaustion. Later Miss Mitchell did suggest, "I guess we can make it if you can."[55]

Thus the show's creators intended for the viewer to appreciate and sympathize with the nursing characters—they were good women who worked hard in the service of others. But the nurses never, with the exception of a public health nurse, appeared as decisive, active contributors to patient welfare. A nurse's true value depended on her obedience to a doctor and her degree of self-sacrifice.

Dr. Hudson's Secret Journal (syndicated, 1955–1957) included moral lessons and miraculous character transformations in every episode. The tone of the series was unmistakably derived from its source, the inspirational novel written by Lloyd C. Douglas, an author popular in the 1940s. The protagonist of the series, Dr. Wayne Hudson, a brilliant surgeon, held that the secret of success in life was to do good secretly, as Jesus taught. To this end, Hudson maintained a secret journal in which he recorded instances of having helped others. The format of each show never varied: the opening scene would depict Hudson, late at night, pondering an incident in his past and taking pen in hand to describe it in his journal; then the incident itself would be shown; the final scene always showed Hudson closing the notebook and replacing it in his safe.

The pace of *Dr. Hudson* differed noticeably from more recent medical drama. The setting lacked the hustle and bustle associated with hospital routine; Center Hospital seemed a sleepy, small-town institution where staff and patients were well-acquainted with each other. Hudson, the chief of staff, assumed a paternal role toward both staff and patients. Medical crises did occur often, but the medical intervention usually took place off camera: the fancy electronic equipment so beloved of 1970s TV medicine and the sweaty atmosphere of the operating room never appeared on *Dr. Hudson*. Dramatic tension arose, usually, from the development of a character who had obviously gone off course in life and needed the guiding hand of Wayne Hudson. Wayward sons and daughters, erring parents, and troubled doctors and nurses were frequently brought back within the fold by Hudson's persuasive power. Given this predominantly psychological and didactic tendency of the show, scenes of intensive patient care rarely appeared, and thus there was little opportunity for decisive or important nursing contributions to patient care. In general, nursing activities were limited to providing comfort measures to the patient, bringing food trays, and administering medications.

The most important nurse character of the series, Ann Talbot (Frances Mercer), appeared to be the perfect nurse and ideal woman. Although she was occasionally referred to as the superintendent of nurses, in fact she was Dr. Hudson's personal assistant. Her virtues were legion: patient, discreet, attractive, competent, loyal, and devoted to Dr. Hudson. Yet she was no mere rubber stamp, and often she offered opinions contrary to Dr. Hudson's and corrected some of his temperamental excesses. Her involvement with patients was infrequent; most of her appearances occurred in Hudson's office, where she typed his lectures, arranged his calendar, and listened to his problems. Hudson considered her his confidante and trusted her with sensitive information about himself and his patients. The show definitely intended that Ann Talbot be considered integral to Hudson's success.

In addition to her official duties at the hospital, Ann assumed the role of surrogate mother to Hudson's motherless daughter, Kathy. One episode told of Kathy's efforts to engineer her father's marriage to Ann. Ann loved Hudson, but some unknown reason prevented him from marrying her. They must have arrived at some mutually satisfying understanding, however, because Ann seemed quite content with her limited role in Hudson's life.

Another recurring nurse character, Tacky Schultz (Blossom Rock), operated the hospital switchboard and relayed information to passers-by. A slightly comic figure, Tacky relieved the heavily sincere and serious tone of the show. In addition to the gossipy Tacky, young and pretty nurse Hakopian appeared in several episodes. A vivacious, dark-haired woman, Hakopian projected girlish innocence and became tongue-tied when asked direct questions by her superiors. Furthermore, she took great liberties with her role as a nurse, intruding her personal opinions into patients' concerns and drafting patients to help her in certain plans. Despite her tendency to meddle, she remained a well-liked and delightful character. Once she managed to parlay some of her inside information into a diamond bracelet and a fur coat

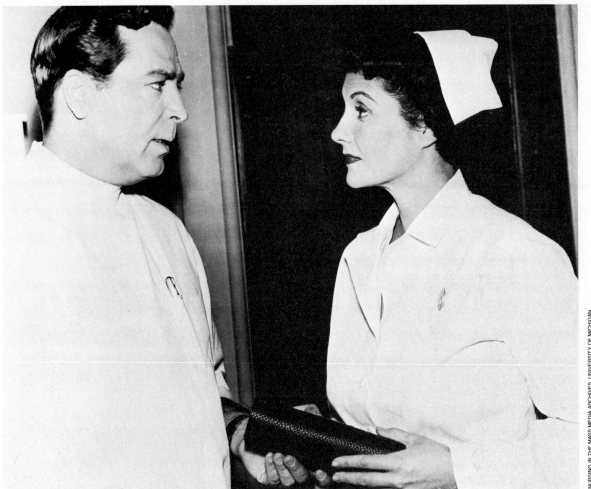

John Howard and Frances Mercer starred as Dr. Wayne Hudson and his faithful nurse Ann Talbot in the television series Dr. Hudson's Secret Journal. *Ann's role in Dr. Hudson's life was to serve as both his professional and personal confidante. Often she served an almost wife-like role, helping with his motherless daughter and giving him a woman's point of view in professional matters.*

from two well-heeled hospital philanthropists. But her wheeling and dealing were deemed matters of womanly wiles rather than questions of professional ethics. Hakopian's last appearance, in "Love in White Shoes," depicted her great romantic frustrations; already an old maid at the age of 23, she decides to campaign avidly to capture the heart of a newly arrived English doctor. After many ups and downs, she gets her man and promises him she'll stay out of the hospital—except to have babies.

A more serious view of a nurse character occurs in "The Livingston Story," in which a middle-aged and grouchy head nurse appears determined to avoid any possible opportunity for friendship. She is a demanding and tyrannical woman, and most staff members feel that she is jealous of the pretty, younger nurses. When Hudson undergoes knee surgery, he has the chance to know her better, but she treats him with the same coldness and insistence upon hospital rules and regulations that she uses for all the staff and patients. In the unfolding of the story, however, it becomes obvious that Livingston is the only nurse who keeps the patient's best interest to the fore at all times. Ann, Hakopian, other doctors and nurses, and Hudson's daughter, in their eagerness to comfort and cheer him, tax his strength with their enthusiasm and cause discomfort by sitting on his bed. Hudson thanks Livingston when she rudely throws everyone out of his room but asks why she had to be so antagonistic. She tells him that in her youth, engaged to a young doctor, she made a terrible mistake in judgment. While nursing her fiancé, he suffered an attack for which he ordered her to administer a drug to him. The injection killed the young man, and Livingston has never forgotten the price of one lapse from hospital procedure. She never should have let a patient, not even a doctor, determine his own care. After a sincere chat with Dr. Hudson, Livingston emerges a changed woman, ready to meet the world on easier terms.

Romantic disappointments and worries did color the personalities of the nurses at Center Hospital. Ann, an admirable and mature woman, settled for a limited relationship with her beloved Dr. Hudson. Hakopian, unsettled by her lack of a mate, set the hospital into turmoil in her search. And Livingston carried a deep and private grief with her for years. Yet the nurses were not simply romantic objects in the series. They provided valuable and appreciated services. Hudson defended Hakopian as a fine nurse, with a special talent for nursing the gravely ill, those on whom Hudson had given up hope. Livingston, although unpopular, made herself the guardian of the patient's welfare. And Ann was seen as a valuable aide to Dr. Hudson, clearly respected by other staff members and by patients; he included her in all his important conferences and discussions.[56]

A few years later, Addy Dalton played nurse Martha Hale, a naval lieutenant, in the comedy *Hennessey* (CBS, 1959-1962). Martha also exuded a clean-cut, wholesome girlishness and enjoyed a long-standing romance with the series' hero, Chick Hennessey, a naval physician; and her romance was also rewarded with marriage in the last year of the series. Martha's main traits arose from her position as female antagonist in the 1950s "battle of the sexes" themes so prevalent in situation comedy: Martha was illogical, gossipy, subject to frequent changes of heart, but intuitive and successful in dealing with people. Martha Hale was a sympathetic, admirable female

character but hardly notable for her intelligence, ambition, or professional expertise.[57]

NURSES IN TV MEDICAL DRAMAS OF THE EARLY-1960s

The early-1960s witnessed the spectacular success of several health care dramas. The introduction and immediate success of two series—*Ben Casey* and *Dr. Kildare*—prompted public attention and enthusiasm similar to the publicity that would surround *Dallas* a generation later. James Moser, who created and wrote *Medic,* introduced *Ben Casey* on ABC in 1961, and this series ran until 1966. The program became an immediate hit because of the instant popularity of Vince Edwards (who played Ben Casey) with adolescent girls. A national mania for things medical ensued, and "Ben Casey shirts" became items of popular fashion. Moser retained both his reverence for the medical profession and his disregard for the contributions of nurses. What Moser did *not* transfer from his *Medic* days was dramatic credibility. Instead of balanced, honest presentations of health care situations, *Ben Casey* opted for melodramatic, often farcical accounts of how Ben snatched yet another patient from the jaws of death.

Because of the series' preoccupation with the surly neurosurgeon, the writers largely underplayed the roles of nurses. Nurses rarely took a major role in the dramatic narrative, and if they did, they never contributed to the patient's recovery. They performed tasks involving minimal skill and no judgment. Nurses were not even deemed worthy of a romantic fling with Ben, who dated his share of other professional women. One episode included a pretty nurse hopelessly in love with her physician employer; he explained why he would not marry her:

> I was married to a nurse, just like you. And she was a romantic dreamer, just like you. Sure. They say it's good for a doctor to marry a nurse because she understands what a difficult life a doctor has. . . . She's supposed to understand the long hours and the failure and the death. . . . Well, that's unadulterated bunk.[58]

Thus an entire profession was dismissed as a group of romantic dreamers, judged unworthy of its divine mission: the provision of suitable wives for doctors. When nurse characters developed serious problems they always turned to a physician for relief rather than to another nurse. One such character, an unmarried, 40-year-old, pregnant nurse, played by Shelley Winters, not only received obstetrical care from the two neurosurgeons, doctors Casey and Zorba, but also turned to them for emotional support rather than to any of her nurse colleagues.

The only continuing nurse character on *Ben Casey* was Miss Wills. She appeared in nearly every episode for 5 years, yet the viewer never knew if she had a first name. She always wore her uniform, even when off duty among other staff members in street clothing. Colorless Miss Wills smiled but never laughed, frowned but never lost her temper, and through it all she answered the phone and delivered messages in a most professional manner.[59]

NBC's entry into the health care trend of the 1960s came in the boyishly charming package of one Dr. James Kildare, portrayed by Richard Chamberlain. *Dr. Kildare,* which also ran from 1961 through 1966, had its origins in the MGM feature films that had achieved great popularity in the late-1930s and early-1940s. The theme was the trials and tribulations of an inexperienced yet idealistic young doctor who depended for advice and wisdom on an older, kindly physician, Dr. Gillespie. *Dr. Kildare* avoided the heavy-handed depiction of a self-righteous medical crusader in the Ben Casey style, but did present the physician-protagonist in glowing, near reverent terms. Jim Kildare, for all his inexperience, was no less heroic than the brooding Ben.

Nurses sometimes appeared in the series as romantic foils for young physicians, and in the final season Head Nurse Zoe Lawton, played by pretty and pert Lee Kurty, became a regular cast member and Kildare's permanent love interest. Occasionally writers did cast sympathetic nurse characters in featured roles—a nurse trying to send her brother to medical school, a nurse coping with a grouchy patient, a nurse recovering from drug addiction, a nurse facing a difficult pregnancy, and so forth. But in all these cases the nurses had to turn to physicians for the resolution of their personal problems.

The professional responsibilities of the nurses of *Dr. Kildare* were similar to those shown on *Ben Casey*—delivering messages, carrying trays, and taking orders. Although *Dr. Kildare* presented more nurse characters, the series was no better than its rival in portraying nurses as decisive, strong individuals or even problem solvers. Often the physicians, including the polite and sensitive Dr. Kildaire, took a

condescending attitude toward the nurses, indicating the physician's superior intelligence or sophistication. When female physicians or medical students appeared, they routinely looked smarter than the nurses; that is, female physicians wore glasses to indicate their education and affected no-nonsense hair styles to indicate their seriousness. Most of the nurses were either young and pretty or old and prim. Nurses never appeared as married women with families; they were either unmarried young women who would undoubtedly quit the profession upon marriage, or else they were older and unmarried—widowed, divorced, or never married—women who had nothing else to do.[60]

Despite the negative images of nursing from these two physician-dominated hit series, the 1960s did offer the highest point for the TV image of the nurse to date. This high point came in CBS's entry into the health care drama competition, an hour-long drama devoted to the nursing profession called *The Nurses* (CBS, 1962–1964). *The Nurses* lasted two seasons before being transformed in its third year to a more conventional physician-dominated format called *The Doctors and The Nurses* (1964–1965). Thanks to producer Herbert Brodkin's commitment to realism and good writing, nurses and nursing emerged in a positive but not exaggerated light. Most of the nurse characters demonstrated balanced, well-rounded personalities. Good nurses had human frailties, and troubled nurses usually had redeeming virtues or extenuating circumstances to mitigate their negative traits.

The character of Liz Thorpe, portrayed by Shirl Conway, was the single best image of the professional nurse in television history. Liz Thorpe, the head nurse in a busy New York hospital, proved to be objective, articulate, disciplined, and concerned with the professional development of herself and her colleagues. More than any other series, *The Nurses* demonstrated the existence of nursing standards and organization: the nurses appeared responsible for their own internal discipline and for defending their rights and privileges. When nurses developed personal and professional problems, they sought advice and help from other nurse characters rather than from physician characters. Most important, the nurses in this series were problem solvers. Rather than waiting for a physician to arrive on the scene and deliver an order, nurses identified problems and found solutions themselves.[61]

NOTES

1. David Reisman, *The Lonely Crowd* (New Haven: Yale University Press, 1950).

2. "A New Look at the American Woman," *Look* 20 (October 16, 1956):35–37.

3. Abbott C. Jones, "Clairol: Quiet Revolution," *Advertising Age* 51 (January 26, 1981):47–48.

4. *Gentlemen Prefer Blondes* (20th Century-Fox, 1953), 91 min. Based on Joseph Fields's and Anita Loos's musical comedy, it was the second highest grossing movie of 1953.

5. L. Baudler and D. G. Patterson, "Social Satus of Women's Occupations," *Occupations* 26 (1948): 421–424.

6. American Nurses' Association, *Facts About Nursing, 1952* (New York: The Association, 1953), pp. 17 and 48.

7. American Nurses' Association, *Facts About Nursing, 1950* (New York: The Association, 1951), pp. 67–71.

8. *The Men* (United Artists, 1950), B & W, 86 min.

9. *Homecoming* (Metro-Goldwyn-Mayer, 1947), B & W, 113 min.

10. *The Hasty Heart* (Warner Brothers, 1949), B & W, 99 min.

11. Ibid.

12. Ibid.

13. *Pinky* (20th Century-Fox, 1949), B & W, 102 min.

14. *The Snake Pit* (20th Century-Fox, 1948), B & W, 108 min.

15. Ibid.

16. Ibid.

17. Ibid.

18. Ibid.

19. P. Kalisch and B. Kalisch, "The Image of Psychiatric Nurses in Motion Pictures," *Perspectives in Psychiatric Care* 19 (1981):116–129.

20. *Fear Strikes Out* (Paramount, 1957), B & W, 100 min.

21. *The Interns* (Columbia, 1962), B & W, 120 min.

22. Ibid.

23. *Battle Circus* (Metro-Goldwyn-Mayer, 1953), B & W, 90 min.

24. *South Pacific* (20th Century-Fox, 1958), 161 min.

25. Ibid.

26. *Captain Newman, M.D.* (Universal, 1963), 126 min.

27. Jeanne Bowman, *Nurse on Pondre Island* (New York: Arcadia House, 1965), p. 120.

28. Marguerite Mooers Marshall, *Wilderness Nurse* (New York: Pocket Books, 1949), p. 228; Kathleen Harris, *Jane Arden: Head Nurse* (New York: Popular Library, 1959), p. 124.

29. Rona Randall, *Nurse Stacey Comes Aboard* (New York: Ace Books, 1958), pp. 157–158.

30. Maud McCurdy Welch, *Nurses Marry Doctors* (New York: Airmont Publishing Company, 1956); Jane Converse, *Nurse in Acapulco* (New York: New American Library, 1964); Marguerite Mooers Marshall, *Nurse Into Woman* (New York: Triangle Books, 1951); Harris, *Jane Arden: Head Nurse,* p. 106.

31. Peggy Gaddis, *The Courtship of Nurse Genie Hayes* (New York: McFadden Books, 1960), p. 127.

32. Ray Dorien, *Noonday Nurse* (New York: Arcadia House, 1957), p. 117.

33. Peggy Dern, *Leona Gregory, R.N.* (New York: Arcadia House, 1961), p. 122.

34. Rosamund Hung, *Nurse Martin's Dilemma* (New York:

Thomas Bouregy and Company, 1961); Marshall, *Wilderness Nurse,* p. 228.

35. Adelaide Humphries, *The Nurse Had A Secret* (New York: Bantam Books, 1960).

36. Adelaide Humphries, *Nurse Landon's Challenge* (New York: Bantam Books, 1952); Welch, *Nurses Marry Doctors,* p. 106.

37. Converse, *Nurse in Acapulco,* p. 93; Georgia Craig, *A Nurse Comes Home* (New York: Arcadia House, 1963); Arlene Hale, *Nurse Shelley Decides* (New York: Pyramid Publications, 1964); Converse, *Nurse in Acapulco,* p. 88.

38. Jane Arbor, *Nurse Atholl Returns* (New York: Harlequin Books, 1952).

39. Marguerite Mooers Marshall, *Nurse With Wings* (New York: Bantam Books, 1952).

40. Welch, *Nurses Marry Doctors,* p. 37; Dorien, *Noonday Nurse,* p. 51.

41. Welch, *Nurses Marry Doctors,* p. 81; Arbor, *Nurse Atholl Returns,* p. 29.

42. Marshall, *Nurse With Wings,* p. 49.

43. Gaddis, *The Courtship of Nurse Genie Hayes,* p. 20.

44. Bowman, *Nurse on Pondre Island,* p. 30.

45. Marshall, *Nurse Into Woman,* p. 27.

46. Humphries, *The Nurse Had a Secret,* p. 105.

47. Arbor, *Nurse Atholl Returns,* p. 60.

48. Marshall, *Wilderness Nurse,* p. 37; Dorien, *Noonday Nurse,* p. 117; Arbor, *Nurse Atholl Returns,* p. 111; Jeanne Judson, *A Doctor for the Nurse* (New York: Avalon Books, 1954).

49. Sears, *Nurse in Acapulco,* p. 31; Marshall, *Nurse with Wings,* p. 74; Arbor, *Nurse Atholl Returns,* p. 40; Rosie Banks, *Navy Nurse* (New York: Permabooks, 1960); Humphries, *The Nurse Had a Secret,* p. 51.

50. Randall, *Lab Nurse,* p. 86.

51. R. V. Cassill, *Nurses' Quarters* (New York: Fawcett Books, 1961); Isobel Moore, *A Challenge for Nurse Melanie* (Sydney, Australia: Star Books, 1961), p. 38; Peggy Dern, *Florida Nurse* (New York: Arcadia House, 1961); Iris Barry, *Nurse Dawn's Discovery* (New York: Monarch Books, 1964); Peggy O'More, *Seacliff Nurse* (New York: Arcadia House, 1966); Gail Jordan, *Student Nurse* (New York: Universal Publishing and Distributing Corp., 1950); Nora Sanderson, *The Two Faces of Nurse Roberts* (New York: Harlequin Books, 1963).

52. Adrian Gray, *Doctor's Passions* (New York: New American Library, 1975).

53. *Mr. Peepers* (30 minutes, Situation Comedy) NBC, July 3, 1952, to June 12, 1955, 96 episodes.

54. *Janet Dean, Registered Nurse* (30 minutes, Nursing Drama) syndicated, 1953 to 1955, 39 episodes.

55. *Medic* (30 minutes, Medical Drama) NBC, September 1954 to November 1956, 60 episodes.

56. *Dr. Hudson's Secret Journal* (30 minutes, Medical Drama) syndicated, 1955 to 1957, 78 episodes.

57. *Hennesey* (30 minutes, Comedy/Drama) CBS, September 28, 1959, to September 17, 1962, 92 episodes.

58. *Ben Casey* (60 minutes, Medical Drama) ABC, October 2, 1961, to March 21, 1966, 153 episodes.

59. Ibid.

60. *Dr. Kildare* (60 minutes, Medical Drama) NBC, September 27, 1961, to August 29, 1966, 190 episodes.

61. *The Nurses (The Doctors and The Nurses)* (60 minutes, Nursing/Medical Drama) CBS, September 27, 1962, to September 17, 1964; as *The Doctors and The Nurses* September 22, 1964, to September 7, 1965, 103 episodes.

CHAPTER EIGHT

SEX OBJECT: MID-SIXTIES TO THE PRESENT

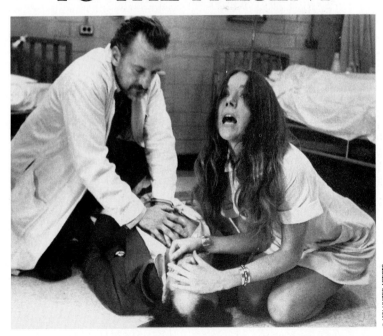

As the image of the nurse as devoted wife and mother declined in the mid-1960s, the vacuum that it left was filled by the most negative media image since Dickens's Sairy Gamp—the nurse as a sex object. During the late-1950s and early-1960s developments were underway that were to burgeon, in a very few years, into a veritable social upheaval. Work for married female nurses had clearly come to stay and as more and more educated nurses experienced the tensions of their complicated dual roles or the frustrations of staying at home, it became evident that this was not simply an individual female dilemma but a widespread social problem.

THE KINSEY REPORT

The acceptance of birth control allowed for the possibility of nonreproductive sexuality within marriage. And Dr. Alfred Kinsey's second report, *The Sexual Behavior of the Human Female* (or the K-bomb, as it was known by the media), forcefully challenged the myth that women did not or could not enjoy sex. As bombshells went, it outclassed Dr. Kinsey's previous findings about males. The sexual behavior referred to turned out to be sexual misbehavior by the standards of the time—and on a widespread scale. Half of the 6,000 women questioned admitted to having intercourse before marriage and a quarter of them to adulterous intercourse after marriage. Pious shock and horror was expressed at this frailty in the face of temptation—far more so than at the evidence that men behaved in the same way. But the really challenging upshot of the report was not this predictable hypocrisy. It was the reaction to the evidence that women were the equals—if not more than the equals—of men in sexual responsiveness and capacity. The established (and now published) fact that women's sexual capacity increases with age and stays at a peak for decades, while men's declines from adolescence on, came as a shock both to men, who suddenly discovered they were the unlucky sex, and to women, who had not realized what they had been missing.[1]

Kinsey and his colleagues had also broken a taboo by openly discussing the female orgasm, a subject still shrouded in misinformation. His finding was that the capacity to experience it was much more highly developed in wives who had indulged in intercourse before marriage than in those who had remained chaste. The report also found that a lot of sexual incompatability and discontent existed. Two thirds of the marriages investigated experienced at least occasional sexual dissatisfaction.

Kinsey himself refrained from moral judgments. But his findings were greeted with dismay and defiant incredulity by professional moralists and church leaders. For the uncommitted public, however, there were two effects of startling importance: sexual frankness took an immense leap forward, and the image of women was changed forever. Any picture America had of its women being shy creatures living sheltered lives, untainted by the world, was shattered by the facts Kinsey reported. Not just the image of women but also the desires of women altered drastically. If women could enjoy sex as much as men, as the report affirmed, then the implication was that they always should; and those who realized they were not achieving Kinsey's statistical norm of orgasm soon asked themselves why not. Those who had accepted the old beliefs about women—slower sexual arousal, natural chastity, and the need for serious emotional involvement to become aroused sexually—were bound to ask themselves whether they had been led up the garden path. Within three years of *The Kinsey Report*'s appearance the limits of permissible sexual explicitness in the arts and entertainment had radically changed, and with them the public image of the ideal nurse. In addition, in 1964 the contraceptive pill arrived and the real possibility of sex free from the fear of pregnancy became apparent. The birthrate also began to decline. And there began to emerge the development of another, new style of feminism—the women's liberation movement.

The work of feminist scholars before the movement took hold was of key significance. The writings on women in the 1950s by feminists and nonfeminists alike tended to take place within a framework that accepted the primacy of the woman's role as wife and mother and tried to fit other aspects of women's lives into that. The emphasis on the dual role of women as wives and mothers and as paid workers was very characteristic of the period, but it was always insisted that the family must come first. Women's entry into employment was understood in the context of a secondary job, preferably to be done part-time, so as to fit in with the needs of husband and children. Ideologies about women in the 1950s were based on the notion of equal but different—

men and women had their special spheres, and women brought different qualities, feminine qualities, to the society that men could not provide.

THE FEMININE MYSTIQUE

A major contribution to the development of a newer philosophy of women's liberation was *The Second Sex* by Simone de Beauvoir, first appearing in translation in the United States in 1952 but belatedly becoming popular in 1961 and 1962.[2] And in 1963 Betty Friedan published *The Feminine Mystique,* a journalistic polemic that was to sell over a million copies. While it wasn't, strictly speaking, a book about liberation and equality, it discussed the discontent that an increasing number of women were experiencing and started the wheels turning in many other women's heads. To Betty Friedan the American home, filled with its creature comforts, was a gilded ghetto, a velvet concentration camp. She wrote, "A baked potato is not as big as the world, and vacuuming the living room floor—with or without makeup—is not work that takes enough thought or energy to challenge a woman's full capacity."[3]

Although Betty Friedan's book is not a historical study, it does offer several hypotheses on the history of women after 1920 that require clarification. Friedan dated the end of the era of the new woman—the woman who searches for her own identity—at around 1950, when a new emphasis on femininity created the feminine mystique of housewife-mother. Her argument is based in large part on analyses of short stories in women's magazines. In 1930 heroines of magazine stories, Friedan found, were proud, adventurous, attractive women, seeking careers and striving to create lives of their own. They were the "new" women with "new" roles. They had spirit, courage, and determination, and they were admired for these qualities by men who understood their commitment to work. But, as Friedan points out, these new women heroines did not reflect the actual work behavior of young women. They were still a part of daydreams of women beginning to express their yearning for an identity that might be realized through work.

During the 1950s virtually all of the stories and articles centered around the housewife, who was told that in her role she was "expert in a dozen fields simultaneously," such as a "business manager, cook, nurse, chauffeur, dressmaker, interior decorator, accountant, caterer, teacher, private secretary . . . [and] philanthropist." She was informed that "great men have great mothers," and warned that careers and higher education led to "masculinization" and concomitant danger "to the home, the children dependent on it and to the ability of the woman as well as her husband to obtain sexual gratification." Typical titles of articles from this era were "Femininity Begins at Home," "Having Babies While You're Young," "How to Snare a Male," "Are You Training Your Daughter to Be a Wife?," "Why G.I.'s Prefer Those German Girls," "Really a Man's World, Politics," "How to Hold On to a Happy Marriage," "Don't Be Afraid to Marry Young," "Cooking to Me Is Poetry," and so on. Friedan notes that "by the end of 1949, only one out of three heroines in the women's magazines was a career woman—and she was shown in the act of renouncing her career and discovering that what she really wanted to be was a housewife." By 1958 Friedan could find no heroines who had a career, a commitment to any work, art, profession, or mission in the world, other than "Occupation: housewife." Moreover, "even the young unmarried heroines no longer worked, except at finding a husband."[4]

Friedan went on to state that the heroines got constantly younger "in looks, and a childlike kind of dependence." Their only vision of the future was to have more babies; the only "active growing figure in their world [was] the child." Their problems consisted of how to get their allowances increased, how to fight those "devil" career women who threatened to steal their husbands, and occasionally, how to squash their own dreams of independence. "The end of the road," writes Friedan, "is the disappearance of the heroine altogether, as a separate self and the subject of her own story. The end of the road is togetherness, where the woman has no independent self; she exists only for and through her husband and children."[5]

Politics, national issues, science, and virtually every idea concerning the world beyond the family were absent from the only material that most females read. Not surprisingly, where the magazine writers and editors of the preceding era were female, in the era of the "feminine mystique," they were replaced by males. As a final, if subtle, insult, "the very size of their print is raised until it looks like a first-grade primer."[6]

Friedan, speaking of white, mostly middle-class, middle-aged, married females, called it "the problem that has no name." She described the female's psychological malaise.

> It was a strange stirring, a sense of dissatisfaction, a yearning that women suffered. . . . Each suburban wife struggled with it alone. As she made beds, shopped for groceries, matched slipcover material, ate peanut butter sandwiches with her children, chauffeured Cub Scouts and Brownies, lay beside her husband at night—she was afraid to ask even of herself the silent question—'Is this all?'[7]

Basically, Friedan's argument was that conformity to stereotyped domesticity had dearly cost large numbers of intelligent, educated, once active and dynamic females. They fled to psychiatrists asking why, with all they had (lovely house, children, loving husband), they were dissatisfied with life, empty, bored, and looking forward to nothing. They complained to their physicians of being tired all the time, a symptom usually regarded as psychosomatic. They turned in large numbers to tranquilizers, barbiturates, and alcohol. And, most tragically, their frustration perhaps resulted in a generation of children who were unable "to endure pain or discipline or pursue any self-sustained goal of any sort," children with "a devastating boredom with life." Friedan's study was important because it revealed a reversal in attitudes about women's roles in the work world. The working woman emerged in the 1920s and 1930s only to retreat in the mid-1940s.[8]

THE WOMEN'S LIBERATION MOVEMENT

When the so-called women's liberation movement emerged in the mid-1960s, therefore, it was in response to a social change that was already in full swing. One of the first rumbles of an active movement came in 1969 when Kate Millet's *Sexual Politics,* a jargony, turgid English thesis offering a historical and cultural analysis of sexism, hit the best-seller list.[9] Germaine Greer's more readable and frequently bawdy book, *The Female Eunuch,* came next, followed by a thundering array of theses, essays, histories, invectives, reprints, exposes, and a new magazine, *Ms,* edited by New York feminist-journalist

Gloria Steinem, all poking and prodding at women's dormant consciousness.[10] About the same time, concern about discrimination against minority groups was widespread, serving to fuel the interest in women's issues. President Kennedy's Commission on the Status of Women made 24 major recommendations to fight sex discrimination and these established the framework for the movement.

Another indication of these changes was seen in responses to the question "Now if you were free to do either, would you prefer to have a job outside the home or would you prefer to stay home and take care of a house and family?" Between 1974 and 1980, the percentage of women who avowed a preference for taking a job rose from 35 to 46 percent. Moreover, sharp differences between the preferences of women under 30 and those over 50 foreshadowed still greater changes to come. Even more striking were generational differences in expectations of women who did not work. The Virginia Slims Poll reported that "Nearly three quarters (73 percent) of non-working women under 30 years of age plan to work in the future. More than three fifths (62 percent) of the non-working women now in their 30s intend to get full-time jobs eventually."[11]

Although national media advertising campaigns continued to assert that a female's proper place was in the home—a cook in the kitchen, a lady in the parlor, a sexual partner in bed—women expressed great dissatisfaction about those conventional roles. The subject of housewife frustration emerged in the early 1970s as a central theme in American fiction. Where traditional male literature placed the major crises of life in late adolescence, a time of career choice and marriage, a series of women's novels emphasized the deep frustration of married heroines. Alice Adams's *Families and Survivors,* Paula Fox's *Desperate Characters,* Joan Didion's *Play It as It Lays,* Alix Kate Shulman's *Memoirs of an Ex-Prom Queen,* Marge Piercy's *Small Changes*—all focused on the collapse of female identity when conventional domestic relations soured.[12]

In addition to the rising divorce rate, social statisticians noted other important changes in American family patterns. The marriage rate, which had steadily increased in the 1960s, began to drop in 1972, reaching a low of 10 marriages per thousand people in 1976. Young adults, wary of marital failure, increasingly delayed their wedding dates, causing a notable rise in the average age of first marriage, to 22.1 for women and 24.6 for men in 1980, a full year older than in 1975 and nearly 2 years older than the averages of the 1950s. These marital decisions also affected the nation's birthrate, which dropped from 18.4 per thousand in 1970 to 14.8 per thousand in 1975. By 1973 the nation's fertility rate slipped below the 2.1 child-per-woman ratio required for the natural replacement of the population and hovered at about 1.8 for the rest of the decade. Among married women in their 20s, the rate of childlessness increased so dramatically that census bureau demographers speculated that a generation of liberated women had not merely delayed motherhood but had chosen to remain forever childless. By mid-decade, the traditional yardstick used by the Department of Labor to define a typical household—a working father, a domesticated mother, and two children— represented only 7 percent of all American families.

The nation's birthrate, which had plummeted steadily for 20 years, stabilized in 1975 and increased slightly in the next 4 years. Surveys by the census bureau in 1980 found that birth expectations among young women aged 18 to 24 had remained constant since 1975, averaging two children each; only 11 percent said they expected to have no children. And the number of women in their early 30s having first children leaped 37 percent, while women in the 35 to 39 age bracket showed a 22 percent increase. "It used to be that when a woman decided not to have a baby at age 35, that was it," explained Kathy Weingarten, coauthor of a study of "late-timing" parents. "Now, women at age 42 are still asking themselves the question."[13]

Meanwhile, the unhappily married increasingly opted for divorce. The national divorce rate, the highest in the world, had grown slowly but steadily since the beginning of the twentieth century; between the mid-1950s and 1970, it leaped by two thirds for women under 45. The highest incidence of divorce occurred in the 20 to 24 age group, an indication that early marriage no longer satisfied a woman's need for identity. More divorced women were now mothers and, unlike an earlier generation of divorced women with children, preferred to support their families rather than seek remarriage. Poor families, which often could not afford the high cost of divorce, simply separated, though frequently women were then left with inadequate means of support.

Female-headed households remained among the poorest in the land.

The willingness of women to merge careers with child rearing revealed not only a shift of values, but also the necessity of earning a living. The great increase in female-headed households simply forced mothers into the workforce. During the 1970s, moreover, the major growth industries of the American economy—health, food, and business services that provided 40 percent of all new private jobs between 1973 and 1980—were traditionally women's work. Such jobs often offered only part-time employment and minimum wages (which explains why women's incomes remained a fraction of male earnings), limited opportunities for advancement, and few union protections. But they did allow flexible schedules, enabling women to juggle family responsibilities with careers. By 1976 only 40 percent of the nation's jobs produced sufficient income to support a family, forcing the employment of married women to bolster household earnings. As a result, half of all American mothers and 43 percent of women with preschool-age children were working.

The increase in the number of working mothers had important consequences for domestic life. Child care, traditionally the responsibility of mothers, moved increasingly beyond the family. In the absence of government programs or workplace facilities, mothers devoted substantial portions of their paychecks to private day-care centers or professional baby-sitters. But in the poorer families, the majority of which were female-headed, children found no more surrogate supervision than the television screen, logging an estimated 12,000 to 16,000 hours by age 16. Working mothers also changed family consumption patterns, preferring fast-food emporiums, convenience products, and microwave ovens to save time.

Despite the need for women to be working, American men were slow to fill the breach in child care. In 1976 Dr. Benjamin Spock, author of America's number-one best seller in the twentieth century (except for the Bible), *Baby and Child Care,* published a major revision "to eliminate the sexist biases that help to create and perpetuate discrimination against girls and women." Responding to the pressures of feminists, Spock insisted that "the father's responsibility is as great as the mother's." But opinion surveys found that while men overwhelmingly approved of working mothers, most continued to define basic domestic chores, such as cleaning toilets, as women's tasks. "All right, you go right ahead and do your thing," Archie Bunker expressed the sentiment. "But you just remember that your thing is eggs over easy and crisp bacon."[14]

IMAGE OF WOMEN

Fashions during the 1960s were increasingly colorful, heterogeneous, varied, and individualized, often to the point of wildness. The look for women of the 1960s was variously characterized as "leggy," "mannish," "total" (meaning coordinated pattern and color from head to toe), "little girl," or "Unisex." The British model Twiggy embodied the mod look and became the idol of fashion-conscious teenagers, with her boyish haircut, big eyes rimmed with painted-on eyelashes, exceedingly slender and flat-chested figure, and gangling grammar-school legs.

It was a decade of tremendous variety in clothing, running the gamut from ultrafeminine to starkly masculine, from Victorian demureness to daring near-nudity. Life seemed to be one long costume party, with every woman for herself, and no wild getup was considered too startling or outrageous to be worn on the street. Hemlines during the 1960s rose and fell; they stood just below the knee in 1961, hovered just at knee height in 1964, went soaring upward to break all previous records in brevity from 1966 through the end of the decade—miniskirts and micro-miniskirts were 3 to 8 inches above the knee. In 1970, just as it appeared that skirts might vanish altogether, the trend reversed, with midi-skirts at mid-calf and maxi-skirts at ankle length.

Pantsuits for women became more and more popular, until by the end of the 1960s they were an almost universal uniform, accepted for business and professional wear as well as for home and street garb. Airline hostesses wore them, and so did their passengers. Nurses appeared in white pants uniforms, female professors as well as students adopted trousers for classroom wear, and secretaries and women executives showed up at their offices in pants. In the hospital and business worlds, this changeover elicited some remonstrance from conservative administrators, but the wearers of pants eventually won the battle.

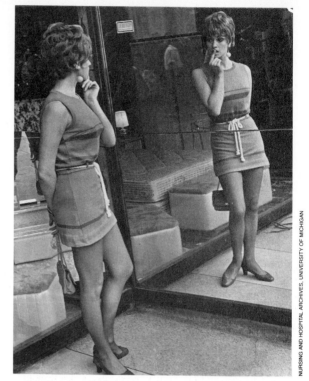

NURSING AND HOSPITAL ARCHIVES, UNIVERSITY OF MICHIGAN

Hemlines went soaring upward to break all previous records from 1966 through the end of the decade—miniskirts and micro-miniskirts were 3 to 8 inches above the knee.

One of the most typical coiffures for women in the 1960s was hair worn long, straight, and flowing, undressed and untrammeled, and often uncombed. Hair streamed out behind a young woman running for a bus, or bounced and swung as she danced the boogaloo. Often she peered out from behind a fringe of bangs or squinted with one eye as a long lock fell across the other. Straight hair was prized over curls, and if a woman's hair was naturally curly, she might use a straightener to correct the condition, or might lay her head on an ironing board and run a warm iron over her tresses to remove unwanted waves. Permanent waves no longer imparted a tight curl to the hair, but simply added "body" or made the hair more tractable and easier to set in huge, sculptured swirls or puffed-out bouffant styles. The hair was often back-combed ("ratted" or "teased") to give it added fullness. The bubble and beehive styles of the late 1950s were still in evidence.

MASS MEDIA IMAGES OF WOMEN AND NURSES

Despite the women's liberation movement, advertisements of the early-1970s accentuated female domesticity, characterizing women primarily as consumers—seldom as workers—whose main purpose in life was to please the opposite sex. American women in advertisements waged endless warfare against sinister subversion, usually portrayed as an invisible conspiracy of germs or dirt. Laundry detergent ads commonly placed women in competition over the whiteness of their clothes. Mainstream mass media products avoided gross sexual expression, but they endorsed the same conservative themes in more subtle ways. At a time when women were challenging the traditional male-female dichotomy, major Hollywood movies continued to define good women as appendages of men (*Straw Dogs,* Cinerama, 1972; *Carnal Knowledge,* Avco-Embassy, 1971), sheltered from worldly affairs (*The Godfather,* Paramount, 1972), while portraying working women as prostitutes (*Klute,* Warner Brothers, 1971). Television's *All in the Family* (CBS, 1971–1983) not only caricatured Edith Bunker as a willing victim to her husband's chauvinism, but also, in the early shows, cast their daughter, Gloria, as a sexy newlywed playing that stereotyped role.

In the majority of media portrayals of nurses from the mid-1960s to the present time, an obsession with nurses's sex lives has dominated all other thematic elements, and yielded a representation of the nursing profession which is often blurred and twisted to fit bizarre objectives. In these portrayals, nurses are depicted as sensual, romantic, hedonistic, frivolous, irresponsible, and promiscuous. And unfortunately, the more the nurse is presented as a sex object, the less she is shown being engaged in actual professional nursing work.

The primary plot development in these stereotypic depictions has the nurse becoming emotionally and sexually involved with her male patients. A patient's welfare becomes the nurse's private mission, and in the process of aiding his physical and psychological recovery, she readily becomes his sexual partner. Another common representation involves the portrayal of sexual liaisons between nurses and physicians. These almost always cast the nurse in a subordinate and usually demeaning role. For instance, in order to assure that the head nurse will not learn of her medication error, a nurse agrees to have sex with a young physician; another nurse allows a psychiatrist to talk her into believing that she is potentially deviant, and then is seduced by him in the name of a cure.

M*A*S*H AND CATCH-22

The most durable nurse of the entertainment media world of the past generation, Margaret "Hot Lips" Houlihan, originated as a sex object character in the 1968 novel and the 1970 motion picture, *M*A*S*H* (20th Century-Fox), which led to the television series of the same title. In physician-author Richard Hooker's *M*A*S*H,* Army surgeons Hawkeye Pierce and Duke Forrest steal a jeep to take them to their new Korean War assignment with a Mobile Army Surgical Hospital. Though close to the combat zone, the camp is peaceful except for disorders caused by the two surgeons' inability to get along with the pious Major Frank Burns. The tensions increase with the arrival of "chest cutter" Trapper John McIntyre, who attacks Burns when he blames a young male orderly for a patient's death.[15]

Major Houlihan, a stunning blonde nurse, joins the hospital to take charge of the nurses and forms a professional alliance with Burns to compel the unruly surgeons to accept military discipline. Their relationship quickly becomes intimate, and Radar O'Reilly, a crony of the surgeons, places a microphone in Burns's tent and broadcasts the sounds of their lovemaking. By the next morning, Major Houlihan is nicknamed Hot Lips and Major Burns suffers a breakdown and is led away in a straightjacket. Painless Pole, the hospital's dentist and a notorious lover, becomes temporarily impotent and threatens suicide after diagnosing himself as a latent homosexual. The staff arranges a "Last Supper" in which Painless is given a suicide pill (actually a tranquilizer). Hawkeye then persuades Lieutenant Dish, a married nurse, to have sex with Painless, thus enabling the dentist to regain his potency. To demonstrate their distaste for her prudery and military manner and in an effort to destroy the last of Hot Lips' self-confidence, the physicians stage the humiliating shower scene in which Hot Lips is exposed in the nude when the shower tent is suddenly yanked off before the assembled

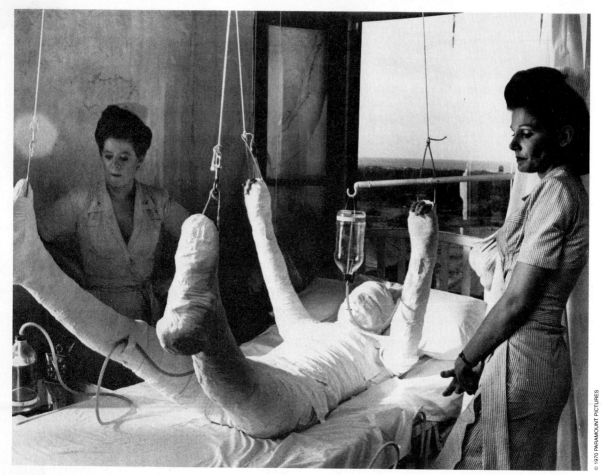

© 1970 PARAMOUNT PICTURES

In Catch-22 *(Paramount, 1970) the nurses' hardened sexuality, their whispering gossip, and their total indifference to their patient all underscore the film's negative perception of nursing.*

audience. This prank was carried out to settle a dispute as to whether Hot Lips is really a natural blonde. The other nurses join in the fun sharing the physicians' delight in witnessing the head nurse's total embarrassment and downfall.

The attractive nurse found in bed with the commanding officer epitomizes what a good nurse should be—sexually attractive and willing to sacrifice herself to a good cause. Outside the operating room, the nurses are just pleasant bodies, to be observed, discussed, handled, and enjoyed like so many pieces of ripe fruit. Except for Hot Lips, who is ridiculed for being a hypocritical "regular Army clown," all the nurses are virtually indistinguishable,

and their importance only as sex objects is underlined by the few names given: Hot Lips, Scorch, Dish, Knocko, and so on. They seem essentially brainless, fit for little more than to relieve the physicians' sexual tensions, sew buttons on the surgeons' shirts, and be cheerleaders at the surgeons' football games.[16]

Joseph Heller's amorphous, surrealistic, satirical antiwar novel, *Catch-22* (Paramount), also came to the large screen in 1970. It starred Alan Arkin as the antihero Yossarian, the only man in the Air Force with enough sense to be scared out of his wits by the dangers of war. The narrative takes place in Allied-occupied Italy during World War II. The film, more than the novel, attempts a chronologically progressive story, in which flashbacks, dreams, and incongruities reveal much of the nightmare-like reality experienced by Yossarian. The premise of the film is simply that madness, once institutionalized into such establishments as the modern military, becomes the norm, and sanity masquerades as madness in order to escape the consequences of this reversal. Everyone associated with the military—or institutionalized insanity—demonstrates some degree of peversity, greed, cowardice, or indifference. The nurses in this film automatically are included in the generalized antipathy for established military institutions. Although they play a minor role in the film, the nurses contribute to the notion that institutions and systems are meaningless at best and life-denying and vicious at worst.[17]

The only scene of nurses delivering professional nursing care occurs during Yossarian's hospitalization when he watches two nurses casually exchange an empty fluid input bottle for the now-filled fluid output bottle. Moving through the ward prettily and whispering something audible but unintelligible and giggling over it, they descend on a patient who is completely bandaged and immobilized. Keeping up their eerie whispering, the two gracefully unhook the bottles attached to the tubes at his arm and groin and reverse them. Having completed this absurd little ballet, they glide back through the ward, arm in arm. The scene is one of the most effective in the film: the sleepy afternoon calm of the ward, drenched in fuzzy white light, the hard-edged, whorish beauty of the nurses in their heavy period makeup, elaborate hairstyles, and tight uniforms, the unsettling not-quite-human sound of their whispering, the absurdity of their action, and the automatic expertise with which they perform it all contribute to the eerie resonance of the scene. It is implied that they do this as a matter of course; their casual demeanor is contrasted with the horror of Yossarian, who does a double take at the switch of glucose and waste and then screams, shocked with disbelief. The nurses' hardened sexuality, their whispering gossip, and their total indifference to their patient all underscore the film's negative perception of nursing.

Even the nurses' sexuality, their most obvious feature, is developed to reveal their lack of warmth and generosity. An amorous Yossarian receives repeated kicks in the groin from sexy Nurse Duckett (Paula Prentiss), who tantalizes the lustful pilot but does not respond to his advances. The nurses are contrasted unfavorably with a more sympathetic group of Italian whores who represent a coarse but real haven for the men and who provide the only natural comfort available in an insane world. The presentation of nurses as sexually provocative—tight uniforms and elaborate makeup—was a recurring theme in many films, novels, and television shows of the 1970s.

THE "CARRY ON" SERIES

This watershed period also saw the birth of a peculiar genre, the British-made "Carry On" films. The seemingly never-ending series of farces produced by Peter Rogers, written by Talbot Rothwell, and directed by Gerald Thomas began innocently enough with *Carry On Sergeant* (Governor, 1958) and then rapidly hit its stride. The health care "Carry Ons"—*Carry On Nurse* (Governor Films, 1959), *Carry On Doctor* (Rank, 1967), *Carry On Again, Doctor* (Rank, 1969), and *Carry On Matron* (Rank, 1972)—span the genre's history. To give a rough idea, *Carry On Nurse* was the third movie in the series and *Carry On Matron* was the twenty-third. Despite the time span, all "Carry Ons" have a fundamental identity. All are thin on plot and heavy on episodic comic crises; all are sexually suggestive (increasingly so as time progressed); and all share a

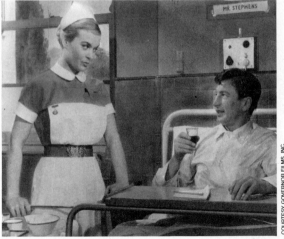

COURTESY GOVERNOR FILMS, INC.

The health care "Carry On" films are full of bedpan humor, doctors and patients lusting after nurses, and jokes about enemas and fear of operations.

team of well-known British performers—Sidney James, Kenneth Williams, Hattie Jacques, Joan Sims, Jim Dale, Charles Hawtrey, Barbara Windsor—consistently appearing in stereotypical roles throughout the entire series.[18]

The health care "Carry Ons," for their part, are full of bedpan humor, doctors and patients lusting after nurses, and jokes about enemas and fear of operations. The comic business of all the medical "Carry Ons" utilizes everyman's notion of what ward life and the relationship between hospital staff and patients—at its most uproarious—is like. Sex, not sickness, is the primary bond between patients, doctors, and nurses, with young nurses synonymous for the most part with beauty and availability. Much of the innuendo derives from childish jokes about nurses dealing with their male patients' bodies. "What a fuss about such a little thing," says a nurse to a bashful patient reluctant to disrobe. Another patient, called a baby when he refuses to be bathed, proves upon undressing that he is no such thing. Obviously, this kind of low-grade humor, when relentlessly iterated throughout the "Carry Ons," sets an appallingly trivial standard and, in an important sense, divides the "Carry On" world from the real world.

The distinction is clearly drawn in *Carry On Nurse,* first and mildest of the health care "Carry Ons," in which good taste and wholesome characters are still present, despite the grade-school humor. Significantly, doctors are noticeably absent from the comic firing line in this first health care "Carry On"; when they appear, which is rarely, they are serious professionals, untainted by the mania to which the rest of the staff and patients are victim. Nurses dominate the goings-on in the men's surgical ward in which the action of *Carry On Nurse* takes place, the nursing personnel themselves (as in all "Carry Ons") being strictly stereotyped, even down to the actress playing the top nurse administrator. Matron, who appears in all four features, was played by England's favorite overweight actress, Hattie Jacques, the personification of unmitigated sternness and uncompromising authority. In *Carry On Nurse* Matron is a wholly dignified nurse, quite unlike the figure of fun into which she degenerated in subsequent features. She is essentially an interloper in the ward's closed comic world, over which the typical "Carry On" head nurse, strict but likable, rules.

Unlike the dreaded Matron, the head nurse (Joan Hickson) is as harassed as her own junior nurses. Slim, middle-aged, efficient, energetic and hardworking, the head nurse constantly strives to present the unappeasable Matron with a perfect ward, but is mostly thwarted in her efforts by the inexorable stupidity of one particular student, Nurse Dawson (Joan Sims), the nursing staff's most incorrigible failure. Clumsy and inept, Student Nurse Dawson spends most of the film knocking over trolleys, bumping into everything imaginable, being late, and creating havoc. She boils catheters dry, summons the fire brigade instead of ringing the visitors' bell, offers a suppository enema to a patient to take orally, and generally behaves like a muddleheaded but well-meaning incompetent.

Above Student Nurse Dawson and doing their best to make up for her idiocy are the staff nurses, capable, forbearing and lovely, turning the heads of patients and doctors alike and dealing urbanely with the coy self-consciousness of their male patients. The leading staff nurse is played by Shirley Eaton, considered a real sex goddess during the ladylike 1950s. Blond, buxom Shirley typifies the attractive nurse who sets the patients in a romantic whirl. One man, who has only just met her, gazes longingly into her eyes as he sighs, "I think you're wonderful." More realistic than he, the nurse replies with the voice of experience, "Hospitals have a strange effect, you know; all the men think they're in love with the nurses. It happens to all the men."[19]

Nurse Shirley is herself more interested in one of the physicians, whom she openly reveres, whispering news of his imminent arrival to her patients as she prepares the ward to greet him, humbly and in awe. The fact that physicians are unaffected by the comedy in *Carry On Nurse*—while nurses stand at the center of it—and are always treated deferentially elevates the physicians' status enormously. Simultaneously, of course, nurses by their very worshipful attitude demean themselves still further. In *Carry On Nurse* physicians are mysterious, dignified and rarely seen, whereas nurses are commonplace and harassed.

Yet for all its juvenile humor and appalling jokes, *Carry On Nurse* retains a freshness and charm, a simplicity and innocence quite lacking in the romps into which the "Carry Ons" declined. Because later health care "Carry Ons," made during more permis-

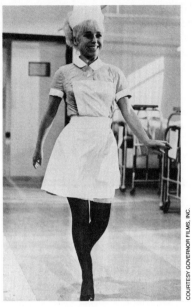

Into the "Carry On" world came a buxom cockney blonde, Barbara Windsor, now the series' sex object in residence.

sive times, relied increasingly on tasteless, unrealistic situations, usually with lewd implications, the comedies became more strained and feverish and all the less endearing. However comic the nurses in *Carry On Nurse* may be, they—and the way they are treated—have a certain class, a vestige of the old traditional British film comedy. This type of nurse depiction soon vanished from the screen.

Eight years intervened between *Carry On Nurse* and *Carry On Doctor,* years during which audience appetite for lewdness, lavatory humor, and exposed bosoms increased enormously as the swinging 1960s influenced mass entertainment. The "Carry On" image of nursing deteriorated accordingly. Into the "Carry On" world came a buxom, cockney blonde, Barbara Windsor, now the series' sex object in residence, who transformed the Shirley Eaton bombshell of old to a nurse character on a new plane of suggestiveness and smut. Over these years the Matron's image altered, too, from that of an impossibly stern authoritarian in *Carry On Nurse* to an utterly nonsensical caricature, pursuing and pursued by doctors, and getting involved in the most demeaning nonsense in the next three features.

In *Carry On Doctor,* for example, Matron thinks unethical thoughts about and lavishes her ample femininity on one Dr. Tinkle (Kenneth Williams) and happily assists him in ruining the career of his younger colleague, Dr. Kilmore (Jim Dale). The entire film is characterized by inanity and sexual innuendo, with Barbara Windsor as Nurse Sandra May [sic], whom Matron plots to get off the hospital premises as she is her romantic rival for Dr. Tinkle.[20]

In *Carry On Matron,* Matron is again ridiculed as an emotional, highly sexed woman, who jealously reacts to a blonde nurse's stealing her chosen doctor by herself running around in a revealing negligee, and participating in such appalling puns as "I want to be wooed," to which her admirer replies, "You can be as wude as you like with me!" The story, if such it can be called, has two strands. The first concerns a maternity hospital in which Kenneth Williams is a physician worried that he is becoming a homosexual who madly pursues Matron to prove that he isn't. The other strand concerns a gang of criminals who break into the hospital to steal a cache of contraceptives; one dresses as a nurse and is billed with the bosomy Barbara Windsor, the sexy nurse, and is himself soon fancied by a groping gynecologist.[21]

The deterioration in Matron's character between 1957 and 1972 is easily discerned. Even in *Carry On Nurse,* the first film in which Matron appears, she is both implicitly and explicitly criticized. Primarily a figure of uncompromising authority, her very appearance is a joke, and her obsession with discipline takes no account of a nurse's proper responsibilities or the needs of patients. This is seen in the way that the daily preparation for her round, one of the film's comic set pieces, wears out the patience of the patient Oliver Reckitt (Kenneth Williams). As Matron approaches his bed, the head nurse warns him not to sit on top of the bedclothes as this is one of Matron's pet hates. When Matron then asks Reckitt if everything is all right, he immediately explodes, "Medically, yes; otherwise, no." He then explains why he refuses to obey a rule that only satisfies her neurosis for disliking men lying about. "Your rule has nothing to do with my cure, therefore it has no meaning here," he tells her. Thus the supreme figure of nursing authority is shown to be an irrational virago, disliked and feared by all, who is primarily driven by personal idiosyncracy rather than rationally based professional principle.[22]

As the character evolves in subsequent pictures, especially *Carry On Doctor* and *Carry On Matron,* things go from stereotypically bad to far worse. Matron's already questionable authority is directly undermined in the cheapest manner by habitually depicting her as a jealous, lovesick fool, the obvious opposite to the stately figure she ought, as a matron, to represent. Though on the most superficial level this is undoubtedly just a great visual gag, on a more fundamental one it nevertheless ridicules the most senior nurse and effectively diminishes her stature and moral fiber. The fun only demonstrates that all nurses are the same—sex mad and easy prey for male physicians, no matter what their age or size.

In a similar manner, the way in which the "Carry On" sexy blonde nurse, originally typified by Shirley Eaton, degenerated into Barbara Windsor's disheveled doxy represents the fundamental alteration in attitude that transpired between the late-1950s and the late-1960s. Barbara Windsor, common and cheerful, is an obvious joke nurse, of far less credibility even than Student Nurse Dawson in *Carry On Nurse.* Instead of laughing *with* the nurses at their lot, over the years the "Carry Ons" inexorably began to laugh *at* them: not as individuals, which in some measure the nurses in *Carry On Nurse* remained, but as stereotypical robots, copied from a sexist world.

NURSE CHARACTERS IN SEXPLOITATION FILMS

The depiction of nurses as the sexual mascots for the medical profession recurs again and again throughout the period after 1965. In sexploitation films nursing has been the most frequent occupational identification used in film titles since the mid-1960s. Of all R- and X-rated films with occupationally linked titles released from 1966 to 1984, *nurse* in some form was used in 21 percent of the titles, followed by wife (16 percent), hooker/prostitute (12 percent), cheerleader (8 percent), and stewardess (8 percent). Furthermore, the word *nurse* in the title of these films scarcely emphasizes nurses' professional aspects. *The Sensuous Nurse* (Cinema Arts, 1980), *Night Call Nurses* (New World, 1972), *Nurses for Sale* (Independent-International, 1977), *Head Nurse* (1979), and *Naughty Nurses* (Target, 1973) are just a few examples. Hence not only theater and cable TV audiences

but also anyone walking by the theater or seeing the newspaper ads and *TV Guide* listings for the films receives the message that nurses are first and foremost sex objects. And this message comes not only from the titles but also from the suggestive captions emblazoned across the ads: "It's what goes on before the anesthesia wears off," "It's always harder at night," "The hospital is one thing, my private life's another," and "What I do with my body is my business!"[23]

Examination of several of these films may suggest answers to three basic questions: How are nurses and nursing exploited in them? Why were these films popular? And, above all, why did they so frequently concentrate on *nurse* characters? Several sets of nurse movies gained popularity in the late-1960s and 1970s: three movies in the *I, A Woman* series, two *Deep Throat* films, five nurse films brought out by Hollywood director-producer Roger Corman, some Russ Meyer movies, and a number of others. Each of these series used recurring ingredients—in effect, a formula—after the first film proved profitable at the box office.

I, A Woman (Audubon Films, 1965) was among the first of the nurse sexploitation films to gain wide popularity. Probably some of the expanded audience came because the movie was touted in some areas as an art film, a claim bolstered by the mere fact that it was a foreign film (from Sweden) and had subtitles. Taken from a rather shallow, pretentious novel of the same name, the movie is the story of a young Swedish nurse, Siv, who rejects her sexually restrained fiancé and her fanatically religious upbringing. She is proclaimed to be sexually "liberated," which is to say she sleeps with any man who stirs her sexual instincts, and she refuses to be tied down by conventional commitments of love and marriage. Hence in the course of the story, she is shown having sex with a patient, with a married doctor, and with a sailor, the latter of whom scorns her when she actually falls in love with him.[24]

There is little emphasis on professional nursing in *I, A Woman,* although Siv is said to be a good nurse. Nursing serves three functions in the film: it enables Siv to be financially independent; it puts her in a position to interact with male physicians and patients; and it elevates her character somewhat, as she is meant to appear to be something better than a common slut. Indeed the film tends to consider Siv almost as the bearer of a new religion, even though

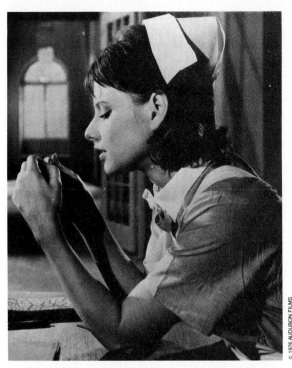

© 1976 AUDUBON FILMS

I, A Woman (Audubon Films, 1965) is the story of a young Swedish nurse, Siv, who rejects her sexually restrained fiancé and her own fanatically religious upbringing.

she is consistently shown as sullen, cruel, and completely self-absorbed. It ends with the preachment that if the viewers have been shocked by the film, then they have forgotten what love is. This pseudo-philosophical gloss probably contributed somewhat to the film's wider public acceptance.

Siv's capabilities as a nurse do little to improve the somewhat unpleasant image she projects. The sexual liberation that the film espouses is ironically undercut by the constant suggestions that women love being submissive and slavish to strong men, that they consciously or unconsciously desire rape and brutality. Since one of Siv's sexual partners is a physician, this sexual submissiveness only increases the usual disparity between the images of the nurse and the doctor, and it further decreases her professional image.

Since the first *I, A Woman* film had shocked the world by portraying then unusual amounts of "normal" sexuality, the second and third stories in the series had no direction to go except toward increasingly deviant topics. The next film, *I, A Woman II* (Chevron Pictures, 1968), shows Siv unhappily married to Hans, a strange, secretive man who makes her pose for pornographic pictures and have sexual relations with his clients while he watches. He will not use the money he makes from these endeavors to pay off their debts, however, so Siv decides to return to nursing and to her affair with the doctor. One of Siv's patients turns out to be Hans's first wife, a woman also forced into prostitution by him. After humiliating her in this fashion, Hans had divorced her, declaring her the guilty party. Ultimately, Siv discovers that her unpleasant husband is a sadistic former Nazi S.S. officer, and she leaves him in disgust.[25]

The third film, *I, A Woman—The Daughter* (Chevron Pictures, 1970), explores the sexual gamut still further, this time concentrating on interracial sex, lesbianism, and hints of incest, with drugs, orgies, and a vicious motorcycle gang stirred in for added titillation. Siv's daughter, Birthe, returns home unexpectedly to find her mother in bed with a lover, and she later discovers their pornographic records, sexual aids, and nude pictures of her mother. Running off in disgust, Birthe gets involved with some hippies, who try to assault her; with Stephen, a black medical student, who falls in love with her; and with Stephen's lesbian sister, who seduces her. This was about as far as the "I, A Woman" story line could go so the series terminated with the third installment.[26]

Meanwhile, even more damage to the image of the nursing profession was done by the heroine of *Deep Throat* (Aquarius, 1972), which was surely one of the most widely attended X-rated movies in history. This is a one-joke film in which the heroine, played by the now famous Linda Lovelace, is unable to find sexual satisfaction until a physician discovers that her clitoris is in her throat and that only fellatio will satisfy her needs. She thanks the doctor by demonstrating her new-found technique on him, whereupon he promptly makes her a nurse in his sex therapy clinic. His regular office nurse also performs various sexual acts with him, often while they are discussing the "scientific" aspects of their sexual research. Most of the movie is taken up by some fifteen sexual acts (mostly oral sex), all of them actual rather than simulated sex.[27]

It was hardly a movie one would predict as a smash hit at the box office, but it played (and is still playing) to unprecedentedly large and diverse audi-

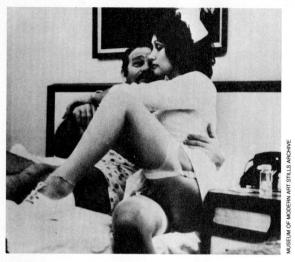

More damage to the image of the nursing profession was done by the heroine of Deep Throat *(Aquarius, 1972), surely one of the most widely attended X-rated movies in history.*

MUSEUM OF MODERN ART STILLS ARCHIVE

ences. At least three factors contributed to its unexpected popularity. First, it was declared to be an artistically made film. Its predecessors in the pornographic field were usually grainy depictions of sexual acts recorded by hand-held cameras in low-budget locations, with little or no attempt at plot, dialogue, or photographic artistry. *Deep Throat*'s thin story line, by sheer contrast, was considered a plot, and the photography, lighting, color, acting, and sets were all proclaimed excellent by early reviews. Second, Al Goldstein, the editor of *Screw* magazine and self-proclaimed king of porn movie reviews, declared *Deep Throat* "the very best porn film ever made, so superior to others that it defies comparison." This pronouncement appeared in almost all the ads for the film and probably stirred the curiosity of many who otherwise might not have considered attending. Finally, the movie probably gained much of its popularity because of its humor. It was one of the first porn films deliberately planned to be a comedy, and the sexual one-liners allowed the audience to laugh at scenes that might embarrass those not accustomed to X-rated films. Many who wouldn't have considered going to a "serious" porn film apparently felt comfortable about viewing comedic pornography.

The sequel, *Deep Throat II* (Bryanson, 1974), was not nearly so popular. It was only R-rated, showing

no actual sex scenes. In addition, the gamut of jokes about nurse Linda Lovelace's amazing talent had been pretty much exhausted by the original film. Nevertheless, the two films had conveyed to millions an image of nursing which was, to say the least, totally unprofessional. The doctor's office nurse seemed to exist only to service his sexual needs. Linda Lovelace was declared a nurse simply on the basis of her abilities to perform fellatio, and she went right to work in the clinic to relieve others of their sexual problems.[28]

THE NURSE FILMS OF ROGER CORMAN AND RUSS MEYER

Such films were not alone. In the early-1970s, producer Roger Corman brought out a special series of R-rated "nurse films," all of them playing heavily on the nurses' sexual lives, although other themes were also broached. Indeed, he had a set formula for the nurse movies, and since it proved financially successfully, he never varied it. The titles of his five nurse films all sounded very much the same: *The Student Nurses* (New World Pictures, 1970), *Private Duty Nurses* (New World Pictures, 1971), *Night Call Nurses* (New World Pictures, 1972), *The Young Nurses* (New World Pictures, 1973), and *Candy Stripe Nurses* (New World Pictures, 1974). These films divided the dramatic and visual interest among three or four nurse characters, showing bits and pieces of their professional and personal lives and concentrating especially on the girls' tendencies to become emotionally and, of course, sexually involved with their patients.

The basic formula that Corman used in these films was as follows: let the nurses include a blonde, a brunette, and a minority woman (Chicano or black); have them become romantically and sexually involved with a patient or physician; let at least one of the nurses take up the cause of her new boyfriend (this is most often the calling of the minority woman); show a lot of undressing and nudity, but keep actual sex scenes at a minimum (this is to ensure an R rather than an X rating in order to play to a target audience of teenagers); bring in a smidgen of contemporary issues, such as drugs, Vietnam veterans, women's rights; and for the benefit of the male audience, include some violent action scenes equipped with motorcycles, trucks, and guns.

The first of this series, *The Student Nurses,* is a loose collection of mostly romantic episodes in the lives of four student nurses who are roommates and classmates: Lynn Verdugo (Brioni Farrell), Sharon Armitage (Elaine Giftos), Phred Stella (Karen Carlson), and Priscilla Kovac (Barbara Leigh). Although all of the student nurses are young, attractive, and friendly, they are not presented as particularly likable individuals. Neither do they contribute to a positive image of nursing. The film is lacking in realistic representations of the demands of study and training experienced by student nurses. The students are shown in the classroom a few times, but the viewer has no idea of the content of the course materials or difficulty of the clinical practice. The student nurses do complain about their hard work and hours, but when these same nurses are seen in the hospital setting, they do little more than carry trays with hypodermic needles on them, swab an arm, or sit with a patient. And although the film raises certain significant social and medical issues—the question of illegal abortions, the issue of better medical services for the poor, and the problem of how to care for the terminally ill—each of these is confronted on a personal rather than a professional level, and their nursing studies never inform their responses to these issues.[29]

The third film of the series, *Night Call Nurses,* was the most outlandish and contrived, containing almost every possible sexual suggestion, activity, and perversion allowable within the confines of its R rating. The very title "Night *Call* Nurses" alludes more to prostitution than nursing. Once again the plot features three attractive and sexually active young nurses: Janis, Sandra, and Barbara. This time the nurses are working at what appears to be a private psychiatric clinic, a situation ripe with potential violence and sexual deviance.[30]

Janis's tale is the least complicated, designed to appeal to those who are more interested in a luscious blonde body than plot. On duty in the emergency room one night, Janis takes care of a young truck driver suffering hallucinations from amphetamines. She devotedly nurses him through the traumatic withdrawal period, and after he is discharged from the clinic they become lovers. As their relationship grows, she tries to get him off speed by interesting him in other stimulating activities: skydiving, waterskiing, and, of course, lovemaking. Nursing aside, Janis is the epitome of the macho, blue-collar

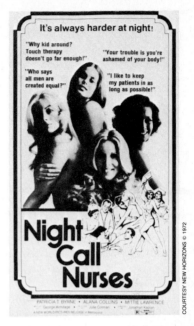

The third film of the Roger Corman series, Night Call Nurses, (New World Pictures, 1972), was outlandish and contrived, containing almost every possible sexual suggestion, activity, and perversion allowable within the confines of its R rating.

male fantasy—blonde, well built, short-skirted, apparently not too smart, interested in men's sports—in short, the perfect decoration for a rolling, thundering semitrailer.

Once again the minority nurse in the trio has the most socially relevant role. The film opens with this nurse, Sandra, trying frantically to save a female patient from taking her own life, but the woman eludes her grasp, jumps nude off the roof of the hospital, and kills herself. Guilt-ridden by the incident, Sandra volunteers to work at the Suicide Prevention Center. In taking care of a militant black leader and convict, Sampson, she learns that his injuries were not the result of a foiled suicide attempt, but were the work of brutal and bigoted prison officials. Together with her boyfriend, Jude (an ex-con), Sandra engineers a plan to smuggle Sampson out of the center. They bandage Sampson up to resemble a burn victim, and then Sandra wheels him out of the hospital to a waiting truck, driven by Janis and her truck-driver boyfriend, that spirits Sampson to a private plane that transports the convict to Africa. The incident is packed with chase scenes, shotgunnings, and close calls, all elements of adventure dramas geared to male tastes. Nurses, insofar as they break away from the establishment and team up with young idealists or radicals, merit a certain amount of esteem in the eyes of the young viewing audience.

Finally, the role of Barbara, the third nurse in the film, is the most blatantly negative due to her utter obsession with kinky sexual behavior. There is no mention of her interacting with patients; instead, she emerges as a woman caught up in her private sexual problems. Barbara is attracted to a handsome but caustic and egotistical psychiatrist, Dr. Bramlett. She joins the encounter group that he directs to learn something more about deviant behavior (a professional interest) and to gain his attention (a personal interest). Barbara's naiveté and openness make her a perfect guinea pig for Bramlett, who is known for his unorthodox methods and theories. Bramlett's pet theory is that any normal person can be pushed into deviant behavior if he is led to believe that he has some subconscious deviant tendencies. Bramlett accordingly rigs an encounter session to convince Barbara that she is a deviant—in this case ashamed of her body—among the other uninhibited group members who readily participate in a nude session. When Barbara is firmly convinced of her deviance, Bramlett proposes to cure her through seduction. Afterward, when he casually admits that he has no feelings for her beyond a scientific curiosity, Barbara threatens to expose him before the medical authorities. Bramlett strikes her, revealing his own deviant tendencies, and they are both suddenly set upon by a psychotic male orderly, dressed in a nurse's uniform and brandishing a cleaver, who has observed their passionate lovemaking. After stunning Bramlett with a blow to the head, the transvestite threatens the bathrobe-clad Barbara. Barbara rescues herself in the corny fashion peculiar to this already preposterous plot: she persuades her attacker that as a real nurse he ought to dedicate himself to saving lives, not destroying them.

Advertising for this series of nurse films focused exclusively on sex, and Corman found a successful formula for the ads nearly as invariable as the plot formula. In virtually all the ads, four naked, beautiful women are pictured, clustered together in such a way that their bare breasts are hidden from sight. All the women, except for the black characters, have

long, loose-flowing, luxuriant hair. Surrounding the four figures are suggestive quotations such as, "What I do with my body is my business!"; "Honestly doctor, I was only giving him a massage!"; "Heartbeat slow . . . I have just the remedy for that!"; "Your trouble is that you're ashamed of your body!"; and "I like to keep my patients in as long as possible!" The ads are also each punctuated with a catchy logo—*The Student Nurses:* "They're learning fast!"; *Private Duty Nurses:* "It's what they do off duty that's *really* private!"; and *Night Call Nurses:* "It's always harder at night!" Finally, beneath the photograph of the four unclad women, most of the ads also have a series of small action sketches that clearly identify the characters as nurses, in case the titles weren't sufficient. The nurses are shown kissing patients, sitting nude in front of a physician, watching (uninvolved) as a physician operates, making love, clinging to a motorcyclist, and so on.[31]

Approaches similar to Corman's were legion during the 1970s and early-1980s. Russ Meyer, for example, wrote, directed, and produced several X-rated movies with nurse characters, the best known of which was probably *Cherry, Harry, and Raquel* (Eve Productions, 1969). The plot of this film can best be summarized by the tag line on the ads: "Ménage à trois . . . contemplate the possibilities. . . ." The viewer need not contemplate for long, because the possibilities for every combination of sexual coupling are soon made quite explicit, not only between Harry, Cherry (the nurse), and Raquel, but also between the women and two other characters named Franklin and Enrique. If the men are not around, the women turn to each other for satisfaction. In between the sexual encounters, some drug smuggling, syndicate killers, and car chases keep the action rolling.[32]

When the sexploitation films did not show the nurses seeking sex, they depicted sex as being forced upon them. Newspaper ads for the film *Nurses for Sale* (Independent-International, 1977) are emblazoned with the tag "Kidnapped, Abused and Tormented—Held for the Highest Price!" The accompanying pictures show one nurse being held by three grinning soldiers who are ripping off the last shreds of her uniform. The other nurse is grimly blasting away with a machine gun; her uniform is strained to the bursting point by an enormous bosom, and the view of her cleavage is interrupted only by one clearly inadequate uniform button.[33]

FILMS FOR GENERAL AUDIENCES

The Honeymoon Killers (Cinerama, 1970) told of the grisly but true romance between registered nurse Martha Beck and con artist Raymond Fernandez, whose scheme of fleecing lonely, wealthy women of their money—and killing whoever intervened— eventually led to their execution at Sing Sing in 1951. The introductory frames of the film capture some of Martha Beck's overweight charms and at the same time offer a classically negative portrayal of a nurse, made worse by the film's claim of documentary authenticity. The most obvious aspects of the nurse's personality are her unattractive appearance and her authoritarianism; indeed, this character recalls the often stereotypic nursing authority figure who, more often than not, is an unattractive and bitter woman. For example, Martha walks into a laboratory and finds an orderly and a nurse in a sexual embrace: rather than simply reprimanding them, she insinuates as much jealousy and hatred as she can into her terse commands. Thus, in the very beginning of the film, the audience knows this nurse character's essential nastiness and her threatening posture. The rest of the film continues in this vein, capturing two frequent nurse presentations of 1970s films—nurses as sexually promiscuous and nurses as sadists or malevolent influences. Martha Beck is seen throughout the film as the jealous paramour of an aging gigolo and as a cold-blooded murderer, capable of drowning little children and bludgeoning unsuspecting women. Aside from constant revulsion at this woman's perverted use of her nurse's training, the audience's only other response to this character would be occasional pity for Beck's pathetic attempts to create a cozy love nest for herself and her bigamous lover.[34]

In *Where Does It Hurt?* (Cinerama, 1972) an entirely corrupt hospital administrator, Mr. Hopfnagel (played by Peter Sellers), runs a profitable racket involving insurance fraud, double-dealing doctors, unnecessary operations, and padded bills. This film presents two highly unattractive and stereotyped nurse characters. Nurse Throttle (Hope Summers) is a dour, older head nurse who conforms to the rules and regulations for their own sake and lacks warmth and sympathy. She is, however, a hypocrite—strictly adhering to the rules for patients, but carelessly and

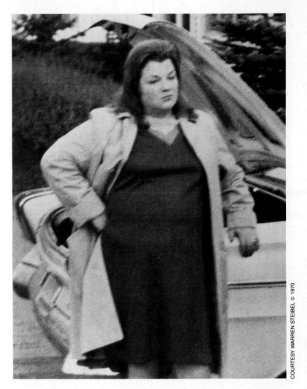

COURTESY WARREN STEIBEL © 1970

The introductory frames of the The Honeymoon Killers *(Cinerama, 1970) capture some of Martha Beck's overweight charms and offer a classically negative portrayal of a nurse.*

deliberately breaking the ethical code of her own profession. Apart from falsifying patient records, she also oversteps her professional bounds by recommending unnecessary surgery and taking a 33 percent cut of any extra charges that are added to her patients' bills as a result. Hers is the popular, lax attitude toward health insurance: spare not the cost since the individual does not have to pay for it anyway. Thus hospital bills are amplified to preposterous levels as patients, physicians, and nurses abuse the system. Nurse Throttle further degrades herself by joining the other nurses, physicians, and hospital staff in a bacchanalian party toward the end of the film: dancing and drinking leave her hair disheveled, her cap askew, her uniform partly unzipped at the back, and her speech slurred. Moreover, in attending the party and permitting her nurses to attend, she grossly neglects the patients in her care: numerous call lights blink as the fun goes on—patients suffer and even die while the staff has a good time. When the hospital commissioner discovers a dead man and asks Nurse Throttle if she knows about it, she responds with complete idiocy, "If I don't write things down it's forgetsville."[35]

A sexy, dumb blond, Nurse La Marr (Eve Bruce), is the other stereotypical nurse: Her body is absurdly large and voluptuous, her breasts and hips ooze out of a low-cut, mid-thigh length nurse's uniform, and her 6-foot height allows the shorter hospital administrator, Hopfnagel, to leer at her bosom at eye level. As a final whorish touch, she wears a curly platinum wig. La Marr is the object of all the men's sexual desires. She and Hopfnagel meet secretly in the linen room, where they are caught in flagrante delicto with the nurse wearing only her panties. One of her two nursing activities is even made into a farce when, after showing her giving a patient a massage, the camera draws back to disclose the man fondling the nurse's legs, as he moans; he then asks if they can do the front side. This sexual relationship between patient and nurse is further emphasized when Nurse Throttle tells the nurses that the big football player patient wants the bottle again: when Nurse La Marr replies, "I'll handle it," another nurse completes the pun by saying, "You'll need both hands."[36]

THE HOSPITAL AND CUCKOO'S NEST

On a more serious note, *The Hospital* (United Artists, 1971) took a satiric, darkly humorous look at the collision between an unwieldy institution and the social convulsions of the late-1960s. The perspective is that of Dr. Herbert Bock (George C. Scott), Director of Medicine at a large public hospital in New York City. The hospital struggles with internal problems caused by its sheer size (pilferage of equipment, staff shortage and absenteeism, impersonality, overcrowding, bureaucratic malfunctions), and is besieged from the outside by malpractice suits and community groups protesting its plans to tear down ghetto housing in order to expand even further. The plot turns on a simple device: writer Paddy Chayevsky asks what would happen if one introduced into this already strained and vulnerable institution a clever paranoid schizophrenic who is knowledgeable about medicine and hospital procedures and who has murderous intentions. The answer is a series of medically

induced deaths that symbolically reveal the institution's fragility: two physicians and a nurse are murdered in the hospital's hands, but in each case the deaths seem to have been caused by the errors of doctors and nurses.[37]

Dr. Bock, representative of the fragmented society that is the film's larger context, is separated from his wife and has rejected his children for their counterculture lifestyles. He is also impotent, constantly tired, drinks heavily and contemplates suicide. In spite of his personal turmoil, Bock is nevertheless a dedicated physician with strong commitments to good patient care and to the preparation of good physicians; in fact, only his professional dedication prevents him from killing himself. When the murders begin to occur, he tries to understand what has happened. His inquiry reveals blunder after blunder by nurses and doctors alike, resulting not only in dead medical personnel but also in an old but healthy man called Drummond falling into a coma. The grotesque errors of the hospital, the institution with which Bock is so deeply identified professionally, rob his last vestiges of dignity and self-respect, and he prepares to kill himself. But Barbara (Diana Rigg), Drummond's daughter, an ex-hippy and inactive registered nurse who has just tried unsuccessfully to seduce Bock, returns as Bock is about to give himself a fatal dose of potassium. Enraged by her interruption and her symbolization of the counterculture he detests, Bock attacks her. But his violence soon turns to sexual passion, and the next morning, restored to potency and self-respect, Bock is something like sane again. Barbara then confronts him with a choice, asking him to go to Mexico with her and her father.

Ex-flower child Barbara, with her cool worldliness and clarity of values, is an interesting counterpart to Bock. She is the representative of the counterculture, whereas Bock is the embodiment of traditional middle-class values. Barbara remains a static character throughout and has the important function of helping Bock discover once again that life is worth living. Obviously the viewer is expected to respond to Barbara the way Bock does—to be attracted to her, to be impressed by her certainty, and to be both repelled and tempted by her escapist values. Though she has been trained as a nurse, nursing seems to be a part of her identity that she has rejected, and indeed she herself represents a more generalized opposition to the system in which nursing plays a part.

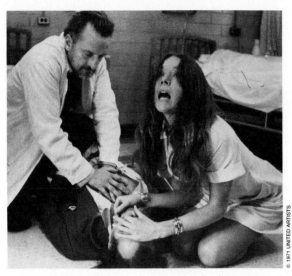

Though Barbara in The Hospital *(United Artists, 1971) has been trained as a nurse, nursing seems to be a part of her identity that she has rejected, and indeed she herself represents a more generalized opposition to the system in which nursing plays a part.*

Nursing is generally represented in this film as an extension of the modern bureaucratic structure. Nurses are the frontline troops, the health care professionals who have the most contact with the public, through whom most of the mistakes, impersonality, and inefficiency of large health care institutions are transmitted. Mrs. Christie (Nancy Marchand), the Director of Nursing, after explaining that a nurse sedated a medical resident instead of the patient who should have been occupying the bed, says, "These things happen," a line which suggests the shared attitude of all the nurses: when nurses make mistakes, there is a denial of personal responsibility or feeling. Nurses do not *do* things; things *happen*. Nurses in *The Hospital* are unable to perceive or appreciate the grotesqueness of the bizarre deaths occurring around them; they seem unshockable. For example, when one finds the medical resident dead in a patient's bed, she registers only mild surprise and then proceeds to check his vital signs. In part, this characteristic lack of reaction is an extension of an observing professional attitude, but since it is entirely free from concern or compassion, it seems cold and indifferent.

In contrast to some of the doctors—notably Dr. Bock—who care deeply about their patients, the composite image of nurses is quite negative. They are consistently depicted as unfeeling, error-prone functionaries in a depersonalized system. Though as individuals they seem ordinarily human, as professionals they seem machinelike. Clearly, by shunting them from floor to floor and shift to shift, the system emphasizes nurses' interchangeability and implicitly diminishes their professional responsibility. *The Hospital* suggests that in large hospitals administrative tasks have preempted direct relationships with patients. Mrs. Christie, for example, speaks almost entirely in terms of the movement of personnel; staff nurses are constantly seen doing paperwork; outside surgery, a nurse carries out the function of a traffic cop or dispatcher, routing patients into (one hopes) the correct operating rooms. Bock ask Drummond how he was able to leave his hospital bed to perform the murders without being detected. Drummond replies that he rang for his nurse, "to insure one full hour of uninterrupted privacy."[38]

The nurses' image suffers worst, however, from the remarks—often ill informed—of the protagonist, Dr. Bock, the character who represents the only "answer" this film has to offer for society's ills. He speaks scornfully of a medical resident named Schaeffer having "talked a nurse into zapping him on the bed." When he questions the director of nursing about Dr. Schaeffer's death, she explains that the high rate of absenteeism among nurses necessitates the use of the float nurses, who do not know the patients or doctors. Again Bock responds scornfully.

> Every time one of [the nurses] has her period, she disappears for three days. My doctors complain regularly that they can't find the same nurse on the same floor two days in a row. . . . Two separate nurses walk into a room and stick needles in a man . . . and it's the wrong poor son of a bitch. I mean, my God, where do you train your nurses, Mrs. Christie? Dachau?[39]

Because Bock still cares deeply about healing, because his anger at the needless deaths is righteous anger, and because he himself is the most likable character in the story, his judgments carry more authority than the actual sight of most of the nurses doing their work as efficiently as they can in the bureaucratic insanity that surrounds them. Whether they work well or whether they commit fatal errors, nurses still function symbolically as part of the cold, unfeeling bureaucracy that the film satirizes and hence elicit a negative response from the viewer.

A much more complicated and frightening image of the nursing profession emerged from Louise

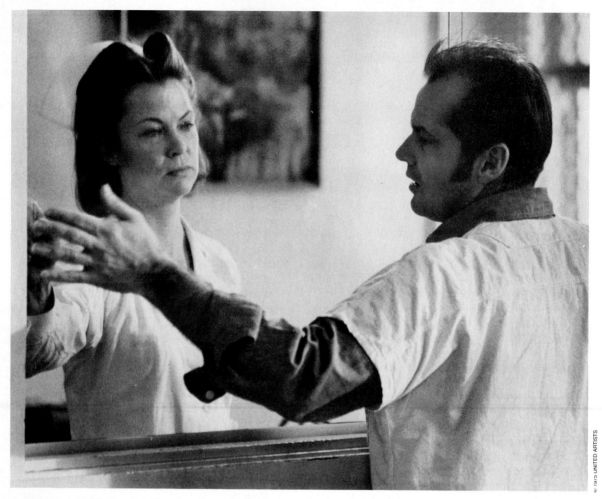

A psychoanalytical look at One Flew Over the Cuckoo's Nest *(United Artists, 1975) would concentrate on Nurse Ratched's role as the all-powerful mother who punishes her male children with guilt and brings about their impotence at all levels.*

Fletcher's interpretation of the role of Nurse Ratched in the highly acclaimed, Academy Award-winning film, *One Flew Over the Cuckoo's Nest* (United Artists, 1975). This film proved to be both a critical and popular success, and as such demands close inspection as to the image of the nursing profession. The complexity of the film challenges one's analytical faculties because it can be approached from so many different perspectives. A psychoanalytical look at the film would concentrate on Nurse Ratched's role as the all-powerful mother who punishes her male children with guilt and brings about their impotence at all levels. By examining all the symbols associated

with Nurse Ratched, one is brought to deeper understanding of her character: blood red nails and mouth contrast with her virginally white, starched uniform; a voluptuous figure is encased in corsets; and a warm, enticing voice comes out of a porcelain face with cold, hard eyes. Nurse Ratched is the perfect mother; she is also the perfect virgin; she is a seductress; and she is a vampire who sucks the life from her charges and turns them into the living dead. *One Flew Over the Cuckoo's Nest* is also an allegory of our technological society, in which sanity and insanity become hopelessly intermingled. Nurse Ratched is the acknowledged authority within the heartless, mechanistic system that orders this allegorical world—the State Mental Hospital.[40]

Louise Fletcher's interpretation of the nurse must have been drawn from an understanding of how mental hospital nurses have often been depicted in popular film and literature. Ratched's character exhibits all the virtues associated with the nursing profession. She demonstrates a warmly voiced concern for her patients' welfare; she imposes organization and discipline in order to provide a secure and well-maintained environment; she is dedicated to her job and has sacrificed her own private life to better serve her patients. Above all, she is maternal in her approach to her patients. All her spoken remarks attest to her desire to help them and to care for them. At the superficial level, Ratched is the perfect nurse. Yet Fletcher's inflections, facial gestures, and her presence undermine all her supposed virtues and expose her as an obsessive-compulsive personality with a need to totally control the lives of her patients. Her need to maintain control and power has brought her to pervert her nursing role. She ruthlessly guarantees that her patients will not recover their autonomy and dignity by her skillful manipulation of her role as therapist. And finally, Ratched stands as a symbol of spiritual death. Throughout the film, her archenemy and rival for control of the patients is McMurphy (Jack Nicholson), an exuberant testimony to life and love. When she brings about his lobotomization by the end of the film, she succeeds in reestablishing her peaceful, well-organized, and utterly sterile world.

One Cuckoo's Nest could reach many people, but unfortunately, this film represented only part of the continuing trend of the 1970s to draw the professional nurse along unflattering and often frightening lines. In Mel Brooks's *High Anxiety* (20th Century-Fox, 1977), a parody of Hitchcock motifs set in a mental institution, Cloris Leachman played a sadistic head nurse named Charlotte Diesel. Among her many abilities, Nurse Diesel had a talent for murder, extortion, and fraud, as well as interests in kinkier forms of sexual experience. Dressed in Nazi uniform and thigh-high boots, Nurse Diesel supplied the discipline and bondage that her lover, Dr. Montague, so craved. Nurse Diesel was a vulgar joke in anyone's opinion, but the effectiveness of this joke rested on the audience's familiarity with the head nurse type parodied by Diesel: the aging, unmarried, megalomaniac, sexually abnormal woman in power.[41]

NURSE SEX OBJECTS ON TELEVISION

Nurses have also been largely portrayed as sex objects in the television entertainment programming since the late-1960s. With the relaxation of censorship standards, television programmers began to exploit their new freedom with liberal use of sexual innuendo and provocative costuming for female nurse characters. The blond, dumb, sexy nurse in a tight, short, low-cut uniform became a stock character in spoofs of the health care establishment. For example, Dan Rowan and Dick Martin rose to fame on the popularity of their television series, *Laugh-In* (NBC), which premiered in 1968 and ran until 1973. *Laugh-In,* a satirical comedy-variety show, became known for its irreverent and boisterous spoofs of every imaginable American tradition, from the cocktail party to the political campaign. In a sketch from 1970, Rowan and Martin attack two venerable institutions: the medical profession and *The Tonight Show* (NBC, 1956–present). While Dick delivers a comic surgical monologue in the mode of Johnny Carson, his assistant chuckles maniacally from the sidelines. Doctors and talk shows may have been the intended targets of the spoof, but the nursing profession appears to have taken the heavy blows. Sexual availability was the single message broadcast about the comic nurses seen. Both before and after the skit, Rowan peeks into a linen closet only to interrupt two different nurses involved in hanky-panky with the same doctor. And the blond nurse who wheeled in a patient looked stupid, sexy, and promiscuous: costume, hairstyle, breathless voice, and body movements combined to bring home the message about the calibre of the nursing profession.[42]

An effort at hospital comedy, *Temperatures Rising,* appeared on ABC off and on from September 1972 until August 1974, when it was cancelled. Throughout its short life (and three formats) the show portrayed the adventures of the fun-loving, wacky staff of a Washington, D.C., general hospital called Capitol General. Cleavon Little played the central character, Dr. Jerry Noland, a fast-talking, streetwise black intern and resident. The series' improbable plot revolved around Noland's schemes to raise money for worthy causes or to solve ridiculous problems. As the Robin Hood of the hospital, Noland counted upon the support of a loyal band of accomplices—

a sexy head nurse; a not-so-sexy, good-sport staff nurse; and a cute, dumb, and eager student nurse.[43]

The salient quality of the nurses shown in this series was their adeptness at following. No matter how stupid, farfetched or illogical Noland's plans, the nurses eagerly joined him and carried out his instructions. The nurses were incapable of handling any situation on their own. For example, when a gangster entered the hospital, the nurses were chased and harassed by a group of unattractive thugs and seemed unable to fend off their unwelcome advances. It took two doctors to rescue one hapless student from an admirer named Nails. The nurses acted as loyal friends and comrades in arms, dedicated to worthy causes. They covered Noland's tracks and participated in his private money-making ventures, but they never initiated anything on their own.

The format of the second year took a more biting approach to nurses; although they maintained their roles as Noland's willing crew, their presentation assumed less-attractive features. In one episode the nurses were shown to be lazy and inattentive to hospital problems, insensitive to patients' concerns, and sexually experienced beyond the general norm. In both formats the professional identities of the nurses remained cloudy: a head nurse sort of stood at the nursing station and answered the phone, a staff nurse sort of did things in the hallways such as delivering mail and running errands, and the student nurse mostly did a little typing, a little patient care, and a lot of dropping things. No hierarchical pattern appeared among the nurses: nurses failed to provide leadership not only within the general framework of the plot but also within their own numbers. Although physicians depicted in the series were greedy, unethical, ineffectual, snide, sarcastic, and silly, they still emerged as problem solvers and natural leaders.

One of the most recent television series showing nurse characters is M*A*S*H (CBS, 1972–1983), the all-time most popular series in television history over its eleven seasons. During the first several seasons, Margaret (then mockingly called Hot Lips), the short-tempered, hypocritical head nurse, was one of the "bad guys." Later, she became fully integrated into the "good guys" camp and generated audience sympathy, as did the irreverent, iconoclastic, yet utterly humane doctors who work in a field hospital during the Korean War. Despite a general improvement, one must not forget the less admirable treat-

ment of nurse characters that marked the show in its first several seasons, for given the great popularity of the series in non-prime-time syndicated reruns, "Hot Lips" is seen just as often as the more recently reformed "Margaret." Although little evidence of professional incompetence ever tarnished the M*A*S*H nurse's image in the early days, the glimmer of nursing skill lay under a heavy layer of sexually oriented jokes and situations that marked the nurses' primary role as leisure-time playmates for the male surgeons. In the operating room, for example, the nurses functioned efficiently, but the surgeons gave their orders with sexual overtones, such as "move your pretty bottom, honey." In one episode Hot Lips is pursued by an amorous plastic surgeon who believes her to be the hot-to-trot nurse promised by Hawkeye in exchange for an off-the-record nose job for a needy soldier. In yet another instance, the nurses do not even become flustered when a man enters their shower looking for another man.[44]

Despite the rocky beginning, as seasons progressed M*A*S*H gradually recognized the distinctive role that nurses play. By the final two seasons, it offered the most professional view of nurses seen on prime-time TV. For example, in one episode the nurses are evacuated, leaving the male doctors to cope for themselves, and it is clear that they miss the nurses, both personally and professionally. Everyone pitches in to help with the nursing chores in the operating room, but it is soon evident that nursing is a special skill, not just something anyone can automatically do. In spite of all his former insubordination, Hawkeye declares fervently that if Margaret were here right now, "I'd kiss her feet." To Father Mulcahy, who is assisting with more goodwill than effectiveness, he says, "Keep those sponges coming, Father. Remember, *nurse* is also a verb. Not only is *nurse* a verb, it is a different verb from *doctor*."[45]

Operation Petticoat (ABC, 1977–1978) and *Black Sheep Squadron* (NBC, 1977–1978) similarly featured military nurses and emphasized their sexual attractiveness. The nurses of *Black Sheep Squadron* were gratuitous characters designed to provide sexual interest, as they were all shapely and young and seemed out of place at a frontline airfield devoid of medical officers or hospital. During the first two seasons, the head nurse character on *Trapper John* (CBS, 1979 to present) served as a general factotum for the chief surgeon; and the comely staff nurse, nicknamed "Ripples," was both a wholesome pal to the male doctors as well as the sexual focus of the series, with her sexually provocative uniform, high heels, and distracting walk. An episode of *House Calls* (CBS, 1979–1982) featured a reputedly good intensive care unit nurse who also worked as a stripper at a nightclub.[46]

SEX OBJECTS AND FRIGID NURSES IN NOVELS

The tradition of the nurse as the physician's sexual plaything carried through the novels of the 1970s. Samuel Shem (the pseudonym for a Boston psychiatrist), who authored *The House of God,* a 1978 novel that has sold over 600,000 copies, claims that the interns' numerous sexual encounters with the nurses in his novel are based on fact. "A nurse gets off at 11 P.M., you're there, and there's a bed. What else do you need?" he asks.[47] *The House of God* shows numerous sexual encounters with nurses to be part of the daily life of an intern who finds himself pitted against the GOMERS, an acronym for the chronically ill, demented, geriatric patients who should die but whose lives are maintained by modern technology. For instance, the following takes place in one of the hospital's on-call rooms.

> There was a knock at the door, and then two more, which was our code. There, in nursing uniform, were Angel and Molly.... In a gomer falsetto I wailed HALP NURSE HALP NURSE, HALP and they came to me. They flung back the curtain covering the lower bunk and bent over me, and the fronts of both their dresses were open, showing four elastical fantastical breasts in a sea froth of lace with two clefts in between. Oh, to nuzzle there, to lay my angry grieving head nuzzling in there and nuzzle and guzzle like a thirsty dumb horse muzzling water. To suck. One two three four nipples.... Up and down and bites and boobs, and just before I blasted off she slipped out of her dress, took down her panties, straddled my face, her lips on my penis again. My olfactory lobe seized up and our machine, spewing camshafts hubcaps and racheted gears slammed out into the wild BLUE YONDERRR!![48]

Shem follows the pronounced trend of physician-authors to depict nurses overwhelmingly as sex objects.

The 1970s ended with the malicious, spiteful, and domineering frigid nurse, presented with various modifications in such novels as *The World According to Garp,* a 1978 best-seller by John Irving. This bizarre and often macabre parable centers on the life and times of nurse Jenny Fields and her muscular and imaginative son, T. S. Garp. As the novel opens, Jenny's parents, possessors of both old money and a profitable shoe factory, are not pleased that Jenny is "slumming her life away as a nurse." Both as a nurse and as a woman, Jenny has little interest in men. For instance, while treating venereal disease patients with the "Valentine treatment" (a method of irrigating the male genital tract that leaves the individual howling in pain), Jenny observes how "appropriate this punishment was for a lover," an attitude that gives this nurse an unmistakably sadistic leaning. When a soldier makes a pass at Jenny in a dark movie theater she reaffirms this impression by slitting his arm from shoulder to wrist with a scalpel, a punishment that she also believes "appropriate" for a man with lust in his heart. After all, the narrator argues, she had no intention of killing the man, for as any nurse knows, it is a horizontal and not a vertical slice that would cause him to bleed to death.[49]

NOTES

1. Alfred C. Kinsey et al., *Sexual Behavior in the Human Female* (Philadelphia: Saunders, 1953); Alfred C. Kinsey, Wardell B. Pomeroy, and Clyde E. Martin, *Sexual Behavior in the Human Male* (Philadelphia: Saunders, 1948).

2. Simone de Beauvoir, *The Second Sex* (New York: Bantam Books, 1961).

3. Betty Friedan, *The Feminine Mystique* (New York: Dell, 1963), pp. 15–32.

4. Ibid., pp. 36–68.

5. Ibid., pp. 67–78.

6. Ibid., pp. 40–42.

7. Ibid., pp. 15–16.

8. Ibid., pp. 310–337.

9. Kate Millet, *Sexual Politics* (New York: Doubleday, 1970).

10. Germaine Greer, *The Female Eunuch* (New York: McGraw-Hill, 1971).

11. The Roper Organization, *The 1980 Virginia Slims American Women's Opinion Poll* (Storrs, Connecticut: The Roper Center, University of Connecticut, 1980), p. 103.

12. Alice Boyd Adams, *Families and Survivors* (New York: Knopf, 1974); Paula Fox, *Desperate Characters* (New York: Harcourt, Brace & World, 1970); Joan Didion, *Play It As It Lays: A Novel* (New York: Farrar, Straus & Giroux, 1970); Alix Kates Shulman, *Memoirs of an Ex-Prom Queen: A Novel* (New York: Knopf, 1972); Marge Piercy, *Small Change* (Garden City, New York: Doubleday, 1973).

13. Pamela Daniels and Kathy Weingarten, *Sooner or Later: The Timing of Parenthood in Adult Lives* (New York: Norton, 1983).

14. Benjamin McLane Spock, *Baby and Child Care* (New York: Pocket Books, 1976), p. 3.

15. *M*A*S*H* (20th Century-Fox, 1970), 116 min.

16. Ibid.

17. *Catch-22* (Paramount, 1970), 122 min.

18. *Carry On Again, Doctor* (Great Britain, RFD, 1979), 89 min.

19. *Carry On Nurse* (Great Britain, Governor Films, 1959), B & W, 90 min.

20. *Carry On Doctor* (Great Britain, Rank, 1972), 90 min.

21. *Carry On Matron* (Great Britain, Rank, 1972), 89 min.

22. *Carry On Nurse,* 1959.

23. Advertising posters for R-rated "Nurse Films," Nursing in the Mass Media Research Project, Ann Arbor, Michigan.

24. *I, A Woman* (Audubon Films, 1965), B & W, 90 min.

25. *I, A Woman Part II* (Chevron Pictures, 1968), 81 min.

26. *The Daughter: Or I A Woman, Part III* (Chevron, 1970), 84 min.

27. *Deep Throat* (Aquarius, 1972), 73 min.

28. *Deep Throat II* (Bryanson, 1974), 00 min.

29. *Student Nurses* (New World Pictures, 1970), 85 min.

30. *Night Call Nurses* (New World Pictures, 1972), 85 min.

31. Advertising posters for R-rated "Nurse Films," Nursing in the Mass Media Research Project, Ann Arbor, Michigan.

32. *Cherry, Harry and Raquel* (Eve Productions, 1969), 61 min.

33. *Nurses For Sale* (Independent-International, 1977), 84 min.

34. *The Honeymoon Killers* (Cinerama, 1970), B & W, 106 min.

35. *Where Does It Hurt?* (Cinerama, 1972), 90 min.

36. Ibid.

37. *The Hospital* (United Artists, 1971), 103 min.

38. Ibid.

39. Ibid.

40. *One Flew Over The Cuckoo's Nest* (United Artists, 1975), 129 min.

41. *High Anxiety* (20th Century-Fox, 1977), 94 min.

42. *Laugh-In* (60 minutes, Comedy-Variety) NBC, 1968–1973.

43. *Temperatures Rising* (30 minutes, Comedy) ABC, September 12, 1972, to August 20, 1974, 42 episodes.

44. *M*A*S*H* (30 minutes, Comedy Drama) CBS, September 17, 1972, to February 28, 1983, 250 episodes.

45. Ibid.

46. *Operation Petticoat* (30 minutes, Comedy) ABC, September 17, 1977, to August 25, 1978, 22 episodes; *The New Operation Petticoat* (30 minutes, Comedy) ABC, September 25, 1978, to October 19, 1978, and June 1, 1979, to August 3, 1979, 9 episodes; *Black Sheep Squadron* (60 minutes, Adventure) NBC, December 14, 1977, to September 1, 1978 (as *Baa Baa Black Sheep,* September 21, 1976, to August 30, 1977), 34 episodes; *Trapper John, M.D.* (60 minutes, Medical Drama) CBS, September 23, 1979, to present, over 170 episodes; *House Calls* (30 minutes, Comedy) CBS, December 17, 1979, to September 13, 1982, 60 episodes.

47. Samuel Shem, *The House of God* (New York: Dell Publishing Company, 1978); "Inside the Quarters of The House of God," *American Medical News* 24:15 (September 11, 1981).

48. Ibid.

49. John Irving, *The World According to Garp* (New York: Pocket Press, 1978).

CHAPTER NINE

CAREERIST: TOWARD A NEW IDEAL

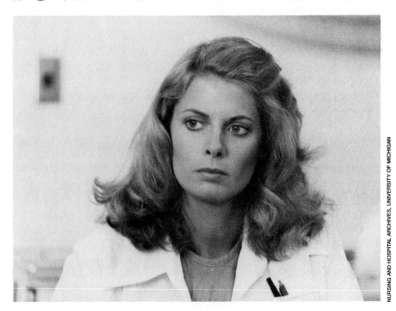

THE REVOLUTION IN HEALTH CARE ORGANIZATION

Today, there is a revolution going on in health care organization, financing, and marketing. Health care has become the subject of numerous articles in such business publications as *Business Week, The Wall Street Journal,* and *Fortune.* The implementation of Medicare's Prospective Payment System (PPS) for hospital inpatient services is having a major effect on health care administration. Payments for illness by the Federal Government's Health Care Financing Administration (HCFA) are now fixed in advance and linked to Diagnostic Related Groups (DRGs). Under the old system, Medicare paid what it considered to be the government's appropriate share of the cost. Under this new system, payments to hospitals are based on the average cost of treating a particular disease. This change was made in an attempt to encourage greater efficiency. The expectation is that hospitals that operate efficiently will benefit from treating Medicare patients, while hospitals that operate inefficiently will lose money. As a result of this change, many hospitals are testing new strategies for controlling costs.

Health Maintenance Organizations (HMOs) are prepaid health insurance plans designed to deliver affordable and comprehensive medical services to enrolled members. There are three types of HMOs. The first, called a group/staff HMO, delivers medical services at one or more locations, using physicians directly employed by the HMO. The second, known as the individual practice association (IPA), makes contractual arrangements with doctors in private practice who treat HMO members in their own offices. The third, the network HMO, involves contractual arrangements between the HMO and two or more group medical practices. The number of HMOs in the United States grew from 39 in 1971 to more than 400 in 1986. Enrollment during that period skyrocketed from 3 million to 15 million.

Meanwhile, private companies that sponsor health plans for their employees are seeking more information about costs from hospitals and physicians, scrutinizing insurance premiums and payments, and studying employee use of health care services. Consumers are also becoming more aware of health care costs, and there are indications that they are using health care services more prudently. The new holistic approach to medicine, which focuses on the whole health of the whole person, epitomizes consumers' heightened personal commitments to their own well-being.

Consumers today are better informed and better able to make their own medical decisions. "Informed consent" rules have provided consumers with the right to learn more from their doctors about their own health. Educational opportunities in the United States have proliferated in recent years. The G.I. Bill of Rights that followed World War II began a trend making higher education available to the masses; greater numbers of people now achieve educational parity with the doctors who treat them. Television has extended its reach into virtually every living room, and medical themes have pervaded television programming. Consumer advocates have employed television and other media to raise viewers' understanding of medicine. Popular magazines such as *Prevention* and *Medical Self-Care,* dealing exclusively with health, abound. Bookstores have established separate "Personal Health" sections in order to accommodate the ever-growing consumer interest. Today's consumers of health care services appear increasingly ready to assume a greater role in shaping medical practice through the exercise of intelligent choice.

Hospitals and physician groups are beginning to advertise extensively to consumers. Traditional advertisers have long realized the importance of advertising that creates mental images in the buyer's mind and now this approach has been extended to health care, the fastest growing segment of the advertising industry. While definite sums on the money that hospitals are putting into advertising are hard to come by, *The Healthcare Marketing Report,* an Atlanta trade publication, put hospitals' advertising expenditures at $600 million in 1984, double the previous year's expenditures, and said they would probably hit $1 billion in 1985 and over $2 billion by 1987. Much of the advertising is image oriented: portraying a hospital as first-rate, caring, or convenient. But as the concept of marketing health care services to consumers takes hold, some hospitals have taken to promoting health care products in much the same way that hamburger moguls promote hamburgers. Few have taken the concept as far as the for-profit investor-owned Republic Health Corporation of Dallas, which has made advertising a cornerstone of its aggressive strategy of packaging medical procedures along with special discounts or financing, giving them a brand name and marketing them directly to consumers. Among its eight branded "products" are "The Gift of Sight"—cataract surgery that includes a waiver by the hospital of medicare deductibles, "You're Becoming"—cosmetic surgery that can include special financing arrangements with certain banks, "Step Lively"—foot surgery, "Soundsense"— hearing exams and device emplacement, "Miracle Moments"—a maternity program; and others designed to treat alcoholism, drug addiction, and eating disorders.

We are witnessing the collectivization of a fragmented industry. Some hospitals and other health care institutions will be organized on a for-profit basis; others will continue to reflect what has been the dominant form of institutional organization over the course of America's medical-care history—the tax exempt, nonprofit model. In some cases, these national and regional organizations will grow through merger and acquisition—a classic industry consolidation process. Others will grow through joint ventures, franchising, and internal growth programs. At the same time there will be a process of vertical integration whereby these health care organizations internalize more and more services: we are already seeing hospitals move into ownership of ambulatory care facilities and after-care programs. If change is a sign of public interest, then today that interest is extraordinary. The structure of the health care system is changing and will continue to do so. As in all revolutions, this is a time of confusion in health care. Old and well-established arrangements are being discarded. New and confusing ones are being instituted. It is hard to sort out how the gains and losses will be distributed.

THE BATTLE AGAINST STEREOTYPES

We are also experiencing what may be the final feminist revolution. In the past, there have been fights for certain specific rights and freedoms for women—the right to own property, to vote, to practice birth control, to enter certain professions, and so forth. But now the movement is toward full equality with men. In language, dress, education, and careers, women have demanded the simple status of "people," rather than that of a separate group— "females." The battles against traditional gender stereotyping based on supposed differences in emotionality, stability, intelligence, rationality, and aggressiveness have been fought on many fronts. The women's liberation movement, therefore, may be more properly called the gender liberation movement. Male and female roles are merging. It is not simply that women are becoming more like men, but that members of both sexes are becoming more alike. Men are now much more likely to turn down overtime work, promotions, or job transfers that will enhance their careers for fear that they will disrupt their family lives. A whole new liberation literature is emerging on the freeing of men from male roles and on the importance of fatherhood to both men and children. A whole new field of study has emerged that transcends the research in sex roles: the area of cognitive or psychological androgyny. This type of androgyny has nothing to do with ambiguous genitalia or appearance. It is concerned, instead, with a blend of the cognitive styles traditionally associated with men and women. An androgyne is a person who is able to be both rational and emotional, strong and nurturant, assertive and compassionate, depending on the demands of the situation.

In the last 15 years, researchers have amassed extensive data on the stereotyped images of men and women in television entertainment and commercials. Studies have shown that male characters far outnumber female characters in television programs. In some programs, the ratio is as high as five males to one female. In many popular adventure series, there have been no significant female characters at all. Male characters are often more exciting and interesting; they portray almost all the professionals, heroes, and criminals. Women characters, in contrast, tend to be dependent on men, less intelligent and competent than men, and more emotional. Women are also portrayed as more passive and less successful in achieving their goals. The sex bias of television content has been clear in adult entertainment, children's programming, and even news and documentaries. There have been some improvements in recent years, but the changes are still minimal, and some observers have argued that the presentation of women has actually worsened even as it has appeared to get better. Researchers have also concluded that the roles played by males and females in television are capable of influencing children's perceptions of appropriate gender roles. In one study, for example, children who saw women portrayed in traditionally male roles were more likely to claim that these roles were appropriate for women than were children who saw only men in these roles. Such studies seem to suggest, therefore, that typical sexist television content not only reflects the current sex biases of the culture but also serves to maintain these biases by passing them on to the next generation.

Today's nurse stereotype promotes negative and wasteful social perceptions of nearly half of all health care providers. Nurse characters are presented as generally less important and capable than physician characters. They are shown to be less committed to and happy with their profession than doctors. Nurses are viewed less positively by other characters; they are portrayed as if they make far fewer contributions to patients' well-being, and as if they are incapable of autonomous judgment. Furthermore, physicians are shown to place little value on their nurse colleagues. Ultimately, there has been little attempt by the media industries, particularly in recent years, to show the central and diverse role the nurse plays in the delivery of health care to the American public.

Furthermore, most of the characterizations of nurses are dominated by what one might call the "medical voice." The definition of nurses' and nursing's most serious problems and the proposed solutions to these problems are really, though often covertly, tailored to meet the needs of fundamentally medical problems. These kinds of characterizations must be termed prejudiced or stereotyped, because they tend always to emphasize one aspect of character while leaving out others of equal or greater importance. Specifically, the biases are carefully chosen to justify certain behavior of physicians toward nurses. The stereotypes of nurses vary, but they vary in response to the needs of physicians. The flattering frequency with which nurses appear in the mass media is ultimately deluding: they appear not as they are, and certainly not as they would define themselves, but as conveniences to the resolution of physicians' dilemmas.

HEALTH CARE GENRE ASSUMPTIONS

Many products of the health care genre incorporate, to some extent, an idealized interpretation of health care that one may call the "miracles of modern med-

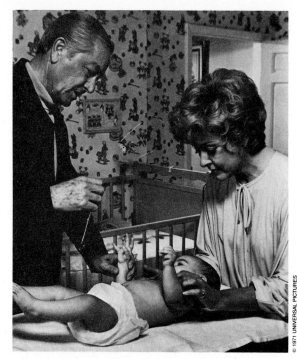

© 1971 UNIVERSAL PICTURES

One of the worst assumptions of the health care genre is that physicians are totally dedicated to a biopsychosocial approach in their delivery of health care, while nurses are simple technicians, clerks, and gofers.

icine" thesis. This set of assumptions can be described as follows.

1. Health care largely manifests itself through its services. The love that paternal physicians and maternal nurses have for their fellow citizens is provided primarily for the benefit of the recipients.
2. While physicians are men of science who are the great healers of modern civilization, nurses are young women who have temporarily (until marriage) dedicated their lives to humanity and to assisting the physicians for whom they work.
3. Physicians are totally dedicated to a biopsychosocial approach in their delivery of health care, while nurses are simple technicians, clerks, and gofers.
4. While males make the best physicians, a few females are specially qualified to deliver outstanding medical care in selected instances; however, men are totally unsuited to nursing roles.
5. Progress in the health care industry results from a deepening sense of physicians' social obligation,

from an increase in findings from biomedical research, and from a more perfect medical technology.

6. Changes are cumulative, and the quality of care evolves constantly and positively in the direction of better health and longer life, even if this life persists at lower and lower thresholds.

7. Improvements are irreversible and the current health care services are of the highest level.

8. While present services are incomplete, the central structure of the health care industry is in splendid condition, and its services are so constituted that the public can confidently look forward to infinite improvement.

This listing constitutes the general framework of the miracles of modern medicine thesis. Not every media product coincides with this thesis, but it is often implicit, if not explicit, in mass media presentations of modern health care.

The final irony is that life often imitates art. When society sanctions or even praises stereotyped images of nurses and physicians, the nurses and physicians who work in our culture form their own self-images accordingly. In the case of nursing, stereotypes may become, by a sort of perversity, an image of reality that even nurses seek to perpetuate. When nurses are constantly portrayed in negatively stereotypical ways, these images affect their lives and their aspirations, and limit the scope of their work. Moreover, authors, producers, directors, scriptwriters, and medical advisors may actually fail to see that the current nurse image is stereotypical and demeaning and that other approaches could work as well or better, because the current approach is ultimately a reinforcement of their own prejudices. To change the current nurse image requires changing the attitudes of the image makers. The mass media industries more than any others have the opportunity to reaffirm these images constantly. The mass media act as molders of outlook and legitimize those roles in which so many nurses find themselves.

Particular assumptions in mass media communications about the division of health care responsibilities among nurses and physicians significantly affect the interests of both professions. These interests are not always entirely coincident. That certain values favoring the interests of physicians have been embodied positively in a variety of health care messages over a long period of time indicates that the

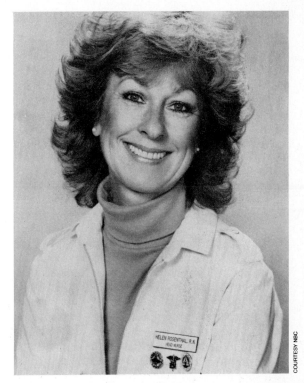

COURTESY NBC

The mass media act as molders of outlook and legitimize those roles in which so many nurses find themselves.

components of the traditional health care genre are an important means by which these values—and hence major inequalities between medicine and nursing—are maintained. That these erroneous stereotypes do not always have to be made explicit in either fictional or actual settings suggests the effects of a powerful set of beliefs concerning nurses and physicians—and that mass media messages are one of the means by which these stereotypes are sustained.

Consequently, the present nature of the health care genre in the mass media constitutes a considerable obstacle to innovation in health care policy, since public policy has its origins in public opinion, whether general or informed. The media offer implicit, persistent, and one-sided interpretative frameworks within which health care events are reported and made sense of. Such frameworks can be mainly accounted for either by organizational factors (for instance, reliance on limited sources of information and the application of media values in selecting content that emphasizes the dramatic, the heroic, and the masculine) or by ideological factors such as stereotypes, archetypes, and myths. While the relation between fiction and fact is invariably subtle, the health care genre communicates, reflects, and justifies practices of traditional medicine, nursing, and health care in the real world outside the mass media. Media create, extend, and confirm the accepted, common sense beliefs and practices of society. And few symbols are of more fundamental importance to a culture than its image and consequent treatment of health care.

The reasons for the past dominance and continuing strength of the miracles-of-modern-medicine thesis in the health care genre must be to some degree speculative. The following factors seem to be important.

1. The development of modern medical technology has been associated with overwhelmingly positive news coverage.
2. Health care has become equated with the practice of scientific medicine incorporating the latest medical technology.
3. The largely male spokespersons of existing medical institutions, who may have a vested interest in supporting the existing media definitions of nursing, are considered the most legitimate.
4. Information supporting the miracles of modern medicine thesis has been more accessible than facts and arguments that would contradict or qualify it.
5. In these circumstances the needs of media message-producers, the values of traditional news and entertainment, and current popular beliefs may operate jointly and harmoniously to deprive the public of an alternative and more historically correct version of health progress, which would relate health more to social environment and to the long-term implementation of health promotion and disease prevention measures.

NEED FOR A NEW DOMINANT IMAGE

We have seen, if only through a glass darkly, the fragmented vision of five dominant images of American nurses. Most of us who have experienced socialization as nurses can readily identify parts of ourselves and our social conditioning in these images. We have all played the angel of mercy, the girl Friday, the heroine, the mother, and the sex object. We have been living with definitions of ourselves and assigned cultural roles in which we have had no hand, yet we have offered amazingly little resistance. Why? This is the real question. At least part of the answer lies in the self-fulfilling nature of stereotypes. Research shows us that members of a stereotyped group often subscribe to the stereotypes about themselves and tend to act in ways that confirm stereotyped expectations. Thus nurses, perhaps on an unconscious level, have contributed to the maintenance of dysfunctional stereotypes. It is perhaps a commentary, however, on our lack of professional self-identity and self-esteem that we have so readily adapted ourselves to images that are so strongly derivative of outmoded military, religious, and female values. What is needed now is to create a new ideal nurse image for the 1980s and 1990s: the careerist—an intelligent, logical, progressive, sophisticated, emphatic, and assertive woman or man who is committed to attaining higher and higher standards of health care for the American public.

The fabrication of a more ideal nurse image for the future, the careerist, is essential to persuade the public (as well as many nurses) that how things are is not how they ought to be, and that the status given nurses in the mass media is much lower than the status nurses ought to have. To the extent that the mass media serve an agenda-setting function, we call for them to effect a transformation of the image of the nurse to one that emphasizes equality, commitment to career, and renunciation of nursing as a physician-dominated occupation demanding an impossible degree of obedience. Substitution of androgyny for traditional, rigid female imagery in media nurse representations would effectively provide alternative role models that would begin to open nursing up as a strong, desirable career option for both sexes.

The implications of equating the nurse with the quintessence of traditional womanhood have come to the fore largely as the result of the woman's movement. There is a parallel assumption that since women have traditionally been subordinated to men, the principal sign of the new woman's emancipation is entrance into the male world of work. Public support through acceptance of new female imagery has helped promote impressive gains: women in 1984 comprised one third of the first-year medical students and one third of all business students, and the percentage of female engineering graduates has soared from one percent in 1970 to 12 percent in 1984. However, the number of male nursing applicants and graduates remains low, despite widespread career opportunities.

Before the turn of the century and during the first half of this century, a woman's decision to become a nurse represented a blow for independence. But for a woman of today, entrance into the nursing profession is too often regarded as one more surrender to the narrowing of personal ambition and as an unadventurous acceptance of the strictures of gender-role specialization. This negative effect is due to the perpetuation of the outmoded occupational stereotype that the ideal nurse is dependent and ineffectual in her attempts to direct her own destiny. Such stereotypes deter prospective nurses from entering the field, and also limit the aspirations and opportunities of active professional nurses, since employers, patients, other health care providers, and nurses themselves are all influenced by media images. The dearth of viable role models of progressive mass media nurses serves to perpetuate the traditional images of nurses as angels of mercy, girls Friday, mothers, and sex objects, while at the same time quietly forgetting the heroine connotations of the 1930s and early-1940s.

WOMEN OF THE 1990s

The transition to a careerist nurse image will necessitate a time of conflict and change. When outmoded images begin to shatter, both old and new alternatives compete for ascendancy. Remember the images of the future we embraced 25 years ago. Optimism was prevalent: the future world would be a technological utopia. Robots would do our work; cars would be steered by remote control; and our appetites would be satisfied by pills. In essence, tomorrow would be bigger, better, and faster. Nurses, of course, would be in the forefront in serving the health care demands of that future society as its members steadily accumulated both health and wealth. But something funny happened on the way to utopia. Our visionary image of the future disappeared under high health care costs, energy shortages, inflation, population explosions, urban decay, and food problems—and with that vision went many

of our hopes for the future. Bit by bit, a new set of images is now evolving that suggests a future radically different from that conceived of in the recent past. The modern world view, predicated on beliefs such as progress being synonymous with amassing greater and greater material abundance and technology being the tool used to provide a limitless future, is being challenged, as are our present health care industry practices. A new world view is about to emerge—one that values restraint and recognizes limits.

Today, in the mid-1980s, it is apparent that the supposedly ideal American family—the husband as sole breadwinner and the wife as full-time housewife taking care of their two children—is now a fading illusion. The Department of Labor predicts that by 1990 more than half of all workers will be women. The numbers serve as evidence that the relations of women to men, children, money, families, politics, and the workplace are shifting quickly and drastically. Perhaps the most compelling reason for women to participate in employment outside the home will be sheer economic necessity. One out of every six families today is headed by a female. The divorce rate has soared and many women are marrying later or not at all. Thus, for those who must support themselves or their families, a job is an unquestioned necessity. In a society in which individuals define their goals and choose their careers, changes in the values associated with specific occupations such as nursing reflect changes in the goals of persons and in the rules governing access to scarce resources.

The principal goal of the career nurse may not be so much to support and advance her family as it is to realize herself as an individual. As with all philosophies, there are those nurses who fully or only partially subscribe to the new, emerging philosophy and those who are adamantly against it. Estimates of women's participation in the labor force in 1990 range between 53.8 percent (if the number of children born to each woman turns upward again) and 60.4 percent (if participation continues to rise at its present rate of growth). It is expected that the proportion of the labor force accounted for by women may reach 45–46 percent of the total by 1990, increasing the economic influence of working women. Married women are expected to account for a larger proportion of the female labor force by the end of the 1980s, due both to an older population and to a continuing increase in participation rates. There is also expected to be a continued increase in the numbers of working mothers with preschool children. By the beginning of the 1990s, two thirds of all married women under 55 may be working, including over half of all mothers of young children.

Women's participation within the family has shifted dramatically. In the process, family forms and domestic relationships have been transformed. New issues have arisen around marriage and family organization. Such questions as whether to live together before marriage, what should be included in the marriage contract, whether to have a second child, when the children are old enough to stay by themselves after school, and who does the laundry or changes the oil in the car are becoming common family decisions. The impact, however, extends beyond individual families to virtually every institution in our society: volunteer work in schools and hospitals; fringe benefits of part-time jobs; social security, pensions, and insurance benefits; child custody and child support; and even census classifications have come under scrutiny. Delaying marriage, planning fertility, participating in the labor market, and heading families indicate women's increasing desire and ability to control the conditions of their lives. Such increasing control challenges the existing assumptions of women's strong tie to wifehood and motherhood. Beliefs that women want and emotionally prefer self-sacrificing behavior, particularly for their husbands and children, are no longer consistent with women's consciousness or behavior.

These sociocultural issues have been postulated to cause changes in men's roles. As more married women enter the work force, more husbands assume responsibility for more household tasks. According to a survey by Benton and Bowles, a well-known advertising agency, 80 percent of young husbands participate in the care of children under age twelve, 53 percent wash dishes, 47 percent cook for the family, 39 percent vacuum the house, 32 percent shop for food, 29 percent do some of the laundry, and 28 percent sometimes clean the bathroom. Significantly, while women opted for more masculine college majors in the 1970s and 1980s, men did not cross over into fields such as nursing, although many occupations once considered limited exclusively to males or females are gaining acceptance by the opposite sex.

NEW FEMALE IMAGERY

As millions of women have moved out of the home into the labor force, they have been accompanied by the creation and diffusion of new female imagery. That new imagery has been provided in part by a host of new magazines. Five of these—*New Woman, Savvy, Self, Spring, Working Woman*—set growth records for women's magazines. It took several years to develop appropriate images for the new working woman. For example, the first issue of *Working Woman* (1976) had not one but nine working women on the cover. How did one stereotype a working woman? With a steno pad? With coveralls? In a uniform? Carrying a briefcase? As a housewife type with horn-rimmed glasses? By the end of the 1970s, however, most of the magazines for working women had settled on an idealized image of a dauntless, attractive business executive in a tailored suit, string tie, and feminine-looking briefcase. Little of this idealized image is appropriate for nurses, who comprise the nation's second largest profession.

Numerous groups such as blacks, native Americans, the handicapped, environmentalists, and feminists have turned to the mass media as one of the most effective means of fostering supportive public opinion. Inherent in these movements, as well as in current efforts to advance nursing, is the need for change, which implies the need for new information to be disseminated to the public. The evolution of nursing as a form of woman's work has been coupled with an outmoded legacy of beliefs, expectations, and myths about nursing. The importance of such a legacy is apparent in Parson's observation that "what persons are can only be understood in terms of a set of beliefs and sentiments which define what they ought to be." In short, the media as political and informational institutions are the central organizing forums for resource-poor groups such as nurses.[1]

That the media image of the nurse in the mid-1980s is at an abysmal low has severe implications for the profession. The mass media reflect and shape the attitudes, values, and needs that the American public has relative to nursing. The images of nursing that are communicated through the media become reality for many people. The mass media show a world of health care that a large portion of the public would otherwise seldom see, and as a result the media help to shape what the public *knows* about nursing, what they *believe* about nursing, and what they *feel* about nursing. Research has shown that the media create such an air of authenticity that disentangling fact from fiction may be almost impossible for many viewers. Consequently, when a negatively stereotyped nursing image is frequently repeated, it becomes accepted as reality.

IMPLICATIONS OF THE NEGATIVE IMAGE OF NURSING

The consequences of a distorted image of nurses and nursing are serious and far-reaching. Perhaps one of the most crucial problems is that this poor image affects the quantity and quality of persons who choose nursing as an occupation. A public constantly fed a demeaning image of nursing will not perceive nursing as a desirable profession. This is especially true for young people, who are very heavy media consumers. The average adolescent graduating from high school has spent more time watching television than in the classroom (15,000 hours in front of the TV versus 12,000 hours in school), and 41 percent of motion picture audiences are between ages 12 and 20. It is particularly troublesome that in a time when young women are choosing traditionally male-dominated professions, nursing is not recruiting a comparable number of young men. Because male nurses are virtually nonexistent in mass-media portrayals of the profession, there is an absence of male nurse role models. This void only increases the barriers to recruiting half the population.

Similarly, the media's portrayal of nursing affects the decisions of policy makers relative to the profession. Decision makers, acting at least in part on the basis of their perceptions of nursing gained through the media, enact legislation that defines the scope and financing of nursing services and allocates the scarce resources that undergird nursing practice, education, and research. If policy makers and their constituents are consistently exposed to images that depict the nurse as merely an unintelligent handmaiden to the physician, more interested in sex than in her profession, then they are much less disposed to pass legislation that gives nurses more autonomy in their practice or to allocate sufficient resources to advance the role of the nurse in health care.

Consumers, too, are affected by the media images that they receive of the profession. Since the media do not portray nurses as instrumental health care providers and have failed to mirror the changing role of the nurse, the public lacks awareness of the many vital services that nurses currently do provide. The physician continues to get nearly all the credit for any positive health care outcomes, and this discrepancy is reinforced in the media.

The negative mass-media images of nurses and nursing also create problems with nurses' self-image. Although some nurses may not consciously recognize the impact of media depictions of their profession, on a subliminal level the effect is unmistakable. Large numbers of nurses declare that they avoid exposure to the media images because they find them painful to watch or read. The effects of media distortion of nurses might be compared to the effects of *Amos and Andy* radio and television portrayals on the self-concepts and aspirations of blacks during the 1930s, 1940s, and early-1950s. Television broadcasting is essentially generated by a few hundred individuals and advertisers, but it is received by more than 200 million Americans. Special interest groups such as nurses have a right to care about how their profession is portrayed in the mass media.

STRATEGIES FOR INTERVENTION

Nurses can intervene to improve the current tarnished image of nursing—not only for the profession itself but especially for the American public it serves. Nurses have the means to voice their objections to the demeaning, one-dimensional, and damaging media portrayals of themselves and their work and to reverse the dangerous downward trend in the quality of their image. The process of intervention involves four key steps: (1) getting organized, (2) monitoring the media, (3) reacting to the media, and (4) fostering an improved image.

GETTING ORGANIZED

The first step in any such effort is organization. To provide leadership, special "image of the nurse" or "nursing in the media" committees or organizations need to be created. These image committees or organizations may be established by nurses in one hospital, health care agency, or school of nursing, or by nurses in a single community, state, or region of the country, as well as by those nurses organized on the national level, either as an independent organization or a sponsored activity by one or more of the nursing associations. Organized efforts are needed on all levels from the institutional to the national level. Several associations have undertaken initial efforts to improve the image of the nurse, including the American Academy of Nursing, the American Nurses' Association, the National League for Nursing, the American Association of Critical Care Nurses, and Sigma Theta Tau.

In the past decade, approximately 250 media watch groups have sprung up on the local and national levels, representing a diversity of special interests and opinions, such as "Black Citizens for a Fairer Media," "Action for Children's Television," "National Organization Against Sexism in the Media," and "National Latino Media Coalition." A national action group designed to deal with the image of the nurse might be called "Nurses for Media Change" or the "National Nurse Media Coalition."

MONITORING THE MEDIA

After such groups are organized, they can embark on a systematic effort to monitor, at both the local and national levels, all the forms of mass communications—television, motion pictures, novels, newspapers, magazines, and radio. While this may seem like a mammoth undertaking, nurses have the advantage of large numbers to share the burden. Since newspapers, radio, and local television programming must be monitored at local levels, there is great need to develop many groups at the local or grassroots level rather than to attempt to handle the entire problem from a national perspective.

Once a media watch group is operational, the basic question to ask is whether or not nurses and nursing are being conveyed by the media in a constructive or destructive manner. A suggested checklist of criteria for monitoring media images of nurses and nursing is offered in Table 9–1. As indicated, nurses should be portrayed with relevance to the current health care scene, with respect, and with recognition of the changing roles and changing values and attitudes of society. The portrayal of nurses as merely the sex objects of the health care world is

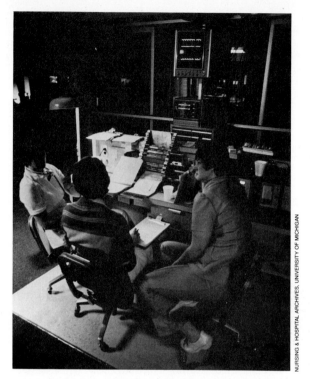

Distorted images of health care professionals in the mass media continue to present obstacles to innovative health care policy because they are potent molders of public opinion.

particularly abhorrent. While most nurses do not reject sensuality per se, there is a very fine line that needs to be drawn between showing that female nurses want to be attractive to the men in their lives and implying that they are objects for sexual exploitation. In addition, even the most traditional nurse resents condescension and deprecation by physicians via mass media depictions.

REACTING TO THE MEDIA

Once the media portrayals are monitored, appropriate and timely reactions by the nursing profession must be forthcoming, reactions that commend or condemn particular portrayals of nurses. This process includes writing letters of protest or praise to producers, directors, editors, writers, sponsors, advertisers, and other persons responsible for the creation and financial support of media depictions.

TABLE 9-1

CHECKLIST FOR MONITORING MEDIA IMAGES
OF NURSES AND NURSING

Prominence in the Plot

1. Are nurse characters seen in leading or supportive roles?

2. Are nurse characters shown taking an active part in the proceedings or are they shown primarily in the background (handing instruments, carrying trays, pushing wheelchairs)?

3. To what extent are nurse characters shown in professional roles, engaged in nursing practice?

4. Is it nurse characters or other characters who provide the actual nursing care?

5. In scenes with non-nurse professionals (physicians, hospital administrators, etc.), who does most of the talking?

Demographics

6. Does the portrayal show that men as well as women may aspire to a career in nursing?

7. Are nurse characters shown to be of varying ages?

8. Are some nurse characters single and others married?

Personality Traits

9. Are nurse characters portrayed as:

a. intelligent	e. sophisticated	i. nurturant
b. rational	f. problem solvers	j. empathic
c. confident	g. assertive	k. sincere
d. ambitious	h. powerful	l. kind

10. If other health care providers are included in the program, what differences are seen in their personality traits as compared with nurse characters?

11. When nurse characters exhibit the personality traits 9a through 9h listed above, do such portrayals show them to be abnormal in some way?

Primary Values

12. Do nurse characters exhibit values for:

    a. service to others, humanism   b. scholarship, achievement

13. If other health care providers are included in the program, what differences are seen in their primary values as compared with nurse characters?

14. When nurse characters exhibit the primary values of scholarship and achievement, do such portrayals show them to be abnormal in some way?

Sex Objects

15. Are nurse characters portrayed as sex objects?

16. Are nurse characters referred to in sexually demeaning terms?

17. Are nurse characters presented as appealing because of their physical attractiveness or cuteness as opposed to their intellectual capacity, professional commitment, or skill?

(continued)

Role of the Nurse

18. Is the profession of nursing shown to be an attractive and fulfilling long-term career?
19. Is the work of the nurse characters shown to be creative and exciting?

Career Orientation

20. How important is the career of nursing to the nurse character portrayed?
21. How does this compare with other professionals depicted in the program?

Professional Competence

22. Are nurse characters praised for their professional capabilities by other characters?
23. Do nurse characters praise other professionals?
24. Do nurse characters exhibit autonomous judgment in professional matters?
25. Is there a gratuitous message that a nurse's role in health care is a supportive rather than central one?
26. Do nurse characters positively influence patient/family welfare?
27. Are nurse characters shown harming or acting to the detriment of patients?
28. How does the professional competence of nurse characters compare with the professional competence of other health care providers?
29. When nurse characters exhibit professional competence, are they shown to be abnormal in some way?

Education

30. Who actually teaches the nursing students?
31. Who appears to be in charge of nursing education?
32. Is there evidence that the practice of nursing requires special knowledge and skills?
33. What is actually taught to nursing students?

Administration

34. Are any roles filled by nurse administrators or managers or are all nurse characters shown as staff nurses or students?
35. Is there evidence of an administrative hierarchy in nursing or are nurses shown answering to physicians or hospital administrators?
36. Are nurse characters shown turning to other nurses for assistance or are they depicted as relying on a physician or other character (generally male) for guidance, strength, and/or rescuing?

Overall Assessment and Comments

37. Overall, is this a positive or negative portrayal of nursing? Why or why not?

Obviously, the larger the number of letters from nurses protesting or supporting a particular TV program, film, or article, the more effective will be the campaign. The development of special media newsletters or a news column in an existing nursing journal would keep a large group of nurses informed about positive and negative images of the profession in the media as well as appropriate actions to take.

It is clear that all media executives and sponsors must pay some attention when a media-conscious organization protests a deficient image: as profit-oriented business ventures, the media must be sensitive to public reaction. There is a special reason for this in the television and radio industries, because broadcasters are obligated by federal law to operate in the public interest. The extraordinary responsibility of the broadcast media exists because the public actually owns the airwaves and each station is granted temporary use of a specific frequency or channel by government license. A triangular relationship thus exists in broadcasting between viewer, sponsor, and broadcaster. The Federal Communications Commission (a six-member team appointed by the President) licenses corporations to use specific channels for 3-year periods. The broadcaster has many obligations to fulfill in order to keep a license. The station's records are subject to review whenever the license comes up for renewal, and these records can also be examined by the public. According to the law, the broadcaster must consult with citizens who are representative of the viewing area to determine their needs. He must present programming of crucial local importance, airing various viewpoints. The broadcaster may and does use the airwaves to make money, but profit must be secondary to the goal of serving the public need.

Several occupational interest groups are currently seeking to influence their media image. For example, the International Association of Machinists deplores how blue-collar workers are depicted on television programs and has joined other labor groups in subsidizing a campaign to monitor network and local programming. They plan to use their findings as evidence to challenge license renewals and to bring pressure on broadcasters. Nurses should not feel that they are meddling in the private business affairs of others by demanding that television and radio stations meet their obligations to the public by providing accurate portrayals of the profession. Responsible action where improvement is needed is better called good citizenship than interference.

When writing about a particular media portrayal, the writer should include in the letter the air or publication date, the title of the program, film, newspaper article, or book, and the reporter's or author's name if listed. It is helpful to make suggestions for improving the image of the nurse rather than simply to criticize the way nurses are depicted. Follow-up letters when improvements do take place are important for building positive relationships. If inaccurate information has been reported in a newspaper, magazine, or television news program, a follow-up story or correction should be suggested.

The top decision makers in the media industry are the key persons to contact. There are more than 9,000 local radio and television stations on the air in the United States today. The latest edition of *Broadcasting Yearbook* contains a complete listing of the address, telephone number, and manager of local stations. Frequently these addresses can also be found in a local telephone book. The letter, telephone call, or visit should be directed to the general manager, who is in the best position to influence locally based programming, and also to the network with which his or her station is linked. Nearly 80 percent of all television programming comes from the major commercial networks, and letters should also be sent to network headquarters.

A reactive strategy that can be used against offensive motion pictures depicting nurses is to picket motion picture theaters that show such films, in order to create negative publicity for the theater and to keep potential consumers from crossing the picket line. Products advertised on radio or television programs containing a negative image of nursing may also be boycotted. This is most successful when accompanied by picketing outside local grocery stores so that the boycott will become known to the public. The product manufacturer should also be notified of the reason for the boycott.

FOSTERING AN IMPROVED IMAGE

In addition to monitoring and reacting to the media as it already exists, nurses need to foster a positive image. One of the first steps in this process is to build strong media contacts and to educate media

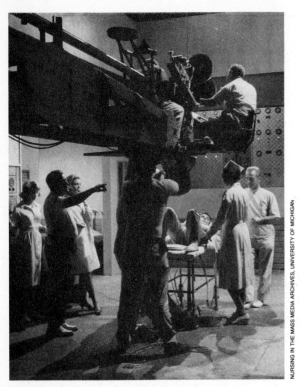

Although nurses have already served as consultants to several media productions, a great deal more could be done in this area.

executives and personnel about today's nursing profession. Arranging conferences that bring nurses, media executives, and legislators together to examine the image of nursing in the media is a particularly effective strategy. It is also important for at least some nurses to learn the technical aspects of the media industries so that they can use their expertise for the advancement of the profession. How the mass media react to nurses and their concerns rests partly on how well nurses understand the role, function, and purpose of the media.

Although nurses have already served as consultants to several media productions, a great deal more could be done in this area. As it stands now, script writers, producers, and researchers tend to contact the office of the American Medical Association's physician advisory groups on Radio, Television, and Motion Pictures in Hollywood, California, using their toll-free telephone number of (800) 621-4115 for

information about accuracy in depicting both medicine and nursing. The AMA has been active in providing a free consultation service since the 1950s, as have numerous other professional groups, such as the National Educational Association and the American Bar Association.

Awards and prizes to media executives, actresses, and actors who facilitate the positive media depiction of nurses and nursing is another important strategy that nursing groups can employ. This is a routine event for such associations as the AMA, which has given awards at their annual conventions to such actors as Raymond Massey and Richard Chamberlain for the representation of physicians on *Dr. Kildare* and to Robert Young for his effective physician portrayal as *Marcus Welby, M.D.* Similarly, the National Commission on Working Women has given special awards to television portrayals of working women. Giving more attention to this type of award would serve the nursing profession well.

Nursing groups can also offer awards or prizes in writing contests for journalists, authors, and producers. Notice of such writing contests is published annually in a special issue of *Editor and Publisher,* where entries are solicited for these annual competitions. These contests carry a substantial cash payment ($250 to $5,000), typically for several categories (books, newspapers, magazines, radio, television, and films). Numerous professional associations have engaged in this activity in recent years, including the American Psychological Association, the American Chiropractic Association, the American Speech-Language-Hearing Association, and the American Bar Association, to name just a few.

In addition to rewarding persons outside of nursing for positive or informative presentations of the profession in the media, nursing groups should reward and encourage nurse authors. It is interesting to note that our study showed nurse authors presented the most positive images of the profession. We have had several outstanding nurse authors, including Mary Roberts Rinehart and Dorothy Deming. A continuation of this important tradition could be facilitated if special grants and awards were established for financial support and recognition of nurse authors of both fiction and health publications for general public consumption.

Many of these strategies might also be incorporated into a regional or national campaign. In addi-

NURSING IN THE MASS MEDIA ARCHIVES, UNIVERSITY OF MICHIGAN

tion, there is a great need to stimulate interest in a prime-time network television entertainment series that communicates a progressive image of the nursing profession. Also needed is a series of one- or two-minute television spots that show nurses in a wide variety of up-to-date roles (for example, as ICU nurses, hospice nurses, nurse-midwives, primary care nurses, or nurse executives). Such spots would demonstrate to the public the true diversity that exists in today's nursing profession and the key role that nurses play in health care. Television documentaries about nursing should also be encouraged.

CONCLUSION

The images of nursing that the public receives from all the media have far-reaching consequences for nurses because these images affect the decisions made about nursing. For instance, on all political levels—local, state, and federal—there are limited health care funds to disperse, and the allocations of the scarce resources that undergird the delivery of nursing services is closely tied to the quality and quantity of the images of nurses and nursing in the mass media. Much of this allocation process is related to the media's ability to make nursing important in the public consciousness. Both entertainment and news media may or may not place nursing issues before the public, and such decisions influence matters of vital importance to the general welfare of the nation.

The quality and quantity of mass communications pertaining to nursing strongly influences the course of the nursing profession by shaping the nature of nursing's relationship with the public it serves. Changes in media portrayals of nurses and nursing are both necessary and possible. Some have already

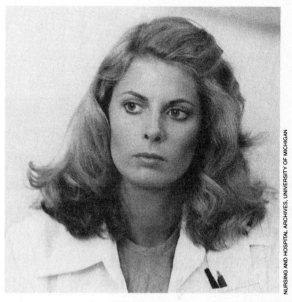

Allocations of the scarce resources that undergird the delivery of nursing services is closely tied to the quality and quantity of the images of nurses and nursing in the mass media.

begun, but they will continue and grow only if nurses nurture those changes by voicing their opinions and by working actively to supplant outdated or negative media images of nurses with vital, positive, and accurate accounts of today's nursing profession.

NOTE

1. Talcott Parsons, "The Superego and the Theory of Social Systems," in eds. Talcott Parsons, Robert F. Bales, and Edward Shils, *Working Papers in the Theory of Action* (New York: The Free Press, 1953), p. 18.

BIBLIOGRAPHY

BOOKS AND ARTICLES

Abbott, Edith. *Women in Industry.* New York: D. Appleton, 1910.

Abdellah, Faye, and Levine, Eugene. "Polling Hospital Patients and Personnel: What Patients Say About Nursing Care." *Hospitals* 31 (Nov. 1, 1957): 44–51.

Abdellah, Faye, and Levine, Eugene. "Polling Patients and Personnel: What Personnel Say About Nursing Care." *Hospitals* 31 (Dec. 1, 1957): 53.

Adams, Elizabeth Kemper. *Women Professional Workers.* New York: Macmillan, 1921.

Adler, Richard, ed. *Television as a Social Force: New Approaches to TV Criticism.* New York: Praeger, 1975.

Adler, Richard, and Cater, Douglass, eds. *Television as a Cultural Force.* Palo Alto, CA: Aspen Institute of Humanistic Studies, 1976

Adoni, H., and Mane, S. "Media and the Social Construction of Reality: Toward an Integration of Theory and Research." *Communication Research* 11, (July 1984): 323–40.

Albrecht, Stan L.; Bahr, Howard M.; and Chadwick, Bruce A. "Public Stereotyping of Sex Roles, Personality Characteristics, and Occupations." *Sociology and Social Research* 61 (January 1977): 223–40.

Alexander, J.W. "How the Public Perceives Nurses and Their Education." *Nursing Outlook* 27, no. 10 (1979): 654.

Alitheide, David. *Creating Reality: How TV News Distorts Events.* Beverly Hills, CA: Sage, 1976.

Altbach, Edith Hoshino, ed. *From Feminism to Liberation.* Cambridge, MA: Schenkman, 1971.

Altbach, Edith Hoshino. *Women in America.* Lexington, MA: D.C. Heath, 1974.

Altman, Charles F. "Psychoanalysis and Cinema: The Imaginary Discourse." *Quarterly Review of Film Studies* 2, no. 3 (1977): 253–67.

American Association of University Women (AAUW). *The Image of Women in Television.* Washington, DC: American Association of University Women, 1974.

American Nurses' Association. *Facts About Nursing, 1950.* New York: American Nurses' Association, 1951.

American Nurses' Association. *Facts About Nursing, 1952.* New York: American Nurses' Association, 1953.

Anderson, Karen. *Wartime Women: Sex Roles, Family Relations, and the Status of Women During World War II.* Westport, CT: Greenwood, 1981.

Andrew, Dudley. *Concepts in Film Theory.* New York: Oxford University Press, 1984.

Andrews, William D., and Andrews, Deborah C. "Technology and the Housewife in Nineteenth-Century America." *Women's Studies* 2, no. 3 (1974): 309–28.

Armstrong, G.A.; Franke, G.R.; and Russ, F.A. "The Effects of Corrective Advertising on Company Image." *Journal of Advertising* 11, no. 4 (1982): 39–47.

Arnheim, R. "World of the Daytime Serial." In *Radio Research,* edited by P.F. Lazarsfeld and F.N. Stanton. New York: Duell, Sloan and Pearce, 1942.

Aronoff, Craig. "Old Age in Prime Time." *Journal of Communication* 24, (Autumn 1974): 86–87.

Aronowitz, Stanley. *False Promises: The Shaping of American Working Class Consciousness.* New York: McGraw-Hill, 1964.

Arons, Leon, and May, Mark A. *Television and Human Behavior.* New York: Appleton-Century-Crofts, 1963.

Aroskar, M.A. "The Fractured Image: The Public Stereotype of Nursing and the Nurse." In *Nursing Images and Ideals,* edited by S. Spicker and S. Gadow. New York: Springer, 1980.

Astin, H.S. "Patterns of Women's Occupations." In *The Psychology of Women: Future Directions in Research,* edited by J. A. Sherman and F.L. Denmark. New York: Wes-Den, 1978.

Austin, Anne L. *The Woolsey Sisters of New York: A Family's Involvement in the Civil War and a New Profession (1860–1900).* Philadelphia: American Philosophical Society, 1971.

Austin, Rita. "Sex and Gender in the Future of Nursing." *Nursing Times* 73 (Aug. 25, and Sept. 1, 1977): 113–16, 117–19.

Bagdikian, Ben. *The Media Monopoly.* Boston: Beacon, 1983.

Bahr, Howard M. "Changes in Family Life in Middletown, 1924–77." *Public Opinion Quarterly* 44 (Fall 1979): 35–52.

Baker, Elizabeth Faulkner. *Technology and Women's Work.* New York: Columbia University Press, 1964.

Bane, Mary Jo. *Here To Stay: American Families in the Twentieth Century.* New York: Basic, 1976.

Banner, Lois W. *Women in Modern America: A Brief History.* New York: Harcourt Brace Jovanovich, 1974.

Baran, S.J. "Sex on TV and Adolescent Sexual Self-Image." *Journal of Broadcasting* 20, (Winter 1976): 61–68.

Barcus, F. Earle. *Images of Life on Children's Television: Sex Roles, Minorities and Families.* New York: Praeger, 1983.

Barker-Benfield, G.J. *The Horrors of the Half-Known Life: Male Attitudes Toward Women and Sexuality in Nineteenth-Century America.* New York: Harper and Row, 1976.

Barnett, James Harwood, and Guren, Rhoda. "Recent American Divorce Novels, 1938–1945: A Study in the Sociology of Literature." *Social Forces* 26 (March 1948): 322–27.

Barnouw, Erik. *A History of Broadcasting in the United States.* 3 Vols. New York: Oxford University Press, 1966–70.

Barnouw, Erik. *Tube of Plenty: The Evolution of American Television.* New York: Oxford University Press, 1975.

Barrett, Michele. "Representation and Cultural Production." In *Ideology and Cultural Production,* edited by Michele Barrett, Philip Corrigan, Annette Kuhn, and Janet Wolfe, 9–24. London: Croom Helm, 1979.

Barrett, Michele; Corrigan, Philip; Kuhn, Annette; and Wolfe, Janet, eds. *Ideology and Cultural Production.* London: Croom Helm, 1979.

Barthes, Roland. *Mythologies.* London: Penguin, 1973.

Barthes, Roland. "Style and Its Image." In *Literary Style: A Symposium,* edited by Seymour Chatman. New York: Oxford University Press, 1971.

Basch, F. *Relative Creatures: Victorian Women in Society and the Novel 1837–1867.* London: Allen Lane, 1974.

Bash, Wendell H. "Changing Birth Rates in Developing America: New York State, 1840–1875." *Milbank Memorial Quarterly* 41 (April, 1963): 161–82.

Basow, S.A. *Sex-Role Stereotypes: Traditions and Alternatives.* Monterey, CA: Brooks/Cole, 1980.

Baudler, L., and Patterson, D.G. "Social Status of Women's Occupations." *Occupations* 26 (May, 1948): 421–24.

Baxandall, Rosalyn; Gordon, Linda; and Reverby, Susan, eds. *America's Working*

Women: A Documentary History, 1600 to the Present. New York: Vintage, 1976.

Baym, Nina. *Woman's Fiction: A Guide to Novels by and About Women in America, 1820–1870.* Ithaca, NY: Cornell University Press, 1978.

Beard, Mary R. *America Through Women's Eyes.* New York: Macmillan, 1933.

Beard, Mary R. *Women as a Force in History.* New York: Macmillan, 1946.

Beasley, Maurine, and Silver, Sheila. *Women in Media: A Documentary Source Book.* Washington, DC: Women's Institute for Freedom of the Press, 1977.

Beauvoir, Simone de. *The Second Sex.* New York: Bantam, 1953.

Becker, Gary S. "Theory of Marriage." *Journal of Political Economy.* July 1973.

Bedell, Sally. "Behind the Scenes at 'Lifeline.' " *TV Guide* 26 (Oct. 7, 1978): 26–31.

Beletz, Elaine. "Is Nursing's Public Image Up to Date?" *Nursing Outlook* 22 (July 1974): 432–35.

Berelson, Bernard. "Content Analysis." Chapter 13 in *Handbook of Social Psychology,* edited by G. Lindzey, vol. 1. Reading, MA: Addison-Wesley, 1954.

Berelson, Bernard. *Content Analysis in Communication Research.* Glencoe, IL: Free Press, 1952.

Berelson, Bernard, and Janowitz, Morris, eds. *Reader in Public Opinion and Communication.* 2nd ed. New York: Free Press, 1966.

Berger, Arthur Asa. *Media Analysis Techniques.* Beverly Hills, CA: Sage, 1982.

Berger, Peter L., and Luckman, Thomas. *The Social Construction of Reality.* Garden City, NY: Doubleday, 1966.

Berk, L.M. "The Great Middle American Dream Machine." *Journal of Communication* 27, (Winter 1977): 27–31.

Berkin, Carol Ruth, and Norton, Mary Beth. *Women of America: A History.* Boston: Hughton-Mifflin, 1979.

Bernays, Edward L. "America Looks at Nursing." *American Journal of Nursing* 46 (September 1946): 590–92.

Bernays, Edward L. "Opinion Molders Appraise Nursing." *American Journal of Nursing* 45 (December 1945): 1005–11.

Bernays, Edward L. "What Government Officials Think About Nursing." *American Journal of Nursing* 46 (January 1946): 22–26.

Bernays, Edward L. "What Patients Say About Nurses." *American Journal of Nursing* 47 (February 1947): 93–96.

Bernstein, L. "The Relationship Between Masculine/Feminine Personality Characteristics and Image of Professional Nursing." Ph.D. diss., Florida Institute of Technology, 1981.

Berry, Gordon L., and Mitchell-Kernan, Claudia, eds. *Television and the Socialization of the Minority Child.* New York: Academic, 1982.

Beuf, Ann. "Doctor, Lawyer, Household Drudge." *Journal of Communication* 24, (Spring 1974): 142–45.

Beurkel-Rothfuss, N.L., and Mayes, S. "Soap Opera Viewing: The Cultivation Effect." *Journal of Communication* 31, (Summer 1981): 108–15.

Bird, Caroline. *Born Female: The High Cost of Keeping Women Down.* New York: Pocket Books, 1972.

Bird, Caroline. "What's Television Doing for 50.9% of Americans?" *TV Guide* 19 (Feb. 27, 1971): 5–8.

Birdwhistell, R.L. "Social Science and Nursing Education: Some Tentative Suggestions." In *National League of Nursing Education Annual Report.* 1949. New York: The League, 1949.

Blake, Nelson Manfred. *The Road to Reno: A History of Divorce in the United States.* New York: Macmillan, 1962.

Blaubergs, M. "On 'The Nurse Was a Doctor.' " In *View on Language,* edited by R. Crdoubadian and W. Engel. Murfreesboro, TN: Inter-University, 1975.

Blood, W. "Agenda Setting: A Review of the Theory." *Media Information* 26 (November 1982): 3–12

Blumer, Herbert. *Movies and Conduct.* New York: Macmillan, 1933.

Blumer, Herbert, and Hauser, Philip M. *Movies, Delinquency and Crime.* New York: Macmillan, 1933.

Blumler, Jay G., and Katz, Elihu, eds. *The Uses of Mass Communication: Current Perspectives on Gratifications Research.* Beverly Hills, CA: Sage, 1974.

Bogart, Leo. *The Age of Television: A Study of the Viewing Habits and the Impact of Television on American Life.* 2nd ed. New York: Ungar, 1958.

Bolin, Winifred D. Wandersee. "The Economics of Middle Income Family Life: Working Women During the Great Depression." *Journal of American History* 65 (June 1978): 60–74.

Boorstin, Daniel J. *The Image: A Guide to Pseudo-Events in America.* New York: Atheneum, 1971.

Boulding, Elise. *The Underside of History: A View of Women Through Time.* Boulder, CO: Westview, 1976.

Boulding, Kenneth E. *The Image: Knowledge in Life and Society.* Ann Arbor: University of Michigan Press, 1956.

Boulton, Harold. "Our Nursing Service in France." *Nineteenth Century* 81 (November 1917): 651–60.

Brady, Anna, et al., eds. *Union List of Film Periodicals: Holdings of Selected American Collections.* Westport, CT: Greenwood Press, 1984.

Brady, G.H.; Stoneman, Z.; and Sanders, A.K. "Effects of Television on Family Interactions: An Observational Study." *Family Relations* 29, no. 2 (1980): 216–20.

Brady, Leo. *The World in a Frame: What We See in Films.* Garden City, NY: Anchor, 1977.

Bressler, Marvin, and Kephart, William. *A Survey of Selected Aspects of the Nursing Profession.* Philadelphia: Pennsylvania State Nurses Association, 1956.

Bridges, W. "Family Patterns and Social Values in America, 1825–1875." *American Quarterly* 17 (Spring 1965): 3–11.

Britain, S.D., and Coker, M. "Recall of Sex-Role Appropriate and Inappropriate Models in Children's Songs." *Sex Roles* 8 (August 1982): 931–34.

Brooks, Tim, and Marsh, Earle. *The Complete Directory to Prime Time Network TV Shows 1946-Present.* New York: Ballantine, 1979.

Brown, Bruce W. *Images of Family Life in Magazine Advertising: 1920–1978.* New York: Praeger, 1981.

Brown, Bruce W. "Wife-Employment and the Emergence of Egalitarian Marital Role Prescriptions: 1900–1974." *The Journal of Comparative Family Studies* 9, no. 1: 5–17.

Brown, Les. *Television: The Business Behind the Box.* New York: Harcourt Brace Jovanovich, 1971.

Brown, Les. *The New York Times Encyclopedia of Television.* New York: New York Times Books, 1977.

Brown Ray, ed. *Children and Television.* Beverly Hills, CA: Sage, 1976.

Brownlee, W. Elliot, and Brownlee, Mary H. *Women in the American Economy: A Documentary History, 1675–1929.* New Haven, CT: Yale University Press, 1976.

Budd, R., and Thorp, K. *Content Analysis of Communications.* New York: Macmillan, 1967.

Buehr, Walter. *Home Sweet Home in the Nineteenth Century.* New York: Thomas Y. Crowell, 1965.

Bullock, Robert P. *What Do Nurses Think of Their Profession?* Columbus: Ohio State University Research Foundation, 1954.

Bumiller, Elisabeth. "America's Working Women: Television Looks a Little Different Now." *TV Guide* 30 (Aug. 21, 1982): 5–6.

Bunkle, Phillida E. "Sentimental Womanhood and Domestic Education,

1830–1870." *History of Education Quarterly* 14 (Winter 1974): 13–30.

Busby, Linda. "Sex-Role Research on the Mass Media." *Journal of Communication* 25 (Autumn 1975): 107–31.

Butler, Matilda, and Paisley, William. *Women and the Mass Media.* New York: Human Sciences, 1980.

Butler-Flora, Cornelia. "The Passive Female: Her Comparative Image by Class and Culture in Women's Magazine Fiction." *Journal of Marriage and the Family* 33 (August 1971): 435–44.

Cain, Glen G. *Married Women in the Labor Force.* Chicago: University of Chicago Press, 1966.

Cantor, Muriel G. *Prime Time Television: Content and Control.* Beverly Hills, CA: Sage, 1980.

Cantor, Muriel G., and Jones, E. "Creating Fiction for Women." *Communication Research* 10 (January 1983): 111–37.

Cantor, Muriel G., and Laurie, Bruce, eds. *Class, Sex and the Woman Worker.* Westport, CT: Greenwood, 1977.

Cantor, Muriel G., and Pingree, Suzanne. *The Soap Opera.* Beverly Hills, CA: Sage, 1983.

Carroll, Berenice A., ed. *Liberating Women's History: Theoretical and Critical Essays.* Urbana: University of Illinois Press, 1974.

Carter, B. "Medicine's Forgotten Women." *Reporter* 26 (1962): 35–37.

Cassara, Beverly Benner, ed. *American Women: The Changing Image.* Boston: Beacon, 1962.

Cassata, M.B.; Anderson, P.A.; and Skill, T.D. "The Older Adult in Daytime Serial Drama." *Journal of Communication* 30, (Winter 1980): 48–49.

Cassata, Mary, and Skill, Thomas. *Life on Daytime Television: Tuning-in American Serial Drama.* Norwood, NJ: Ablex, 1983.

Cassata, Mary; Skill, T.D.; and Boadu, S.O. "In Sickness and in Health." *Journal of Communication* 29 (Autumn 1979): 73–80.

Castleman, H., and Podrazik, W.J. *Watching TV: Four Decades of American Television.* New York: McGraw-Hill, 1982.

Cawelti, John G. *Adventure, Mystery and Romance.* Chicago: University of Chicago Press, 1976.

Chafe, William H. *The American Woman: Her Changing Social, Economic and Political Roles, 1920–1970.* New York: Oxford University Press, 1972.

Chafe, William H. *Women and Equality: Changing Patterns in American Culture.* New York: Oxford University Press, 1977.

Chermesh, R. "Press Criteria for Strike Reporting: Counting or Selective Presentation?" *Social Science Research* 11 (March 1982): 88–101.

Chodorow, Nancy. *The Reproduction of Mothering: Psychoanalysis and the Sociology of Gender.* Berkeley and Los Angeles: University of California Press, 1978.

Christ, Carol. "Marcus Welby or Archie Bunker: Will the Real Chauvinist Pig Please Stand Up?" *Christian Century* 92 (March 12, 1975): 260–62.

Christiansen, J.B. "Television Role Models and Adolescent Occupational Goals." *Human Communication Research* 5, (Summer 1979): 335–37.

Churchill, G.A., and Moschis, G.P., Jr. "Television and Interpersonal Influences on Adolescent Consumer Learning." *Journal of Consumer Research* 6, (June 1979): 23–35.

Clark, R.L. "How Women's Magazines Cover Living Alone." *Journalism Quarterly* 58 (Summer 1981): 291–94.

Clinton, Catherine. *The Other Civil War: American Women in the Nineteenth Century.* New York: Hill and Wang, 1984.

Cohn, Victor. *Sister Kenny: The Woman Who Challenged the Doctors.* Minneapolis: University of Minnesota Press, 1975.

Cole, Barry G. "Women on the Screen." In *Television.* New York: Free Press, 1970.

Collins, Doris L., and Joel, Lucille A. "The Image of Nursing Is Not Changing." *Nursing Outlook* 19 (July 1971): 456–59.

Comstock, George A. "The Mass Media and Social Change." In *Handbook of Social Intervention,* edited by E. Seidman, 268–88. Beverly Hills, CA: Sage, 1983.

Comstock, George A. *Television and Human Behavior: The Key Studies.* Santa Monica, CA: Rand, 1975.

Comstock, George A. *Television in America.* Beverly Hills, CA: Sage, 1980.

Comstock, George A., and Fisher, M. *Television and Human Behavior: A Guide to the Pertinent Scientific Literature.* Santa Monica, CA: Rand, 1975.

Comstock, George A., and Linsey, G. *Television and Human Behavior: The Research Horizon, Future and Present.* Santa Monica, CA: Rand, 1975.

Comstock, George A.; Chaffee, S.; Katzman, N.; McCombs, M.; and Roberts, D. *Television and Human Behavior.* New York: Columbia University Press, 1978.

Cook, Edward. *The Life of Florence Nightingale.* 2 vols. London: Macmillan, 1913.

Coombe, Jack D. "Public Relations: The TV Medical Show: That's Entertainment,

But Is That Harmless?" *Hospitals* 56, no. 15 (Aug. 1, 1982): 71–75.

Cott, Nancy F. *The Bonds of Womanhood: "Woman's Sphere" in New England, 1780–1835.* New Haven, CT: Yale University Press, 1977.

Cott, Nancy F. "Divorce and the Changing Status of Women in Eighteenth-Century Massachusetts." *William and Mary Quarterly* 33 (October 1976): 586–614.

Cott, Nancy F., and Pleck, Elizabeth H. *A Heritage of Her Own: Toward a New Social History of American Women.* New York: Simon and Schuster, 1979.

Courtney, Alice E., and Lockeretz, Sara Wernick. "A Woman's Place: An Analysis of the Roles Portrayed by Women in Magazine Advertisements." *Journal of Marketing Research* 8, no. 1 (1971): 92–95.

Courtney, Alice E., and Whipple, Thomas W. *Sex Stereotyping in Advertising.* Lexington, MA: Lexington, 1983.

Courtney, Alice E., and Whipple, Thomas W. "Women in TV Commercials." *Journal of Communication* 24, (Spring 1974): 110–18.

Coveney, Peter. *The Image of Childhood.* Rev. ed. Baltimore: Penguin, 1967.

Cowan, Geoffrey. *See No Evil: The Backstage Battle over Sex and Violence on Television.* New York: Simon and Schuster, 1979.

Cross, Donna W. *Media-Speak: How Television Makes Up Your Mind.* New York: New American Library, 1984.

Cuber, John F. "Changing Courtship and Marriage Customs." *Annals of the American Academy of Political and Social Science* 229 (September 1943): 30–38.

Cust, R.N. "Scutari Hospital." *Notes and Queries* 9 (Aug. 25, 1908), 337.

Czitrom, Daniel J. *Media and the American Mind: From Morse to McLuhan.* Chapel Hill: University of North Carolina Press, 1982.

Dahlstrom, Edmund, ed. *The Changing Roles of Men and Women.* Boston: Beacon, 1971.

Daniels, Pamela, and Weingarten, Kathy. *Sooner or Later: The Timing of Parenthood in Adult Lives.* New York: Norton, 1983.

Davidson, William. "Jack Klugman of 'Quincy.'" *TV Guide* 25 (March 26, 1977): 29–34.

Davidson, William. "Medical Center." *TV Guide* 19 (July 17, 1971): 12–16.

Davis, Howard, and Walton, Paul, eds. *Language, Image, Media.* Oxford: Basil Blackwell, 1983.

Davis, J. "Sexist Bias in Eight Newspapers." *Journalism Quarterly* 49 (Autumn 1982): 456–60.

Davis, Katherine B. *Factors in the Sex Life of Twenty-Two Hundred Women*. New York: Harper, 1929.

Davison, W.P., et al. *Mass Media: Systems and Effects*. New York: Praeger, 1976.

De Fleur, Melvin. "Occupational Roles as Portrayed on Television." *Public Opinion Quarterly* 28 (Spring 1964): 57–74.

De Fleur, Melvin. *Theories of Mass Communication*. New York: David McKay, 1970.

De Fleur, Melvin, and De Fleur, L. "The Relative Contribution of Television as Learning Source for Children's Occupational Knowledge." *American Sociological Review* 32 (October 1967): 777–89.

Degler, Carl N. "What Ought To Be and What Was: Women's Sexuality in the Nineteenth Century." *American Historical Review* 79 (December 1974): 1467–90.

Delano, Jane A. "Thirty Thousand Nurses Needed: What American Women and Girls Can Do." *McCall's* 45 (July 1918): 18.

Deming, Barbara. *Running Away from Myself: A Dream Portrait of America Drawn from the Films of the Forties*. New York: Grossman, 1969.

Dempsey, Mary V. *The Occupational Progress of Women, 1910 to 1930*. U.S. Women's Bureau Bulletin no. 104. Washington, DC: U.S. Department of Labor, 1933.

Deutscher, Irwin. *A Study of the Registered Nurse in a Metropolitan Community*. Parts 1, 5. Kansas City: Community Studies, 1957.

Devereux, George, and Weiner, Florence. "The Occupation Status of Nurses." *American Sociological Review* 15 (October 1950): 628.

Dickens, Charles. "Hospitals." *Household Words* 12 (Dec. 15, 1855): 457–71.

Dickens, Charles. "The Nurse in Leading Strings." *Household Words* 12 (Jan. 15, 1855): 601–6.

Dingwall, Eric John. *The American Woman: An Historical Study*. New York: Rinehart, 1956.

Dinnerstein, Dorothy. *The Mermaid and the Minotaur: Sexual Arrangements and Human Malaise*. New York: Harper and Row, 1976.

Ditzion, Sidney. *Marriage Morals and Sex in America: A History of Ideas*. New York: Bookman, 1953.

Dominick, J.R. "Business Coverage in Network Newscasts." *Journalism Quarterly* 58 (Summer 1981): 179–85.

Donegan, Jane B. *Women and Men Midwives: Medicine, Morality, and Misogyny in Early America*. Westport, CT: Greenwood, 1978.

Douglas, Ann. *The Feminization of American Culture*. New York: Knopf, 1977.

Douglas, Emily Taft. *Margaret Sanger: Pioneer of the Future*. New York: Holt, Rinehart and Winston, 1970.

Downing, Mildred. "Heroine of the Daytime Serial." *Journal of Communication* 24, (Spring 1974): 130–37.

Downs, Florence, and Brooten, Dorothy. *New Careers in Nursing*. New York: Arco, 1983.

Dublin, Thomas. *Women at Work: The Transformation of Work and Community in Lowell, Massachusetts, 1826–1860*. New York: Columbia University Press, 1979.

Durdeen-Smith, Jo. "Daytime TV: Soft Soaping the American Woman." *The Village Voice* 18 (Feb. 8, 1973): 19.

Earnest, Ernest. *The American Eve in Fact and Fiction, 1775–1914*. Urbana: University of Illinois Press, 1974.

Edmondson, Madeleine, and Rounds, David. *The Soaps: Daytime Serials of Radio and TV*. New York: Stein and Day, 1973.

Efron, Edith. "Is Television Making a Mockery of the American Woman?" *TV Guide* 18 (Aug. 8, 1970): 7–9.

Efron, Edith. "The Soap Opera Nurses." *TV Guide* 19 (Feb. 19, 1972): 24–25.

Efron, Edith. "The Soaps—Anyting but 99 44/100 Percent Pure." *TV Guide* 13 (March 13, 1965): 6–11.

Efron, Edith. "Taking the Pulse of 'The Nurses.'" *TV Guide* 10 (Dec. 15, 1962), 22–26.

Elder, Glen H., Jr., and Rockwell, Richard C. "Marital Timing in Women's Life Patterns." *Journal of Family History* 1 (Spring 1976): 34–53.

Eliot, Marc. *American Television: The Official Art of the Artificial*. Garden City, NY: Doubleday, 1981.

Elliott, P. *The Making of a Television Series: A Case Study in the Sociology of Culture*. New York: Hastings House, 1973.

Elliott, William Y. *Television's Impact on American Culture*. East Lansing: Michigan State University Press, 1956.

Ellison, J.C. "I've Had a Thousand Babies." *Saturday Evening Post* 225 (June 6, 1953): 22–23.

Elms, R.E., and Moorehead, J.M. "Will the 'Real' Nurse Please Stand Up: The Stereotype vs. Reality." *Nursing Forum* 16, no. 2 (1977): 113.

England, P.; Kuhn, A.; and Gardner, T. "The Ages of Men and Women in Magazine Advertisements." *Journalism Quarterly* 58 (Fall 1981): 468–71.

England, R.W., Jr. "Images of Love and Courtship in Family Magazine Fiction."

Marriage and Family Living 22 (November 1960): 162–65.

Epstein, Cynthia Fuchs. *Woman's Place*. Berkeley and Los Angeles: University of California Press, 1970.

Etaugh, C., and Stern, J. "Person Perception—Effects of Sex, Marital Status, and Sex-Typed Occupation." *Sex Roles* 11, nos. 5–6 (September 1984): 413–24.

Ewen, Stuart, and Ewen, Elizabeth. *Channels of Desire: Mass Images and the Shaping of American Consciousness*. New York: McGraw-Hill, 1982.

Fennell, Geraldine. *Avoiding Sex Role Stereotypes in Advertising: More Questions than Answers*. Advances in Consumer Research, vol. 11. Ann Arbor, MI: Association for Consumer Research, 1984.

Ferguson, M. *Images of Women in Literature*. Boston: Houghton Mifflin, 1973.

Ferguson, M. "The Woman's Magazine Cover Photograph." In *The Sociology of Journalism and the Press*, edited by H. Christian, 219–38. Totowa, NJ: Rowman and Littlefield, 1980.

Fernandez, R.C. "Let's Turn Off the Soap Opera Image of Nursing!" *RN* 43, (September 1980): 77.

Ferriss, Abbott L. *Indicators of Change in the American Family*. New York: Russell Sage Foundation, 1970.

Festinger, L. *A Theory of Cognitive Dissonance*. Stanford, CA: Stanford University Press, 1962.

Filene, Peter Gabriel. *Him/Her/Self: Sex Roles in Modern America*. New York: Harcourt Brace Jovanovich, 1974.

Fishbein, M. "Nursing as a Career." *Hygeia* 25 (December 1947): 915.

Flexner, Eleanor. *Century of Struggle: The Woman's Rights Movement in the United States*. Cambridge, MA: Harvard University Press, 1959.

Foner, Philip S. *Women and the American Labor Movement: From Colonial Times to the Eve of World War I*. New York: Free Press, 1979.

Fonesca, J.D. "The Public and Not So Public Image of Nursing." *Nursing Outlook* 28, (September 1980): 539.

Ford, Thomas R., and Stephenson, Diane D. *Institutional Nurses: Roles, Relationships and Attitudes in Three Alabama Hospitals*. Tuscaloosa, AL: University of Alabama Press, 1954.

Fottler, M.D., and Bain, T. "Realism of Occupational Choice Among High School Seniors—Implications for Quality of Work Life." *Journal of Occupational Behaviour* 5, no. 4 (October 1984): 237–52.

Fowles, Jib. *Mass Advertising as Social Forecast: A Method for Future Research*. Westport, CT: Greenwood, 1976.

Fox, David J.; Diamond, Lorraine K.; and Jocobowsky, Nadia. *Career Decisions and Professional Expectations of Nursing.* New York: Columbia Teachers College, 1961.

Frankfort, Roberta. *Collegiate Women: Domesticity and Career in Turn-of-the-Century America.* New York: New York University Press, 1978.

Franzblau, S.; Sprafkin, J.N.; and Rubinstein, E.A. "Sex on TV: A Content Analysis." *Journal of Communication* 27 (Spring 1977): 164–71.

Franzwa, Helen H. *The Image of Women in Television: An Annotated Bibliography.* Washington, DC: U.S. Commission on Civil Rights, 1976.

Freedman, Estelle B. "The New Woman: Changing Views of Women in the 1920's." *Journal of American History* 61 (September 1974): 372–93.

Freeman, Jo. *The Politics of Women's Liberation: A Case Study of an Emerging Social Movement and Its Relation to the Social Policy Process.* New York: McKay, 1975.

Freuh, T., and McGhee, P.E. "Traditional Sex Role Development and Amount of Time Spent Watching Television." *Developmental Psychology* 11, no. 1, (1975): 109.

Frey, Linda, et al., eds. *Women in Western European History: A Select Chronological, Geographical, and Topical Bibliography: The Nineteenth and Twentieth Centuries.* Westport, CT: Greenwood, 1984.

Friedan, Betty. *The Feminine Mystique.* New York: Dell, 1963.

Friedan, Betty. *It Changed My Life: Writings on the Women's Movement.* New York: Random House, 1976.

Friedan, Betty. "Television and the Feminine Mystique." *TV Guide* 12 (Feb. 1, Feb. 8, 1964): 6–11, 19–24.

Friedman, Jean E., and Shae, William O., eds. *Our American Sisters: Women in American Life and Thought.* 2d ed. Boston: Allyn and Bacon, 1976.

Friedman, Leslie J. *Sex Role Stereotyping in the Mass Media: An Annotated Bibliography.* New York: Garland, 1977.

Frieze, Irene H., et al. *Women and Sex Roles: A Social Psychological Perspective.* New York: Norton, 1978.

Fritz, Leah. *Dreamers and Dealers: An Intimate Appraisal of the Women's Movement.* Boston: Beacon, 1979.

Fryer, Judith. *The Faces of Eve: Women in the Nineteenth-Century American Novel.* New York: Oxford University Press, 1976.

Gade, E.M. "Representation of the World of Work in Daytime Television Serials." *Journal of Employment Counseling* 8 (March 1971): 37–42.

Gallagher, Margaret. *Unequal Opportunities: The Cases of Women and the Media.* Paris: UNESCO Press, 1981.

Gallup, George H., ed. *The Gallup Poll: Public Opinion, Nineteen Eighty-One.* Wilmington, DE: Scholarly Research, 1982.

Gandy, H., Jr. *Beyond Agenda Setting: Information Subsidies and Public Policy.* Norwood, NJ: Ablex, 1982.

Gans, Herbert J. *Popular Culture and High Culture: An Analysis and Evaluation of Taste.* New York: Basic, 1974.

Garlington, W.K. "Drinking on Television: A Preliminary Study with Emphasis on Method." *Journal of Studies on Alcohol* 38 (November 1977): 2199–2205.

Garrett, C.; Ein, L.; and Tremaine, L. "The Development of Gender Stereotyping of Adult Occupations in Elementary School Children." *Child Development* 48 (June 1977): 507–12.

Gerbner, George. "Content Analysis and Critical Research in Mass Communication." *AV Communication Review* 6 (Spring 1958): 85–108.

Gerbner, George, and Gross, Larry, "The Scary World of TV's Heavy Viewer." *Psychology Today* 10 (April 1976): 41–46.

Gerbner, George, and Signorielli, Nancy, "Women and Minorities in Television Drama, 1969–1978." Unpublished manuscript, University of Pennsylvania, 1979.

Gerbner, George, et al. "Scientists on the TV Screen." *Society* 18 (May/June 1981): 41–44.

Gerbner, George, et al., eds. *The Analysis of Communication Content.* New York: Wiley, 1969.

Gerbner, George; Gross, Larry; Morgan, Michael; and Signorielli, Nancy. "Health and Medicine on Television." *The New England Journal of Medicine* 305 (Oct. 8, 1981): 901–4.

Gerbner, George; Gross, Larry; Signorielli, Nancy; and Morgan, Michael. "Aging with Television: Images on Television Drama and Conceptions of Social Reality." *Journal of Communication* 30, (Winter 1980): 37–47.

Gerbner, George; Morgan, Michael; and Signorielli, Nancy. *Programming Health Portrayals: What Viewers See, Say, and Do.* Philadelphia: The Annenberg School of Communications, University of Pennsylvania, 1981.

Gertner, Richard, ed. *International Motion Picture Almanac.* New York: Quigley, 1980.

Geyman, Richard. "Caseyitis." In *TV Guide: The First 25 Years*, edited by Jay S. Harris. New York: Simon and Schuster, 1978.

Giele, Janet Zollinger. *Women and the Future: Changing Sex Roles in Modern America.* New York: Free Press, 1978.

Ginzberg, Eli, et al. *Educated American Women: Life Styles and Self Portraits.* New York: Columbia University Press, 1966.

Gitlin, Todd. *Inside Prime Time.* New York: Pantheon, 1983.

Glennon, L.M., and Butsch, R. "The Family as Portrayed on Television 1946-1978." In *Television and Behavior: Ten Years of Scientific Progress and Implications for the Eighties,* edited by D. Pearl, et al. Washington, DC: U.S. Government Printing Office, 1980.

Glick, Paul C. "Family Trends in the U.S., 1890-1940." *American Sociological Review* 7 (August 1942): 505–14.

Glick, Paul C. "The Life Cycle of the Family." *Marriage and Family Living* 17 (February 1955): 3–9.

Glick, Paul C. "Updating the Life Cycle of the Family." *Journal of Marriage and the Family* 39 (February 1977): 3–13.

Goethals, Gregor T. *The TV Ritual: Worship at the Video Altar.* Boston: Beacon, 1981.

Goffman, Erving. "Gender Advertisements." *Studies in the Anthropology of Visual Communication* 3, no. 2 (1976): 69–154.

Goldberg, Marshall. "A Doctor Examines TV's Health Shows." *TV Guide* 25 (May 14, 1977): 4–8.

Golding, Peter, and Murdock, Grahan. "Ideology and the Mass Media: The Question of Determination." In *Ideology and Cultural Production,* edited by Michele Barrett, et al. New York: St. Martin's, 1979.

Goldsen, Rose. *The Show and Tell Machine: How Television Works and Works You Over.* New York: Dial, 1975.

Goodman, Jack, ed. *While You Were Gone: A Report on Wartime Life in the United States.* New York: Simon and Schuster, 1946.

Gordon, Michael, ed. *The American Family in Social-Historical Perspective.* New York: St. Martin's. 1978.

Gordon, Michael, and Bernstein, M. Charles. "Mate Choice and Domestic Life in the Nineteenth Century Marriage Manual." *Journal of Marriage and the Family* 32 (August 1970): 665–75.

Gornick, Vivian, and Moran, Barbara K. *Woman in Sexist Society: Studies in Power and Powerlessness.* New York: Basic, 1971.

Goslin, D.A., ed. *Handbook of Socialization Theory and Research.* Chicago: Rand McNally, 1969.

Graves, S.B. "Psychological Effects of Black Portrayals on Television." In *Television and Social Behavior: Beyond Violence and Children*, edited by S.B. Withey and R.P. Abeles. Hillsdale, NJ: Lawrence Erlbaum Associates, 1980.

Greenberg, Bradley S. *Life on Television: Content Analyses of United States TV Drama*. Norwood, NJ: Ablex, 1980.

Greenberg, Bradley S. "Television and Role Socialization." In *Television and Behavior: Ten Years of Scientific Progress and Implications for the Eighties*, edited by D. Pearl, et al. Washington DC: U.S. Government Printing Office, 1980.

Greenberg, Bradley S.; Abelman, R; and Neuendorf, K. "Sex on the Soap Operas: Afternoon Delight." *Journal of Communication* 31 (Summer 1981): 83–89.

Greenberg, Bradley S., and Reeves, B. "Children and Perceived Reality of Television." *Journal of Social Issues* 32, no. 4, (1976): 86–97.

Greenleaf, N.P. "Coming to Terms with Nurse Ratched." *Supervisor Nurse* 7, (June 1976): 48.

Gross, Larry, and Jeffries-Fox, Susan. "What Do You Want To Be When You Grow Up, Little Girl?" In *Hearth and Home: Images of Women in the Mass Media*, edited by G. Tuchman, et al. New York: Oxford University Press, 1978.

Gross, Leonard, "Why Can't a Woman Be More Like a Man?" *TV Guide* 21 (Aug. 11, 1973): 6–8.

Groves, Ernest R. *The American Woman*. New York: Emerson, 1944.

Gutcheon, Beth R. "Look for Cop-Outs on Prime Time, Not on 'Soaps.'" *New York Times* 122 (Dec. 16, 1973): D-21.

Gutcheon, Beth R. "There Isn't Anything Wishy-Washy About Soaps." *Ms.* 3 (August 1974): 42–43.

Guttentag, M., and Bray, H. *Undoing Sex Stereotypes*. New York: McGraw-Hill, 1976.

Haas, A., and Sherman, M.A. "Reported Topics of Conversation Among Same-Sex Adults." *Communication Quarterly* 30 (Fall 1982): 332–52.

Hacker, Helen. "Women as a Minority Group." *Social Forces* 30 (October 1951): 60–69.

Halberstam, Michael J. "An M.D. Reviews Dr. Welby of TV." *New York Times Magazine* 121 (Jan. 16, 1972): 12.

Haller, John S., and Haller, Robin M. *The Physician and Sexuality in Victorian America*. Urbana: University of Illinois Press, 1974.

Halloran, James D., ed. *Mass Media and Socialization*. Leicester, England: IAMCR/UNESCO, 1976.

Handel, Leo. *Hollywood Looks at Its Audience: A Report of Film Audience Research*. Urbana, IL: University of Illinois Press, 1950.

Handlin, David P. "Efficiency and the American Home." *Architectural Quarterly* 5 (Winter 1972): 50–54.

Hareven, Tamara K. "Modernization and Family History: Perspectives in Social Change." *Signs: A Journal of Women in Culture and Society* 2 (Autumn 1976): 190–207.

Harris, Barbara J. *Beyond Her Sphere: Women and the Professions in American History*. Westport, CT: Greenwood, 1978.

Hart, Irving Harlow. "The One Hundred Leading Authors of Best Sellers in Fiction From 1895–1944." *Publishers Weekly* 149 (Jan. 19, 1946): 285–90.

Hart, James D. *The Popular Book: A History of America's Literary Taste*. New York: Oxford University Press, 1950.

Hartman, Mary, and Banner, Lois, eds. *Clio's Consciousness Raised: New Perspectives on the History of Women*. New York: Harper, 1974.

Hartmann, Susan. *The Home Front and Beyond: American Women in the 1940s*. Boston: Twayne, 1982.

Harvey, S.E.; Sprafkin, J.N.; and Rubinstein, E. "Prime Time Television: A Profile of Aggressive and Prosocial Behaviors." *Journal of Broadcasting* 23, (Spring 1979): 179–89.

Haskell, Molly. *From Reverence to Rape: The Treatment of Women in the Movies*. New York: Holt, Rinehart and Winston, 1973.

Haskell, Molly. "Women in the Movies Grow Up." *Psychology Today* 17 (January 1983): 18–27.

Hastings, Donald W., and Robinson, J. Gregory. "Incidence of Childlessness for U.S. Women, Cohorts Born 1891–1945." *Social Biology* 21, no. 2 (1974): 178–84.

Havens, Elizabeth M. "Women, Work and Wedlock: A Note on Female Marital Patterns in the United States." *American Journal of Sociology* 78 (January 1973): 975–81.

Hawkins, R.P., and Pingree, S. "TV Influence on Social Reality and Conceptions of the World." In *Television and Behavior: Ten Years of Scientific Progress and Implications for the Eighties*, edited by D. Pearl, et al. Washington, DC: U.S. Government Printing Office, 1980.

Hawkins, R.P., and Pingree, S. "Using Television to Construct Social Reality." *Journal of Broadcasting* 25 (Fall 1981): 347–64.

Heidgerken, Loretta. "Nursing as a Career: Is It Relevant?" *American Journal of Nursing* 69 (June 1969): 1217–22.

Heilbrun, Carolyn G. *Toward A Recognition of Androgyny*. New York: Knopf, 1973.

Hess, Thomas B., and Nochlin, Linda. *Woman as Sex Object: Studies in Erotic Art, 1730–1970*. New York: Newsweek Books, 1972.

Hewitt, Nancy A. *Women's Activism and Social Change: Rochester, New York, 1822–1872*. Ithaca, NY: Cornell University Press, 1984.

Hodges, K.K.; Brandt, D.A.; and Kline, J. "Competence, Guilt, and Victimization: Sex Differences in Attribution of Causality in Television Dramas." *Sex Roles* 7 (May 1981): 537–46.

Hogeland, Ronald W. "The Female Appendage: Feminine Life-Styles in America, 1820–1960." *Civil War History* 17 (June 1971): 102–14.

Holcombe, Lee. *Victorian Ladies at Work: Middle-Class Working Women in England and Wales 1850–1914*. Newton Abbot, Devon, England: David and Charles, 1973.

Hole, Judith, and Levine, Ellen. *Rebirth of Feminism*. New York: Quadrangle, 1971.

Holsti, O. "Content Analysis." Chap. 16 in *The Handbook of Social Psychology*, edited by G. Lindzey and E. Aronson, vol. 2. 2d ed. Reading, MA: Addison-Wesley, 1968.

Holsti, O. *Content Analysis for the Social Sciences and Humanities*. Reading, MA: Addison-Wesley, 1969.

Honey, Maureen. "Images of Women in the *Saturday Evening Post*, 1931–1936." *Journal of Popular Culture* 10 (Fall 1976): 352–58.

Hooks, Janet M. *Women's Occupations Through Seven Decades*. U.S. Women's Bureau Bulletin no. 218. Washington, DC: U.S. Department of Labor, 1947.

Hott, J.R. "Updating Cherry Ames." *American Journal of Nursing* 77, (October 1977): 1581.

Howe, Louise Kapp. *Pink Collar Workers: Inside the World of Women's Work*. New York: Putnam's, 1977.

Howitt, D. *The Mass Media and Social Problems*. Elmsford, NY: Pergamon, 1982.

Hughes, L. "The Public Image of the Nurse." *Advances in Nursing Science* 2, (April 1980): 55.

Humphrey, Ronald, and Schuman, Howard. "The Portrayal of Blacks in Magazine Advertisements: 1950–1982." *Public Opinion Quarterly* 48, (Autumn 1984): 551–63.

Hynes, T. *Magazine Portrayals of Women, 1911–1930.* Journalism Monograph no. 72. Minneapolis, MN: Association for Education in Journalism, 1981.

Irwin, Inez Haynes. In *Angels and Amazons: One Hundred Years of American Women,* 267–75. Garden City: Doubleday, Doran, 1933.

Jackson, Anthony W., ed. *Black Families and the Medium of Television.* Ann Arbor: Bush Program in Child Development and Social Policy, University of Michigan, 1982.

Jacobs, Norman, ed. *Culture for the Millions: Mass Media in Modern Society.* Boston: Beacon, 1964.

Janowitz, M. "Content Analysis and the Study of Sociopolitical Change." *Journal of Communication* 26 (Autumn 1976): 10–21.

Jeffrey, Kirk. "Marriage, Career, and Feminine Ideology in Nineteenth-Century America: Reconstructing the Marital Experience of Lydia Maria Child, 1828–1874." *Feminist Studies* 2 (June 1975): 113–30.

Jensen, Oliver. *The Revolt of American Women. A Pictorial History of the Century of Change from Bloomers to Bikinis—from Feminism to Freud.* New York: Harcourt, Brace, 1952.

Johns-Heine, Patricke, and Gerth, Hans. "Values in Mass Periodical Fiction, 1921–1940." *Public Opinion Quarterly* 13 (Spring 1949): 105–13.

Johnston, Claire. "Myths of Women in the Cinema." In *Women and the Cinema: A Critical Anthology,* edited by Karyn Kay and Gerald Peary. New York: E.P. Dutton, 1977.

Johnston, David. "Teamwork M*A*S*H-style." *TV Guide* 28 (Jan. 5, 1980): 22–26.

Johnston, Jerome, and Ettema, James S. *Positive Images: Breaking Stereotypes with Children's Television.* Beverly Hills, CA: Sage, 1982.

Johnston, Jerome; Ettema, James S.; and Davidson, T. *An Evaluation of "Freestyle: A Television Series Designed to Reduce Sex Role Stereotypes."* Ann Arbor, MI: Institute for Social Research, 1980.

Jones, Abbott C. "Clairol: Quiet Revolution." *Advertising Age* 51 (Jan. 26, 1981). 46–49.

Kalisch, B., and Kalisch, P. "An Analysis of News Coverage of Maternal-Child Nurses." *Maternal-Child Nursing Journal* 13, no. 2 (Summer 1984): 77–90.

Kalisch, B., and Kalisch, P. "An Analysis of the Impact of the Authorship on the Image of the Nurse Presented in Novels." *Research in Nursing and Health* 6 (March 1983): 17–24.

Kalisch, B., and Kalisch, P. "Anatomy of the Image of the Nurse: Dissonant and Ideal Models." In *Image Making in Nursing,* 3–22. Kansas City, MO: American Academy of Nursing, 1983.

Kalisch, B., and Kalisch, P. "Communicating Clinical Nursing Issues to the Public Through the News Media." *Nursing Research* 30 (May/June 1981): 132–38.

Kalisch, B., and Kalisch, P. "The Dionne Quintuplets Legacy: Establishing the 'Good Doctor and His Loyal Nurse' Image in American Culture." *Nursing and Health Care* 5, no. 5 (May 1984). 242–51.

Kalisch, B., and Kalisch, P. "Good News, Bad News, or No News: How Nurses Can Improve Radio and TV Coverage of Nursing Issues." *Nursing and Health Care* 6 no. 5 (May 1985) 255–60.

Kalisch, B., and Kalisch, P. "Heroine Out of Focus: Images of Florence Nightingale on Stage, Screen, Radio and Television, Part One." *Nursing and Health Care* 4 (April 1983): 181–87.

Kalisch, B., and Kalisch, P. "Heroine Out of Focus: Images of Florence Nightingale on Stage, Screen, Radio and Television, Part Two." *Nursing and Health Care* 4 (May 1983): 270–78.

Kalisch, B., and Kalisch, P. "Improving the Image of Nursing." *American Journal of Nursing* 83 (January 1983): 48–52.

Kalisch, B., and Kalisch, P. "Improving the Image of the Nurse Through Nurse Authored Novels." *Stanford News* 6, no. 3 (Fall 1984): 6–9.

Kalisch, B., and Kalisch, P. *Politics of Nursing.* Philadelphia: J.B. Lippincott, 1982.

Kalisch, B., and Kalisch, P. "The U.S. Cadet Nurse Corps and World War II." *American Journal of Nursing* 76 (February 1976): 240–42.

Kalisch, B., and Kalisch, P. "When Americans Called for Dr. Kildare: Images of Physicians and Nurses in the Dr. Kildare and Dr. Gillespie Movies, 1937–1947." *Medical Heritage* 1 (Summer 1985): 348–63.

Kalisch, B.; Kalisch, P.; and Belcher, B. "Forecasting for Nursing Policy: A News-Based Image Approach." *Nursing Research* 34 no. 1, (January/February, 1985) 44–49.

Kalisch, B.; Kalisch, P.; and Clinton, J. "An Analysis of News Flow on the Nation's Nurse Shortage." *Medical Care* 19 (September 1981): 938–50.

Kalisch, B.; Kalisch, P.; and Clinton, J. "How the Public Sees Nurse-Midwives: 1978 News Coverage of Nurse-Midwifery in the Nation's Press." *Journal of*

Nurse-Midwifery 26 (July–August 1980): 31–39.

Kalisch, B.; Kalisch, P.; and Clinton, J. "Minority Nurses in the News." *Nursing Outlook* 29 (January 1981): 49–65.

Kalisch, B.; Kalisch, P.; and McHugh, M. "Content Analysis of Film Stereotypes of Nurses." *International Journal of Women's Studies* 3, no. 6 (November-December 1980): 531–58.

Kalisch, B.; Kalisch, P.; and McHugh, M. "The Nurse as a Sex Object in Motion Pictures, 1930 to 1980." *Research in Nursing and Health* 5 (September 1982): 147–54.

Kalisch, B.; Kalisch, P.; and McHugh, M. "School Nursing in the News." *Journal of School Health* 53, no. 9 (November 1983): 3–22.

Kalisch, B.; Kalisch, P.; and Scobey, M. "Reflections on a Television Image: *The Nurses,* 1962–1965." *Nursing and Health Care* 2, 53 (May 1981, November 1983): 248–55, 3–22.

Kalisch, B.; Kalisch, P.; and Young, R. "Television News Coverage of Nurse Strikes: A Resource Management Perspective." *Nursing Research* 32, no. 3 (May–June 1983): 175–79.

Kalisch, B.; Livesay, E.; and Kalisch, P. "When Nurses Are Accused of Murder." *Nursing Life* 2 (September–October 1982): 44–47.

Kalisch, P. and Kalisch, B. "Gerontological Nursing Gets Expert Help in Using the News." *Journal of Gerontological Nursing* 11 no. 5 (May 1985) pp. 31–35.

Kalisch, P., and Kalisch, B. "Heroine Out of Focus: Media Images of Florence Nightingale, Popular Biographies and Stage Productions, Part One." *Nursing and Health Care* 4 (April 1983): 181–87.

Kalisch, P., and Kalisch, B. "Heroine Out of Focus: Media Images of Florence Nightingale on Stage, Screen, Radio and Television, Part Two." *Nursing and Health Care* 4 (May 1983): 270–78.

Kalisch, P., and Kalisch, B. "The Image of the Nurse in Motion Pictures." *American Journal of Nursing* 82 (April 1982): 605–11.

Kalisch, P., and Kalisch, B. "The Image of the Nurse in Novels." *American Journal of Nursing* 82 (August 1982): 1220–24.

Kalisch, P., and Kalisch, B. "The Image of the Psychiatric Nurse in Motion Pictures." *Perspectives in Psychiatric Care* 19, nos. 3 and 4 (1981): 116–29.

Kalisch, P., and Kalisch, B. "Images of Nurses and Physicians in the Mass Media Health Care Genre." In *The Media, Communication and Health Policy: Proceedings of the 4th Annual Nor-*

fleet Forum, Memphis: University of Tennessee (Summer 1984), 129–55.

Kalisch, P., and Kalisch, B. "The Nurse-Detective in American Film." *Nursing and Health Care* 3 (March 1982): 146–53.

Kalisch, P., and Kalisch, B. "The Nurse Shortage, the President, and the Congress." *Nursing Forum* 19, no. 2 (1980): 138–64.

Kalisch, P., and Kalisch, B. "Nurses on Primetime Television." *American Journal of Nursing* 82 (February 1982): 264–70.

Kalisch, P., and Kalisch, B. "Perspectives on Improving Nursing's Public Image." *Nursing and Health Care* 11 (July–August 1980): 10–15.

Kalisch, P., and Kalisch B. "Policy Perspectives on Newspaper Reports of Nurse Strikes." *Research in Nursing and Health* 8 (September 1985), 243–51.

Kalisch, P., and Kalisch, B. "The Press Image of Community Health Nurses." *Public Health Nursing* 1, no. 1 (March 1984): 3–15.

Kalisch, P., and Kalisch, B. "Psychiatric Nurses and the Press: A Troubled Relationship." *Perspectives in Psychiatric Care* 22, no. 1 (January–March 1984): 5–15.

Kalisch, P., and Kalisch, B. "Reflections on Marcus Welby's First Practice, 1969–1976." *Medical Heritage* (1986). In press.

Kalisch, P., and Kalisch, B. "Sex Role Stereotyping of Nurses and Physicians on Prime Time Television: A Dichotomy of Occupational Portrayals." *Sex Roles* 10 nos. 7/8 (1984): 533–53.

Kalisch, P., and Kalisch, B. "When Nurses Were National Heroines: Images of Nursing in American Film, 1942–1945." *Nursing Forum* 20, no. 1 (1981): 15–61.

Kalisch, P.; Kalisch, B.; and Clinton, J. "World of Nursing on Prime Time Television, 1950–1980." *Nursing Research* 31 (November–December 1982): 358–63.

Kalisch, P.; Kalisch, B.; and Livesay, E. "'The Angel of Death' Case: The Anatomy of 1980's Major News Story." *Nursing Forum* 19, no. 3 (1980): 212–41.

Kalisch, P.; Kalisch, B.; and Scobey, M. *Images of Nurses on Television.* New York: Springer, 1983.

Kalisch, P.; Kalisch, B.; and Young, R. "Television News Coverage of Nurse Strikes: A Resource Management Perspective." *Nursing Research* 32 (May/ June 1983): 175–79.

Kane, Paula. *Sex Objects in the Sky.* Chicago: Follett, 1974.

Kaplan, F. I. "Intimacy and Conformity in American Soap Operas." *Journal of Popular Culture* 9 (Winter 1975): 622–25.

Katzman, David M. *Seven Days a Week: Women and Domestic Service in Industrializing America.* New York: Oxford University Press, 1978.

Katzman, N. "Television Soap Operas: What's Been Going On Anyway?" *Public Opinion Quarterly* 36 (Summer 1972): 200–12.

Kaufman, H.J. "The Appeal of Specific Daytime Serials." In *Radio Research, 1942–43,* edited by P.F. Lazarfeld and F.N. Stanton. New York: Duell, Sloan, and Pearce, 1944.

Kaufman, L. "Prime Time Nutrition." *Journal of Communication* 30, no. 3 (Summer 1980): 37–46.

Kay, Karyn, and Peary, Gerald. *Women in the Cinema.* New York: E.P. Dutton, 1977.

Kelley, Mary. *Private Woman, Public Stage: Literary Domesticity in Nineteenth-Century America.* New York: Oxford University Press, 1984.

Kennedy, Anne. "History of the Development of Contraceptive Materials in the United States." *American Medicine* 41 (March 1935): 159–61.

Kennedy, David M. *Birth Control in America: The Career of Margaret Sanger.* New Haven, CT: Yale University Press, 1970.

Kennedy, Susan Estabrook. *If All We Did Was To Weep at Home: A History of White Working-Class Women in America.* Bloomington: Indiana University Press, 1979.

Kenny, Elizabeth. *And They Shall Walk: The Life Story of Sister Elizabeth Kenny.* New York: Dodd, Mead, 1943.

Kessler, Ronald C., and Stipp, Horst. "The Impact of Fictional Television Suicide Stories on U.S. Fatalities: A Replication." *American Journal of Sociology* 90, no. 1 (July 1984): 102–67.

Kessler-Harris, A. *Out to Work: A History of Wage-Earning Women in the United States.* New York: Oxford University Press, 1982.

Key, Wilson B. *Media Sexploitation.* New York: Signet, 1976.

Kilbourne, Jean. "Images of Women in TV Commercials." In *TV Book,* edited by Judy Fireman, 293–96. New York: Workman, 1977.

Kilbourne, William E. "An Exploratory Study of Sex Roles in Advertising and Women's Perceptions of Managerial Attributes in Women." In *Advances in Consumer Research,* edited by Thomas C. Kinnear, vol. 11. Ann Arbor, MI: Association for Consumer Research, 1984.

Kilgus, Anne F. "Using Soap Operas as a Therapeutic Tool." *Social Casework* 55 (November 1974): 525–30.

King, Josephine, and Stott, Mary, eds. *Is This Your Life? Images of Women in the Media.* London: Virago/Quartet, 1977.

Kinsey, Alfred; Pomeroy, Wardell B.; and Martin, Clyde E. *Sexual Behavior in the Human Female.* Philadelphia: Saunders, 1953.

Kinsey, Alfred; Pomeroy, Wardell B.; and Martin, Clyde E. *Sexual Behavior in the Human Male.* Philadelphia: Saunders, 1948.

Kinzer, Nora Scott. "Soapy Sin in the Afternoon." *Psychology Today* 7 (August 1973): 46–48.

Kirsch, J.W. "The Ethics of Going Public: Communicating Through Mass Media." *American Behavioral Scientist* 26 (November/December 1982): 251–64.

Klapper, J.T. *The Effects of Mass Communication.* Glencoe, IL: Free Press, 1960.

Klavan, E. *Turn that Damned Thing Off: An Irreverent Look at TV's Impact on the American Scene.* New York: Bobbs-Merrill, 1972.

Klein, P. "The Men Who Run Television Aren't That Stupid. . . . They Know Us Better Than You Think." *New York* 120 (Jan. 25, 1971): 20–31.

Kleinberg, Susan J. "Technology and Women's Work: The Lives of Working Class Women in Pittsburgh, 1870–1900." *Labor History* 17 (Winter 1976): 58–72.

Klemesrud, Judy. "TV's Women Are Dingbats." *New York Times* 122 (May 27, 1973): D-15.

Klemesrud, Judy. "The Year of the Lusty Woman." *Esquire* 19 (December 1978): 33.

Kline, F. Gerald, and Tichenor, Philip J., eds. *Current Perspectives in Mass Communication Research.* Beverly Hills, CA: Sage, 1972.

Knudsen, D.D. "The Declining Status of Women: Popular Myths and the Failure of Functionalist Thought." *Social Forces* 48 (September 1969): 183–93.

Komarovsky, Mirra. *Women in the Modern World: Their Education and Their Dilemmas.* Boston: Little, Brown, 1953.

Komisar, Lucy. "The Image of Women in Advertising." In *Women in Sexist Society,* edited by V. Gornick and B.K. Moran, 207–17. New York: New American Library, 1972.

Kraditor, Aileen S. *The Ideas of the Woman Suffrage Movement 1890–1920.* New York: Columbia University Press, 1965.

Kraditor, Aileen S., ed. *Up from the Pedestal: Selected Writings in the History of*

American Feminism. Chicago: Quadrangle, 1968.

Kreps, Juanita. *Sex in the Marketplace: American Women at Work.* Baltimore: Johns Hopkins University Press, 1971.

LaGuardia, Robert. *The Wonderful World of TV Soap Operas.* New York: Ballantine, 1974.

Lake, S., ed. *Television's Impact on Children and Adolescents.* Phoenix, AZ: Oryx, 1981.

LaMotte, E.N. "American Nurse in Paris." *Survey* 34 (July 10, 1915): 333–34.

Larson, T.A. "Women's Role in the American West." *Montana Magazine of Western History* 24 (Winter 1974): 3–11.

Lasch, Christopher. *Haven in a Heartless World: The Family Besieged.* New York: Basic Books, 1977.

Lasswell, Harold D. "The Structure and Function of Communication in Society." In *The Communication of Ideas*, edited by Norman Byrson, 37–51. New York: Harper and Row, 1948.

Lazarsfeld, Paul F., and Merton, Robert K. "Mass Communication, Popular Taste, and Organized Social Action." In *Mass Culture*, edited by Bernard Rosenberg and David Manning White. Glencoe, IL: Free Press, 1957.

Lee, A.A. "Nursing's Shopworn Image: How It Hurts You . . . How It Helps You." *RN* 42, (September 1979): 42.

Lemons, J. Stanley. "Dominant or Dominated? Women on Prime Time Television." In *Hearth and Home: Images of Women in the Mass Media*, edited by T. Tuchman, et al., 51–68. New York: Oxford University Press, 1978.

Lemons, J. Stanley. *The Woman Citizen: Social Feminism in the 1920's.* Urbana: University of Illinois Press, 1973.

Lerner, Gerda. "The Lady and the Mill Girl: Changes in the Status of Women in the Age of Jackson." *American Studies* 10 (Spring 1969): 5–14.

Lerner, Gerda. *The Majority Finds Its Past: Placing Women in History.* New York: Oxford University Press, 1979.

Lerner, Gerda. *The Woman in American History.* Menlo Park, CA: Addison-Wesley, 1971.

Levine, H.J. *I Knew Sister Kenny: A Story of a Great Lady and Little People.* Boston: Christopher, 1954.

Levinson, Richard, and Link, William. *Stay Tuned: An Inside Look at the Making of Prime-Time Television.* New York: St. Martin's, 1981.

Lewis, E. "Dialogue on a Train." *Nursing Outlook* 21 (July 1973): 439.

Lewis, E. "So Many Images, So Many Voices." *Nursing Outlook* 14 (April 1966): 14.

Lewis, Richard Warrington Bladwin. *Edith Wharton: A Biography.* New York: Harper and Row, 1975.

Leymore, Varda Langholz. *Hidden Myth: Structure and Symbolism in Advertising.* New York: Basic, 1975.

Liebert, Robert M.; Neale, Joyce M.; and Davidson, Emily S. *The Early Window: Effects of Television on Children and Youth.* New York: Pergamon, 1973.

Lingeman, Richard. *Don't You Know There's a War On? The American Homefront, 1941–1945.* New York: Putnam's, 1970.

Lippman, Walter. *Public Opinion.* New York: Macmillan, 1922.

Longfellow, H.W. "Santa Filomenna." *Atlantic Monthly* 1 (November, 1857): 22–23.

Lopata, Helena Znaniecki. "The Life Cycle of the Social Role of the Housewife." *Sociology and Social Research* 51 (October 1966): 5–22.

Lopate, Carol. "Daytime Television: You'll Never Want To Leave Home." *Radical America* 11 (January–February 1977): 33–51.

Lopate, Carol. *Women in Medicine.* Baltimore: Johns Hopkins University Press, 1968.

Lowenthal, Leo. *Literature, Popular Culture and Society.* Englewood Cliffs, NJ: Prentice-Hall, 1961.

Lowery, Shearon. "Soap and Booze in the Afternoon: An Analysis of Alcohol Use in Daytime Serials." *Journal of Studies on Alcohol* 41 (September 1980): 829–38.

Lowery, Shearon, and De Fleur, Melvin L. *Milestones in Mass Communication Research: Media Effects.* New York: Longman, 1983.

Lowry, D.T.; Love, G.; and Kirby, M. "Sex on the Soap Operas: Patterns of Intimacy." *Journal of Communication* 31 (Summer 1981): 90–96.

Lull, James. "Family Communication Patterns and the Social Uses of Television." *Communications Research* 7 (Spring 1980): 319–34.

Lull, James. "Girl's Favorite TV Females." *Journalism Quarterly* 57 (July 1980): 146–50.

Lull, James. "The Social Uses of Television." *Human Communication Research* 6 (Spring 1980): 197–209.

Lupri, E., ed. *The Changing Position of Women in Family and Society.* Atlantic Highlands, NJ: Humanities Press, 1983.

Luttbeg, N.R., ed. *Public Opinions and Public Policy.* Itasca, IL: Peacock, 1981.

Lynch, William. *The Image Industries.* New York: Sheed and Ward, 1959.

Lynd, Robert S., and Lynd, Helen Merrell. *Middletown: A Study in American Culture.* New York: Harcourt and Brace, 1929.

Lynd, Robert S., and Lynd, Helen Merrell. *Middletown in Transition: A Study in Cultural Conflicts.* New York: Harcourt and Brace, 1937.

Lyson, Thomas A. "Sex Differences in the Choice of a Male or Female Career Line: An Analysis of Background Characteristics and Work Values." *Work and Occupations* 11, no. 2 (May 1984): 131–46.

Maccoby, E.E., and Wilson, W.C. "Identification and Observational Learning from Films." *Journal of Abnormal and Social Psychology* 55 (Winter 1957): 76–87.

McClare, M. "A Nurse Leads a Human Life." *Charm* 10 (September 1956): 67–68.

McConnell-Ginet, S.; Borker, R.; and Furman, N., eds. *Women and Language in Literature and Society.* New York: Praeger, 1980.

MacCulloch, Campbell. "Movies Are Helping America." *Theatre Arts* 11 (October 1927): 23–27.

McGhee, P.E., and Frueh, T. "Television Viewing and the Learning of Sex-Role Stereotypes." *Sex Roles* 6, no. 2 (1980): 179–88.

McGovern, James R. "The American Woman's Pre-World War I Freedom in Manners and Morals." *Journal of American History* 55 (September 1968): 315–33.

Machlup, F. *Knowledge: Its Creation, Distribution, and Economic Significance.* Vol. 1, *Knowledge and Knowledge Production.* Princeton, NJ: Princeton University Press, 1980

MacKuen, M.B., and Coombs, S.L. *More than News: Media Power in Public Affairs.* Beverly Hills, CA: Sage, 1981.

McLaughlin, James M. "The Doctor Shows." *Journal of Communication* 25 (Summer 1975): 182–84. (Originally "Characteristics and Symbolic Functions of Fictional Televised Medical Professionals and Their Effect on Children." Master's thesis, University of Pennsylvania, 1975.)

McNeil, Jean C. "Feminism, Femininity and the Television Series: A Content Analysis." *Journal of Broadcasting* 19 (Summer 1975): 259–71.

McQuail, Denis. *Towards a Sociology of Mass Communications.* London: Collier-Macmillan, 1969.

Makosky, Donald R. *The Portrayal of Women in Wide Circulation Magazine Short Stories.* Ph.D. diss., University of Pennsylvania, 1966.

Maltin, Leonard. *TV Movies, 1985–86.* New York: New American Library, 1984.

Mankiewicz, Frank, and Swerdlow, Joel. "Sex Roles in TV: Co-Opted Liberation." *Television Quarterly* 14 (Winter, 1977–78), 7–12.

Mannes, Marya. "Everything's Up-to-Date in Soap Operas." *TV Guide* 17 (March 15, 1969): 16–21.

Marc, David. *Demographic Vistas: Television in American Culture.* Philadelphia: University of Pennsylvania Press, 1984.

Margulies, Lee. "The Second Time Around." *Emmy: The Magazine of Television Arts and Sciences* 1 (Fall 1979): 39–40, 55–56.

Martel, Martin. "Age-Sex Roles in American Magazine Fiction 1890–1955." In *Middle Age and Aging,* edited by B. Neugarten, 47–57. Chicago: University of Chicago Press, 1968.

Marting, Leeda Pollock. "An Empirical Study of the Images of Males and Females During Prime-Time Television Drama." Ph.D. diss., Ohio State University, 1973.

Mason, K.O.; Czajka, J.L.; and Arber, S. "Change in U.S. Women's Sex-Role Attitudes, 1964–1974." *American Sociological Review* 41 (August 1976): 573–96.

"The Medium Is Macho." *Human Behavior* 4 (August 1975): 71.

Meehan, Diana M. *Ladies of the Evening: Women Characters of Prime-Time Television.* Metuchen, NJ: Scarecrow, 1983.

Mellen, Joan. *Women and Their Sexuality in the New Film.* New York: Horizon, 1973.

Melosh, B. *The Physician's Hand.* Philadelphia: Temple University Press, 1982.

Mendelsohn, Harold. *Mass Entertainment.* New Haven, CT: College and University Press, 1966.

Merrill, Frances E., and Truxal, Andrew G. *Marriage and Family in American Culture.* New York: Duell, Sloan and Pearce, 1953.

Middleton, Russell. "Fertility Values in American Magazine Fiction, 1916–1956." *Public Opinion Quarterly* 24 (Summer 1960): 139–43.

Miles, Betty. *Channeling Children: Sex Stereotyping in Prime Time TV.* Princeton, NJ: Women on Words and Images, 1975.

Miller, Mark M., and Reeves, Byron. "Dramatic TV Content and Children's Sex-Role Stereotypes." *Journal of Broadcasting* 20 (Winter 1976): 35–50.

Millet, Kate. *Sexual Politics.* New York: Doubleday, 1970.

Mills, Kay. "Fighting Sexism on the Airwaves." *Journal of Communication* 24, (Spring 1974): 150–53.

Millum, Trevor. *Images of Woman: Advertising in Women's Magazines.* Totowa, NJ: Rowan and Littlefield, 1975.

Miner, Madonne M. *Insatiable Appetites: Twentieth-Century American Women's Bestsellers.* Westport, CT: Greenwood, 1984.

Mitchell, Juliet. *Psychoanalysis and Feminism.* New York: Random House, 1974.

Monaco, James. *American Film Now: The People, the Power, the Money, the Movies.* New York: New American Library, 1984.

Moody, K. *Growing Up on Television.* New York: New York Times Books, 1980.

Morantz, Regina. "Making Women Modern: Middle Class Women and Health Reform in Nineteenth-Century America." *Journal of Social History* 10 (June 1977): 490–508.

"More Glamour, Pay, Glory Needed To Attract Nurses." *Science Newsletter* 88 (March 1965): 89.

Mueller, Claus. *The Politics of Communication.* New York: Oxford University Press, 1973.

Murray, John P. *Television and Youth: 25 Years of Controversy.* Omaha, NE: Boys Town Center for the Study of Youth Development, 1980.

Naisbitt, John. *Megatrends: Ten New Directions Transforming Our Lives.* New York: Warner, 1982.

"NCWW Studies 10 Years of TV Portrayal of Working Women: Rarely Reflects Reality." *Media Report to Women* 11 (January–February 1982): 16–18.

Nelson, Martha. "The Sex Life of the Romance Novel." *Ms.* 12 (February 1983): 97–103.

Neuman, W.R., ed. *The Social Impact of Television: A Research Agenda for the 1980s.* Queenstown, MD: Aspen Institute for Humanistic Studies, 1981.

Newcomb, Horace, ed. *Television: The Critical View.* New York: Oxford University Press, 1976.

Newcomb, Horace, and Alley, Robert S. *The Producer's Medium: Conversations with Creators of American TV.* New York: Oxford University Press, 1983.

"A New Look at the American Woman." *Look* 20 (Oct. 16, 1956): 16–43.

Nichols, D.; Knox, A.; and McCarthy, M. *Sister Kenny: A Screen Play.* Los Angeles: RKO, 1945.

Nightingale, Florence. "Cassandra." Appendix to *"The Cause:" A Short History of the Women's Movement in Great Britain,* by Ray Strachey. Reprint. Port Washington, NY: Kennikat, 1969.

Nightingale, Florence. *Notes on Nursing: What It Is and What It Is Not.* London: Harrison, 1860.

Nimmo, D.D., and Sanders, K.R., eds. *Handbook of Political Communication.* Beverly Hills, CA: Sage, 1981.

Norback, Craig T., and Norback, Peter G., eds. *TV Guide Almanac.* New York: Ballantine, 1980.

Northcott, Herbert C.; Seggar, John F.; and Hinton, James L. "Trends in TV Portrayal of Blacks and Women." *Journalism Quarterly* 52 (Winter 1975): 741–44.

"Notes on Nursing." *Saturday Review* 2 (Jan. 21, 1860): 84–85.

"Nurse's Experiences: Incidents of Life in a French Hospital." *Current Opinion* 64 (February 1918): 136.

"Nursing and the Popular Press." *American Journal of Nursing* 58 (December 1958): 1665.

Nye, F. Ivan. *Role Structure and Analysis of the Family.* Beverly Hills, CA: Sage, 1976.

Oakley, Ann. *Woman's Work: The Housewife, Past and Present.* New York: Pantheon, 1974.

O'Bryant, S.L., and Corder-Bolz, C.R. "The Effects of Television on Children's Stereotyping of Women's Work Roles." *Journal of Vocational Behavior* 12 (Spring 1978): 233–44.

Ogburn, William F., and Nimkoff, Meyer F. *Technology and the Changing Family.* Boston: Houghton Mifflin, 1955.

O'Neill, William. *Divorce in the Progressive Era.* New Haven, CT: Yale University Press, 1967.

O'Neill, William. *Everyone Was Brave: A History of Feminism in America.* Chicago: Quadrangle, 1971.

Oppenheimer, Valerie Kincade. *The Female Labor Force in the United States: Demographic and Economic Factors Governing Its Growth and Changing Composition.* Berkeley and Los Angeles: Institute of International Studies, University of California Press, 1970.

Orden, Susan R., and Bradburn, Norman M. "Working Wives and Marital Happiness." *American Journal of Sociology* 74 (January 1969): 392–407.

Osmund, Marie Withers, and Martin, Patricia Yancey. "Sex and Sexism: A Comparison of Male and Female Sex-Role Attitudes." *Journal of Marriage and the Family* 37, no. 4 (November 1975): 744–59.

Papashvily, Helen Waite. *All the Happy Endings: A Study of the Domestic Novel in America, the Women Who Wrote It, the Women Who Read It, in the Nineteenth Century.* New York: Harper and Brothers, 1956.

Parsons, Talcott. "The Superego and the Theory of Social Systems." In *Working*

Papers in the Theory of Action, edited by Talcott Parsons, et al. New York: Free Press, 1953.

Patterson, Thomas. *The Mass Media Example.* New York: Praeger, 1980.

Paul, J.R. *A History of Poliomyelitis.* New Haven, CT: Yale University Press, 1971.

Pearse, Susan R. *Body, Mind and Soul: An Annotated Bibliography of U.S. Woman's History.* Mesquite, Texas: Ide House, 1984.

Peevers, B.N. "Androgyny on the TV Screen? An Analysis of Sex-Role Portrayal." *Sex Roles* 5, no. 6 (1979): 797–809.

Perry, G.S. "Nurses Are Lucky Girls." *Saturday Evening Post* 226 (March 27, 1954): 24–25.

Perry, Jeb H. *Universal Television: The Studio and Its Programs, 1950–1980.* Metuchen, NJ: Scarecrow, 1983.

Peterson, M. Jeanne. *The Medical Profession in Mid-Victorian London.* Berkeley and Los Angeles: University of California Press, 1978.

Peterson, Richard, ed. *The Production of Culture.* Beverly Hills, CA: Sage, 1976.

Peterson, Theodore. *Magazines in the Twentieth Century.* Urbana: University of Illinois Press, 1964.

Phelan, John M. *Mediaworld: Programming the Public.* New York: Seabury, 1977.

Phelps, Elizabeth Stuart. "Her Shadow." *Atlantic Monthly* 49 (July 1906), 608.

Phillips, D.P. "The Impact of Fictional Television on U.S. Adult Fatalities: New Evidence on the Effect of the Mass Media on Violence." *American Journal of Sociology* 87 (May 1982): 1340–59.

Pidgeon, Mary Elizabeth. *Women in the Economy of the United States of America.* U.S. Women's Bureau Bulletin no. 155. Washington, DC: U.S. Department of Labor, 1937.

Pingree, S. "The Effects of Nonsexist Television Commercials and Perceptions of Reality on Children's Attitudes About Women." *Psychology of Women Quarterly* 2 (Spring 1978): 262–77.

Pion, G.M., and Lipsey, M.W. "Public Attitudes Toward Science and Technology: What Have the Surveys Told Us?" *Public Opinion Quarterly* 45 (Fall 1981): 303–16.

Pitz, Henry. "Charles Dana Gibson: Delineator of an Age." Introduction to *The Gibson Girl and Her America,* edited by Edmund V. Gillon, Jr. New York: Dover, 1969.

Plamentz, John. *Ideology.* London: Macmillan, 1971.

Ploghoft, Milton E., and Anderson, James A. *Teaching Critical Television*

Viewing Skills: An Integrated Approach. Springfield, IL: Charles C. Thomas, 1982.

Poindexter, P.M., and Stroman, C.A. "Blacks and Television: A Review of the Research Literature." *Journal of Broadcasting* 25 (Spring 1981): 103–22.

Polenberg, Richard. *War and Society: The U.S., 1941–1945.* New York: J.B. Lippincott, 1972.

President's Research Committee On Social Trends. *Recent Social Trends.* New York: McGraw-Hill, 1933.

Prisco, D.D. "Women and Social Change as Reflected in a Major Fashion Magazine." *Journalism Quarterly* 59 (Spring 1982): 131–35.

Pryluck, Calvin. *Sources of Meaning in Motion Pictures and Television.* New York: Arno, 1976.

Raddatz, Leslie. "The Destiny of *The Bold Ones.*" *TV Guide* 17 (Oct. 25, 1969): 40–46.

Raddatz, Leslie. "Let's Play Father Image." *TV Guide* 12 (May 23, 1964): 24–27.

Ragan, J.M. "Gender Displays in Portrait Photographs." *Sex Roles* 8 (January 1982): 33–44.

Rainwater, Lee; Coleman, Richard; and Handel, Gerald. *Workingman's Wife: Her Personality, World, and Life Style.* New York: Oceania Publications, 1959.

Ramsdell, M.L. "The Trauma of Television's Troubled Soap Families." *Family Coordinator* 22 no. 3 (1973): 299–304.

Real, Michael R. *Mass-Mediated Culture.* Englewood Cliffs, NJ: Prentice-Hall, 1977.

Rees, B.L. "Television Talk Shows: An Untapped Resource for Nursing." *Nursing Outlook* 28, (September 1980): 562.

Reisman, David. *The Lonely Crowd.* New Haven, CT: Yale University Press, 1950.

Reissman, Leonard, and Rohrer, John. *Change and Dilemma in the Nursing Profession: Studies of Nursing Service in a Large Urban Hospital.* New York: Putnam's, 1957.

Richardson, Herbert. *Nun, Witch, and Playmate: The Americanization of Sex.* New York: Harper, 1971.

Richter, L., and Richter, E. "Nurses in Fiction." *American Journal of Nursing* 74, (July 1974):1280.

Rickel, A., and Grant, L. "Sex Role Stereotypes in the Mass Media and Schools: Five Consistent Themes." *International Journal of Women's Studies.* 2, (March/April 1979): 164–79.

Riley, J.W., Jr., and Riley, Matilda W. "Mass Communication and the Social System." In *Sociology Today: Problems and Prospects,* edited by Robert K. Merten. New York: Basic, 1959.

Rinehart, Mary Roberts. *My Story.* New York: Farrar and Rinehart, 1931.

Robinson, Paul A. *The Modernization of Sex.* New York: Harper, 1976.

Rock, Gail. "Same Time, Same Station, Same Sexism." *Ms.* 2 (December 1973): 24–26.

Roiphe, Anne. "The Waltons." *New York Times Magazine* 122 (Nov. 18, 1973): 40.

Rollins, Mable A. "Monetary Contributions of Wives to Family Income in 1920 and 1960." *Marriage and Family Living* 25 no. 2 (1963): 226–27.

Roper, Brent S., and LaBeff, Emily. "Sex Roles and Feminism Revisited: An Intergenerational Attitude Comparison." *Journal of Marriage and the Family* 39, no. 1 (1977): 113–19.

Roper Organization, comp. *The 1980 Virginia Slims American Women's Opinion Poll.* Storrs, CT: The Roper Center, University of Connecticut, 1980.

Rosaldo, Michelle Zimbalist, and Lamphere, Louise. *Woman, Culture and Society.* Stanford, CA: Stanford University Press, 1974.

Rosen, Diane. "TV and the Single Girl." *TV Guide* 19 (Nov. 6, 1971): 13–14.

Rosen, Harvey S. "The Monetary Value of a Housewife: A Replacement Cost Approach." *American Journal of Economics and Sociology* 33 no. 1 (1974): 65–73.

Rosen, Marjorie. *Popcorn Venus: Women, Movies and the American Dream.* New York: Coward, McCann, and Geoghahan, 1973.

Rosenblatt, P.C., and Cunningham, M.R. "Television Watching and Family Tension." *Journal of Marriage and the Family* 38 (February 1976): 105–11.

Rosengren, K.E. *Advances in Content Analysis.* Sage Annual Reviews of Communication Research, vol. 9. Beverly Hills, CA: Sage, 1981.

Rosenthal, D., and Chapman, D. "The Lady Spaceman: Children's Perceptions of Sex-Stereotyped Occupations." *Sex Roles* 8, no. 9: 959–65.

Ross, L.; Anderson, D.R.; and Wisocki, P.A. "Television Viewing and Adult Sex-Role Attitudes." *Sex Roles* 8 (June 1982): 589–92.

Roszak, Betty, and Roszak, Theodore, eds. *Masculine/Feminine: Readings in Sexual Mythology and the Liberation of Women.* New York: Harper and Row, 1969.

Rothman, Sheila. "The Mass Media in Post-Industrial Society." In *The Third Century: America as a Post-Industrial Society,* edited by S.M. Lipset, 346–88. Chicago: University of Chicago Press, 1979.

Rothman, Sheila. *Women's Proper Place: A History of Changing Ideals and Practices, 1870 to the Present.* New York: Basic, 1978.

Rubens, W.S. "Sex and Violence on TV." *Journal of Advertising Research* 21 (December 1981): 13–20.

Ruffing, Mary Ann. "Literature by Consumers for Nursing." *Nursing Forum* 14 (1975): 87–93.

Runco, Mark A., and Pezdek, Kathy. "The Effect of Television and Radio on Children's Creativity." *Human Communication Research* 11, no. 1 (Autumn 1984): 109–20.

Russell, R. *Life Is a Banquet.* New York: Random House, 1977.

Ruthstein, Pauline Marcus. "Women: A Selected Bibliography of Books." *Bulletin of Bibliography and Magazine Notes* 32, no. 2 (1975): 45–54.

Ryan, Mary P. *Womanhood in America: From Colonial Times to the Present.* New York: Franklin Watts, 1975.

Safilios-Rothschild, Constantino. "The Study of Family Power Structure: A Review 1960–1969." *Journal of Marriage and the Family* 32 (November 1970): 539–52.

Sanderson, Warren. "The Fertility of American Woman Since 1920." *Journal of Economic History* 30 (June 1970): 271–88.

Sapir, J. David. "The Anatomy of a Metaphor." In *The Social Use of Metaphor,* edited by J.D. Sapir and J.C. Crocker. Philadelphia: University of Pennsylvania Press, 1977.

Saxton, Martha. *Louisa May: A Modern Biography of Louisa May Alcott.* Boston: Houghton Mifflin, 1977.

Scanzoni, Letha, and Scanzoni, John. *Men, Women, and Change: A Sociology of Marriage and the Family.* New York: McGraw-Hill, 1976.

Schiffman, L.G., and Kanuk, L.L. *Consumer Behavior.* Englewood Cliffs, NJ: Prentice-Hall, 1978.

Scholes, Robert. *Structuralism in Literature.* New Haven, CT: Yale University Press, 1974.

Schorr, Thelma. "Nursing's TV Image." *American Journal of Nursing* 63 (October 1963): 119–21.

Schram, Rosalyn Weinman. "Marital Satisfaction over the Family Life Cycle: A Critique and Proposal." *Journal of Marriage and the Family* 41, no. 1 (1979): 7–12.

Schramm, Wilbur. *The Process and Effects of Communication.* Urbana: University of Illinois Press, 1961.

Schwartz, Meg, ed. *TV and Teens: Experts Look at the Issues.* Reading, MA: Addison-Wesley, 1982.

Schwartz, Tony. *Media: The Second God.* New York: Random House, 1981.

Schwichtenberg, C. "The Love Boat: The Packaging and Selling of Love, Heterosexual Romance, and Family." *Media Culture and Society* 6, no. 3 (July 1984): 301–12.

Scott, Anne Firor. "Women's Perspective on the Patriarchy in the 1850's." *Journal of American History* Vol. 61 (January 1974): 52–64.

Scott, Anne Firor, ed. *The American Woman: Who Was She?* Englewood Cliffs, NJ: Prentice-Hall, 1971.

Sees, Mary C. "Image of Nursing: Its Relationship to Characteristics of Students and Faculty in Baccalaureate Nursing Programs." Ph.D. diss., Syracuse University, 1974.

Seggar, J.F. "Imagery of Women in Television Drama: 1974." *Journal of Broadcasting* 19, (Summer 1975): 273–82.

Seggar, John F. "Television's Portrayal of Minorities and Women." *Journal of Broadcasting* 21 (Fall 1977): 435–46.

Seggar, John F. "Women's Imagery on TV: Feminist, Fair Maiden or Maid? Comments on McNeil." *Journal of Broadcasting* 19, no. 3 (1975): 289–94.

Seggar, J.F., and Wheeler, P. "World of Work on TV: Ethnic and Sex Representation in TV Drama." *Journal of Broadcasting* 17 (Spring 1973): 201–14.

Seidenberg, Robert. *Marriage in Life and Literature.* New York: Philosophical Library, 1970.

Shils, E., and Finch, H.A. *Max Weber on the Methodology of the Social Sciences.* Glencoe, IL: Free Press, 1949.

Shover, Michele. "Roles and Images of Women in World War I Propaganda." *Politics and Society* 5, no. 3 (1975): 469–89.

Showalter, Elaine. "Victorian Women and Insanity." *Victorian Studies* 23 (Winter 1980): 176–79.

Signorielli, Nancy. "Men and Women in Television Drama: The Use of Two Multi-Variate Techniques for Isolating Dimensions of Characterization." Ph.D. diss., University of Pennsylvania, 1975.

Signorielli, Nancy. "Patterns in Prime Time." *Journal of Communication* 24 (Spring 1974): 119–24.

Silverman, L.T.; Sprafkin, J.N.; and Rubinstein, E.A. "Physical Contact and Sexual Behavior on Prime-Time TV." *Journal of Communication* 29 (Winter 1979): 33–43.

Simmons, Leo W. "Images of the Nurse: Theory" and "Images of the Nurse: Studies." In *Nursing Research: A Survey and Assessment,* by Leo W. Simmons and Virginia Henderson, 167–223. New York: Appleton-Century-Crofts, 1964.

Simmons, Leo W. "Past and Potential Images of the Nurse." *Nursing Forum* 1 (Summer 1962): 19.

Skill, Thomas. "Television's Families: Real by Day, Ideal by Night." In *Life on Daytime Television,* edited by M. Cassata and T. Skill. Norwood, NJ: Ablex, 1983.

Sklar, Robert. *Movie-Made America: A Social History of American Movies.* New York: Random House, 1975.

Sklar, Robert. *Prime-Time America: Life on and Behind the Television Screen.* New York: Oxford University Press, 1982.

Skornia, Harry J. *Television and Society: An Inquest and Agenda for Improvement.* New York: McGraw-Hill, 1965.

Smith, Alfred B. *Communication and Culture.* New York: Holt, Rinehart and Winston, 1966.

Smith, Daniel Scott. "The Dating of the American Sexual Revolution: Evidence and Interpretation." In *The American Family in Social-Historical Perspective,* edited by Michael Gordon, 321–35. New York: Random House, 1973.

Smith, Page. *Daughters of the Promised Land: Women in American History.* Boston: Little, Brown, 1970.

Smith, R. "Images and Equality: Women and the National Press." In *The Sociology of Journalism and the Press,* edited by H. Christian, 239–58. Totowa, NJ: Rowan and Littlefield, 1980.

Smith, Thelma. "Feminism in Philadelphia, 1790–1850." *Pennsylvania Magazine of History and Biography* 68 (Spring 1944): 243–68.

Smith-Rosenberg, Carroll. "The Hysterical Woman: Sex Roles and Role Conflict in Nineteenth-Century America." *Social Research* 39 no. 4 (1972): 652–78.

Smith-Rosenberg, Carroll, and Rosenberg, Charles. "The Female Animal: Medical and Biological Views of Woman and Her Role in Nineteenth-Century America." *Journal of American History* 60 (September 1973): 332–56.

Smuts, Robert. *Women and Work in America.* New York: Columbia University Press, 1959.

Smythe, Dallas W. "New Directions for Critical Communications Research." *Media Culture and Society* 6, no. 3 (July 1984): 205–18.

Smythe, Dallas W. "Reality as Presented by Television." *Public Opinion Quarterly* 18 (Summer 1954): 143–56.

Smythe, Dallas W. *Three Years of New York Television: 1951–1953.* New York: National Association of Educational Broadcasters, 1953.

Snitow, Ann Barr. "Mass Market Romance: Pornography for Women Is Different." *Radical History Review* 19 (Spring 1979): 141–61.

Snow, R.P. *Creating Media Culture.* Beverly Hills, CA: Sage, 1983.

Sochen, June. *Herstory: A Woman's View of American History.* New York: Alfred, 1974.

Sochen, June. *Movers and Shakers: American Women Thinkers and Activists 1900–1970.* New York: Quadrangle, 1973.

Soltow, Martha Jane. *Women in American Labor History, 1825–1935: An Annotated Bibliography.* East Lansing, MI: Michigan State University, 1972.

Somers, A.R. "Violence, Television, and the Health of American Youth." *New England Journal of Medicine* 294, no. 15 (1976): 811–17.

Sonenschein, David. "Love and Sex in the Romance Magazines." *Journal of Popular Culture* 4, no. 2 (Fall 1970): 398–409.

Sorokin, Pitirim. *The American Sexual Revolution.* Boston: Porter Sargeant, 1956.

Spacks, Patricia Meyer. *The Female Imagination.* New York: Knopf, 1975.

Spock, Benjamin McLane. *Baby and Child Care.* New York: Pocket Books, 1976.

Sprafkin, Joyce; Swift, Carolyn; and Hess, Robert, eds. *Rx Television: Enhancing the Preventive Impact of TV.* New York: Haworth, 1983.

Sprigge, S. Squire. "The Medicine of Dickens." *The Cornhill Magazine* 35 (March 1877): 258–67.

Stein, Benjamin. *The View from Sunset Boulevard: America as Brought to You by the People Who Make TV.* New York: Basic, 1979.

Steinberg, Cobbett. *TV Facts.* New York: Facts on File, 1984.

Steiner, Gary A. *The People Look at Television.* New York: Knopf, 1963.

Stempel, Guido H., and Westley, Bruce H., eds. *Research Methods in Mass Communication.* Englewood Cliffs, NJ: Prentice-Hall, 1981.

Sternglanz, S.H., and Serbin, L.A. "Sex Role Stereotyping in Children's Television Programs." *Developmental Psychology* 10, no. 6 (1974): 710–15.

Stouffer, Samuel A., and Lazarsfeld, Paul F. *The Family in the Depression.* New York: Social Science Research Council, 1937.

Strainchamps, Ethel, ed. *Rooms with No View: A Woman's Guide to the Man's World of the Media.* Compiled by the Media Women's Association. New York: Harper and Row, 1974.

Strouse, J.C. *The Mass Media, Public Opinion and Public Policy Analysis.*

Political Science Series. Columbus, OH: Merrill, 1975.

Sweet, James A. *Women in the Labor Force.* New York: Seminar Press, 1973.

Tan, A.S. "Television Use and Social Stereotypes." *Journalism Quarterly* 59 (Spring 1982): 118–22.

Tannenbaum, P.H., ed. *The Entertainment Functions of Television.* Hillsdale, NJ: Lawrence Erlbaum Associates, 1980.

Tebbel, John. *The Media in America.* New York: Crowell, 1974.

Tedesco, Nancy S. "Patterns in Primetime." *Journal of Communication* 24, no. 2 (Spring 1974): 119–24.

Tentler, Leslie Woodcock. *Wage-Earning Women: Industrial Work and Family Life in the United States, 1900–1930.* New York: Oxford University Press, 1979.

Terrace, Vincent. *The Complete Encyclopedia of Television Programs 1947–1976.* 2 vols. New York: Barnes, 1976.

Theberge, L.J., ed. *Crooks, Con Men and Clowns: Businessmen in TV Entertainment.* Washington, DC: Media Institute, 1981.

"There's a Doctor in the House." *TV Guide* 18 (April 18, 1970): 41–44.

Thomas, Sari, ed. *Film/Culture: Explorations of Cinema in Its Social Context.* Metuchen, NJ: Scarecrow, 1982.

Thomsom, Patricia. *The Victorian Heroine—A Changing Ideal: 1837–1873.* London: Oxford University Press, 1956.

"Through the Years with Dr. Kildare." *TV Guide* 21 (Jan. 20, 1973): 15–18.

Tuchenor, P.J., et al. "Mass Media Flow and Differential Growth in Knowledge." *Public Opinion Quarterly* 34 (1979): 159–70.

Tuchman, Gaye. "Assembling a Television Talk Show." In *The TV Establishment: Programming for Power and Profit,* edited by Gaye Tuchman. Englewood Cliffs, NJ: Prentice-Hall, 1974.

Tuchman, Gaye. "The Impact of the Mass-Media Stereotypes upon the Full Employment of Women." In *American Women Workers in a Full Employment Economy,* 249–68. Washington, DC: U.S. Government Printing Office, 1977.

Tuchman, Gaye. *Making News: A Study in the Construction of Reality.* New York: Free Press, 1978.

Tuchman, Gaye. "Women's Depiction in the Mass Media." *Signs* 4, (Spring 1979): 528–42.

Tuchman, Gaye, and Fortin, Nina E. "Fame and Misfortune: Edging Women Out of the Great Literary Tradition." *American Journal of Sociology* 90, no. 1 (July 1984): 72–96.

Tully, J.; Stephan, C.; and Chance, B. "The Status and Sex-Typed Dimensions of Occupational Aspirations in Young Adolescents." *Social Science Quarterly* 56, no. 4 (1976): 638–49.

U.S. Bureau of Labor. *Report on the Condition of Women and Child Wage Earners in the United States* 61st Cong, 2d ses, 1910. S. Doc. 645.

U.S. Bureau of Labor Statistics. *Handbook of Labor Statistics, 1967.* Washington, DC: U.S. Government Printing Office, 1967.

U.S. Bureau of the Census. *Fourteenth Census of the United States, 1920, Population, 1920.* Vol. 2. Washington, DC: U.S. Government Printing Office, 1922.

U.S. Bureau of the Census. *Marriage and Divorce: 1867–1907.* Washington, DC: U.S. Government Printing Office, 1908.

U.S. Bureau of the Census. *U.S. Census of the Population: 1900.* Vol. 1, pt 1; vol. 2, pt 2. Washington, DC: U.S. Government Printing Office, 1901.

U.S. Bureau of the Census. *U.S. Census of the Population: 1910.* Vol. 1. Washington, DC: U.S. Government Printing Office, 1913.

U.S. Bureau of the Census. *U.S. Census of the Population, 1920.* Vols. 2, 3, 4. Washington, DC: U.S. Government Printing Office, 1922.

U.S. Bureau of the Census. *U.S. Census of the Population, 1930.* Vol. 3, pt 1; vol. 4. Washington, DC: U.S. Government Printing Office, 1932.

U.S. Bureau of the Census. *U.S. Census of the Population, 1940.* Vol. 2, pt 2. Washington, DC: U.S. Government Printing Office, 1943.

U.S. Bureau of the Census. *U.S. Census of the Population, 1950.* Vol. 2, pt 2. Washington, DC: U.S. Government Printing Office, 1952.

U.S. Bureau of the Census. *U.S. Census of the Population, 1950.* Vol. 2, pt 14. Washington, DC: U.S. Government Printing Office, 1952.

U.S. Bureau of the Census. *U.S. Census of the Population, 1960.* Vol. 1, pt 16. Washington, DC: U.S. Government Printing Office, 1961.

U.S. Bureau of the Census. *U.S. Census of the Population, 1970. General Social and Economic Characteristics.* Washington, DC: U.S. Government Printing Office, 1971.

U.S. Commission on Civil Rights. *Social Indicators of Equality for Minorities and Women.* Washington, DC: U.S. Government Printing Office, 1979.

U.S. Commission on Civil Rights. *Window Dressing on the Set: Women and*

Minorities in Television. Washington, DC: U.S. Government Printing Office, 1977.

U.S. Congress, House Committee on Interstate and Foreign Commerce, Subcommittee on Communications. *Sex and Violence on TV.* Hearings, 95th Cong, 1st ses, 1977. Washington, DC: U.S. Government Printing Office, 1977.

U.S. Congress, Senate Committee on Commerce, Subcommittee on Communications. *Impact of Television on Children.* Hearings, 94th Cong, 2d ses. Washington, DC: U.S. Government Printing Office, 1976.

U.S. Congress, Senate Committee on Commerce, Subcommittee on Communications. *Surgeon General's Report by the Scientific Advisory Committee on Television and Social Behavior.* Hearings, 92d Cong, 2d ses, 1972. Washington, DC: U.S. Government Printing Office, 1972.

U.S. Department of the Interior, Census Division. *Compendium of the Eleventh Census: 1890.* Pt 1. Washington, DC: U.S. Department of the Interior, 1896.

U.S. Public Health Service, Alcohol, Drug Abuse and Mental Health Administration, National Institute of Mental Health. *Television and Behavior: Ten Years of Scientific Progress and Implications for the Eighties.* Washington, DC: U.S. Government Printing Office, 1982.

U.S. Public Health Service, Surgeon General's Scientific Advisory Committee on Television and Social Behavior. *Television and Social Behavior.* Vol 1, *Media Content and Control.* Washington, DC: U.S. Government Printing Office, 1972.

Venkatesan, M., and Losco, Jean. "Women in Magazine Ads: 1959–1971." *Journal of Advertising Research* 15, no. 5 (May 1975): 49–54.

Versteeg, D. "The Fictional Nurse: Is She for Real?" *Nursing Outlook* 16 (August 1968): 20–25.

"Violence on TV: Why People Are Upset." *U.S. News & World Report* 75 (Oct. 29, 1973): 34.

Volgy, T., and Schwartz, T. "Television Entertainment Programming and Sociopolitical Attitudes." *Journalism Quarterly* 57 (Spring 1980): 150–54.

Wade, Serena, and Schramm, Wilbur. "The Mass Media as Sources of Public Affairs, Science and Health Knowledge." *Public Opinion Quarterly* 33 (Summer 1969): 197–209.

Wahl, Otto. "TV Myths About Mental Illness." *TV Guide* 24 (March 13, 1976): 4–8.

Waite, Linda J. "Working Wives: 1940–1960." *American Sociological Review* 41, no. 1 (February 1976): 65–79.

Wald, Carol. *Myth America: Picturing Women, 1865–1945.* New York: Pantheon, 1975.

Walker, Alexander. *The Celluloid Sacrifice: Aspects of Sex in the Movies.* London: Joseph, 1966.

Walsh, Mary Roth. *"Doctors Wanted; No Women Need Apply": Sexual Barriers in the Medical Profession, 1835–1975.* New Haven, CT: Yale University Press, 1977.

Walters, Ronald, ed. *Primers for Prudery: Sexual Advice to Victorian America.* Englewood Cliffs, NJ: Prentice-Hall, 1974.

"War Letters of an American Woman." *Outlook* 113 (Aug 20, 1916): 794–99.

Warner, W. Lloyd. *American Life: Dream and Reality.* Chicago: University of Chicago Press, 1953.

Warshow, Robert. *The Immediate Experience: Movies, Comics, Theatre and Other Aspects of Popular Culture.* Garden City, NY: Doubleday, 1962.

Wasserstrom, William. *Heiress of All the Ages: Sex and Sentiment in the Genteel Tradition.* Minneapolis, MN: University of Minnesota Press, 1959.

Waters, Harry. "Life According to TV." *Newsweek* 100 (Dec. 6, 1982): 136–140.

Watkins, P.R. "Perceived Information Structure: Implications for Decision Support System Design." *Decision Sciences* 13 (January 1982): 38–59.

Weibel, Kathryn. *Mirror Mirror: Images of Women Reflected in Popular Culture.* Garden City, NY: Anchor, 1977.

Weigel, R.H., and Howes, P.W. "Race Relations on Children's Television." *Journal of Psychology* 3 (May 1982): 109–12.

Weigel, R.H., and Loomis, J.W. "Televised Models of Female Achievement Revisited: Some Progress." *Journal of Applied Social Psychology* 11 (January/February 1981): 58–63.

Wein, Roberta. "Women's Colleges and Domesticity, 1875–1918." *History of Education Quarterly* 14 (Spring 1974): 31–48.

Welch, R.L.; Huston-Stein, A.; Wright, J.C.; and Plehal, R. "Subtle Sex-Role Cues on Children's Commercials." *Journal of Communication* 29, no. 3 (Summer 1979): 202–9.

Wells, Robert V. "Demographic Change and the Life Cycle of American Families." *Journal of Interdisciplinary History* 2 (Autumn 1971): 273–82.

Welter, Barbara. "The Cult of True Womanhood: 1820–1860." *American Quarterly* 18 (Summer 1966): 151–74.

Welter, Barbara, ed. *Dimity Convictions: The American Woman in the Nineteenth Century.* Columbus: Ohio University Press, 1975.

Werner, A. "The Effects of Television on Children and Adolescents: A Case of Sex and Class Socialization." *Journal of Communication* 25, no. 4 (1975): 45–50.

Wertheimer, Barbara. *We Were There: The Story of Working Women in America.* New York: Praeger, 1975.

Wertz, Richard W., and Wertz, Dorothy C. *Lying-In: A History of Childbirth in America.* New York: Free Press, 1977.

Wexler, Marvin, and Levy, Gilbert. "Women on Television: Fairness and the 'Fair Sex.'" *Yale Review of Law and Social Action* 2 (Winter 1971): 59–68.

"What Factors Affect Patients' Opinions of Their Nursing Care." *Hospitals* 31 (November, 1957): 61–64.

Wheelock, A. "The Tarnished Image." *Nursing Outlook* 24, (August 1976): 509.

Whipple, T.W., and Courtney, A.E. "How to Portray Women in TV Commercials." *Journal of Advertising Research* 20, no. 2 (1980): 53–60.

White, Cynthia. *Women's Magazines: 1693–1968.* London: Michael Joseph, 1970.

White, Llewellyn. *The American Radio.* Chicago: University of Chicago Press, 1947.

"The White Parade." *Trained Nurse and Hospital Review* 93 (June 1934): 563–65.

"Who Has Heard the Nightingale?" *Ladies' Home Journal* 65 (May 1948): 11.

"Who's Running America." *U.S. News & World Report* 92 (May 10, 1982): 34–45.

Wilk, Max. *The Golden Age of Television: Notes from the Survivors.* New York: Delacorte, 1976.

Willey, G. "The Soap Operas and the War." *Journal of Broadcasting* 7 (Fall 1963): 339–52.

Williams, C.T. "It's Not So Much 'You've Come a Long Way, Baby,' as 'You're Gonna Make It After All.'" *Journal of Popular Culture* 7 (Spring 1974): 981–89.

Wimmer, Roger D., and Dominick, Joseph R. *Mass Media Research: An Introduction.* Belmont, CA: Wadsworth, 1983.

Winick, C., and Winick, M.P. "Courtroom Drama on Television." *Journal of Communication* 24 (Winter 1974): 67–73.

Winick, M.P., and Winick, C. *The Television Experience: What Children See.* Beverly Hills, CA: Sage, 1979.

Winn, M. *The Plug-in Drug.* New York: Viking, 1979.

Withey, Stephen B., ed. *Television and Social Behavior: Beyond Violence and Children.* Hillsdale, NJ: Lawrence Erlbaum Associates, 1980.

Wolf, M.A.; Hexamer, A.; and Meyer, T.P. "Research on Children and Television: A Review of 1980." In *Communication Yearbook 5,* edited by M. Burgoon. New Brunswick, NJ: Transaction, 1982.

Wolff, Ilse S. "As Others See Us." *Nursing Outlook* 2 (August 1954): 408–12.

Wolfenstein, Martha, and Leites, Nathan. *Movies: A Psychological Study.* Glencoe, IL: Free Press, 1950.

Woodham-Smith, Cecil. *Florence Nightingale: 1820–1910.* London: Constable, 1950.

Woolley, A. "Nursing's Image on Campus." *Nursing Outlook* 29 (August 1981): 460–66.

Wright, Carroll D. *A Report on Marriage and Divorce in the U.S., 1867–1886.* Washington, DC: U.S. Government Printing Office, 1897.

Wright, Charles. *Mass Communication: A Sociological Perspective.* New York: Random House, 1959.

Wright, James D. "Are Working Women Really More Satisfied? Evidence from Several National Surveys." *Journal of Marriage and the Family* 40 (May 1978): 301–13.

Yellis, Kenneth A. "Prosperity's Child: Some Thoughts on the Flapper." *American Quarterly* 21 (Spring 1969): 44–64.

Zaltman, G. "Knowledge Utilization as Planned Social Change." *Knowledge: Creation, Diffusion, Utilization* 1 (Spring 1979): 82–105.

Zukin, Cliff, and Synder, Robin. "Passive Learning: When the Media Environment Is the Message." *Public Opinion Quarterly* 48, no. 3 (Autumn 1984): 629–38.

NOVELS

In this section of the bibliography, paperback books are identified at the end of the citation by (P).

Abbott, Eleanor Hallowell. *The White Linen Nurse.* New York: Century, 1913. 276 pp.

Abraham, J. Johnston. *The Night Nurse.* New York: E. P. Dutton, 1914. 311 pp.

Ackworth, Robert. *Dr. Kildare.* New York: Lancer, 1962. 159 pp. (P)

Ackworth, Robert. *Dr. Kildare Assigned to Trouble.* Racine, WI: Whitman, 1963. 212 pp.

Ackworth, Robert. *Dr. Kildare: The Magic Key.* Racine, WI: Whitman, 1964. 210 pp.

Ackworth, Robert. *Mary Winters, Student Nurse.* New York: Prestige, 1966. 205 pp. (P)

Ackworth, Robert. *North Country Nurse.* New York: Dell, 1965. 157 pp. (P)

Adams, Alice Boyd. *Families and Survivors.* New York: Knopf, 1974. 381 pp.

Adams, Tracy. *Spotlight on Nurse Thorne.* New York: Ace, 1962. 127 pp. (P)

Adams, Tracy. *Washington Nurse.* New York: Avon, 1963. 128 pp. (P)

Adlon, Arthur. *Private Nurse.* New York: Universal, 1964. 155 pp. (P)

Airlie, Catherine. *Doctor Overboard.* New York: Harlequin, 1966. 191 pp. (P)

Alan, Jane. *Doctor Jonathan.* New York: Harlequin, 1965. 191 pp. (P)

Alden, Sue. *Nurse of St. John.* New York: Avalon, 1958. 217 pp.

Alexander, Jean. *Nurse in South America.* New York: Prestige, 1968. 223 pp. (P)

Allen, Grant. *Hilda Wade: A Woman with Tenacity of Purpose.* Completed by Sir Arthur Conan Doyle. New York: Putnam's, 1900. 653 pp.

Ames, Jennifer. *Dr. Brad's Nurse.* New York: Prestige, 1968. 255 pp. (P)

Ames, Jennifer. *Nurse's Holiday.* New York: Beagle, 1965. 159 pp. (P)

Ames, Jennifer. *Overseas Nurse.* New York: Ace, 1951. 159 pp. (P)

Anderson, Betty Baxter. *Ann Porter Nurse.* New York: Cupples and Leon, 1924. 246 pp.

Anderson, Peggy. *Nurse.* New York: Berkley, 1978. 344 pp. (P)

Andrews, Jane. *Problem at St. Peter's.* London: Mills & Boon, 1982. 156 pp. (P)

Andrews, Lucilla. *Nurse Errant.* New York: Lenox Hill, 1975. 216 pp.

Andrews, Lucille. *The Secret Armour.* London: Corgi, 1955. 158 pp. (P)

Angellotti, Marion. *The Firefly of France.* New York: Century, 1918. 363 pp.

Arbor, Jane. *Flower of the Nettle.* New York: Harlequin, 1959. 157 pp. (P)

Arbor, Jane. *Nurse Atholl Returns.* New York: Harlequin, 1952. 190 pp. (P)

Armstrong, Juliet. *Nurse at Saint Monique.* London: Mills & Boon, 1966. 192 pp. (P)

Ash, Pauline. *Doctor Napier's Nurse.* New York: Harlequin, 1967. 188 pp. (P)

Ash, Pauline. *The Much-Loved Nurse.* New York: Harlequin, 1967. 188 pp. (P)

Ash, Pauline. *Student Nurse at Swale.* New York: Harlequin, 1966. 190 pp. (P)

Ash, Pauline. *With Love from Dr. Lucien.* New York: Harlequin, 1966. 191 pp. (P)

Avallone, Michael. *The Doctors.* New York: Ace, 1970. 143 pp. (P)

Avallone, Michael. *Sinners in White.* New York: Tower, 1962. 190 pp. (P)

Bailey, Temple. *The Pink Camellia.* New York: Dell, 1952. 240 pp. (P)

Baldwin, Faith. *Breath of Life.* New York: P. F. Collier, 1941. 282 pp.

Baldwin, Faith. *District Nurse.* New York: Grossett and Dunlap, 1932. 310 pp.

Baldwin, Faith. *He Married a Doctor.* New York: Triangle, 1943. 236 pp.

Baldwin, Faith. *Medical Center.* New York: Triangle, 1939. 369 pp.

Baldwin, Faith. *Private Duty.* New York: Triangle, 1935. 338 pp.

Baldwin, Faith. *The Rest of My Life with You.* New York: P. F. Collier, 1942. 290 pp.

Baldwin, Faith. *The Velvet Hammer.* New York: Popular Library, 1969. 192 pp. (P)

Banfill, B. J. *Labrador Nurse.* Philadelphia: Macraw Smith, 1953. 256 pp.

Bangert, Ethel. *Nurse in Spain.* New York: Thomas Bouregy, 1974. 191 pp.

Bangert, Ethel. *Nurse of the Sacramento.* New York: Avalon, 1971. 189 pp.

Bangert, Ethel. *Nurse Suzanne's Bold Journey.* New York: Avalon, 1975. 186 pp.

Bangert, Ethel. *Nurse Under Suspicion.* New York: Avalon, 1973. 181 pp.

Bangert, Ethel. *Reservation Nurse.* New York: Valentine, 1970. 174 pp. (P)

Banks, Rosie. *Navy Nurse.* New York: Permabooks, 1960. 170 pp. (P)

Banks, Rosie. *Settlement Nurse.* New York: Pocket Books, 1959. 183 pp. (P)

Banks, Rosie. *Ship's Nurse.* New York: Pocket Books, 1962. 117 pp. (P)

Banks, Rosie. *Surgical Nurse.* New York: Pocket Books, 1959. 152 pp. (P)

Barclay, Virginia. *Crisis.* New York: New American Library, 1981. 187 pp. (P)

Barclay, Virginia. *Double Face.* New York: New American Library, 1982. 177 pp. (P)

Barclay, Virginia. *Emergency.* New York: New American Library, 1981. 184 pp. (P)

Barclay, Virginia. *High Risk.* New York: New American Library, 1981. 185 pp. (P)

Barclay, Virginia. *Life Support.* New York: New American Library, 1982. 183 pp. (P)

Barclay, Virginia. *Trauma.* New York: Signet, 1981. 185 pp. (P)

Barrie, Susan. *A Case of Heart Trouble.* New York: Harlequin, 1963. 160 pp. (P)

Barry, Iris. *Nurse Dawn's Discovery.* New York: Monarch, 1964. 127 pp. (P)

Beach, Rex. *The Net*. New York: Harper and Brothers, 1912. 333 pp.

Beauchamp, Loren. *Nurse Carolyn*. New York: Tower, 1960. 157 pp. (P)

Begner, Edith. *Surgeon's Ordeal*. New York: Lancer, 1963. 255 pp. (P)

Bellamann, Henry. *Kings Row*. New York: Simon and Schuster, 1942. 674 pp.

Benn, Matthew. *Private Practice*. New York: Berkley Medallion, 1975. 316 pp. (P)

Berg, Louis. *Prison Nurse*. New York: Bantam, 1934. 182 pp. (P)

Bird, Caroline. *Enterprising Women*. New York: New American Library, 1976. 216 pp. (P)

Blair, Joan. *Course of True Love*. New York: Harlequin, 1974. 224 pp. (P)

Blair, Marcia. *The Final Lie*. New York: Kensington, 1978. 156 pp. (P)

Blaustein, Phyllis, and Blaustein, Albert, eds. *Doctor's Choice*. New York: Wilfred Funk, 1957. 310 pp.

Bleneau, Adele. *Nurse's Story: In Which Reality Meets Romance*. New York: Bobbs-Merrill, 1915. 291 pp.

Bligh, Norman, *Wayward Nurse*. New York: Venus, 1953. 129 pp. (P)

Boltar, Russell. *M.D.* New York: Dell, 1964. 254 pp. (P)

Boltar, Russell. *The Operation*. New York: Dell, 1962. 254 pp. (P)

Bonham, Barbara. *Army Nurse*. New York: Pyramid, 1965. 125 pp. (P)

Bonham, Barbara. *Diagnosis: Love*. Derby, CT: Monarch, 1964. 123 pp. (P)

Boothe, Clare. *The Women*. New York: Random House, 1937. 90 pp. (P)

Bottome, Phyllis. *Private Worlds*. Boston: Houghton Mifflin, 1934. 342 pp.

Bowers, Mary C. *Nurse Beckie's New World*. New York: Avalon, 1982. 192 pp.

Bowers, Mary C. *Nurse Charly's New Love*. New York: Avalon, 1982. 186 pp. (P)

Bowers, Mary C. *Nurse in Australia*. New York: Avalon, 1981. 192 pp. (P)

Bowers, Mary C. *Nurse in Peru*. New York: Avalon, 1981. 197 pp. (P)

Bowers, Mary C. *Nurse Karen's Masquerade*. New York: Avalon, 1982. 186 pp. (P)

Bowman, Jeanne. *City Hospital Nurse*. New York: Arcadia House, 1967. 192 pp. (P)

Bowman, Jeanne. *Conflict for Nurse Elsa*. New York: Arcadia House, 1968. 175 pp. (P)

Bowman, Jeanne. *Doomed to Hate*. New York: Arcadia House, 1969. 192 pp. (P)

Bowman, Jeanne. *Door to Door Nurse*. New York: Lancer, 1967. 159 pp. (P)

Bowman, Jeanne. *Harmony Hospital*. New York: Arcadia House, 1967. 191 pp. (P)

Bowman, Jeanne. *Neighborhood Nurse*. New York: Arcadia House, 1968. 188 pp. (P)

Bowman, Jeanne. *Nurse à la Mode*. New York: Arcadia House, 1968. 174 pp. (P)

Bowman, Jeanne. *Nurse Betrayed*. New York: Arcadia House, 1966. 126 pp. (P)

Bowman, Jeanne. *Nurse of Polka Dot Island*. New York: Manor, 1968. 176 pp. (P)

Bowman, Jeanne. *The Nurse on Medicine Mountain*. New York: Arcadia House, 1966. 189 pp. (P)

Bowman, Jeanne. *Nurse on Pondre Island*. New York: Arcadia House, 1965. 128 pp. (P)

Bowman, Jeanne. *Nurse's Heritage*. New York: Lancer, 1965. 192 pp. (P)

Bowman, Jeanne. *Ready to Love*. New York: Tower, 1965. 141 pp. (P)

Bowman, Jeanne. *Shoreline Nurse*. New York: Pyramid, 1971. 158 pp. (P)

Bowman, Jeanne. *Trust in Love*. New York: Arcadia House, 1966. 125 pp. (P)

Boylan, Rowena. *Medic in Love*. New York: Ace, 1962. 128 pp. (P)

Boylston, Helen Dore. *Clara Barton*. New York: Scholastic, 1966. 154 pp. (P)

Boylston, Helen Dore. *Sue Barton: Neighborhood Nurse*. Boston: Little, Brown, 1949. 236 pp.

Boylston, Helen Dore. *Sue Barton: Rural Nurse*. Boston: Little, Brown, 1939. 254 pp.

Boylston, Helen Dore. *Sue Barton: Senior Nurse*. Boston: Pocket Books, 1950. 226 pp. (P)

Boylston, Helen Dore. *Sue Barton: Staff Nurse*. Boston: Little, Brown, 1952. 204 pp.

Boylston, Helen Dore. *Sue Barton: Student Nurse*. New York: Comet, 1947. 160 pp. (P)

Boylston, Helen Dore. *Sue Barton: Superintendent of Nurses*. Boston: Little, Brown, 1949. 239 pp. (P)

Boylston, Helen Dore. *Sue Barton: Visiting Nurse*. New York: Popular Library, 1966. 173 pp. (P)

Brand, Max. *Calling Dr. Kildare*. New York: Dell, 1939. 159 pp. (P)

Brand, Max. *Dr. Kildare's Crisis*. New York: Dell, 1940. 160 pp. (P)

Brand, Max. *Dr. Kildare Takes Charge*. New York: Dell, 1962. 159 pp. (P)

Brand, Max. *Dr. Kildare's Trial*. New York: Dell, 1962. 160 pp. (P)

Brand, Max. *The Secret of Dr. Kildare*. New York: Dell, 1962. 160 pp. (P)

Brand, Max. *Young Dr. Kildare*. New York: Avon, 1938. 126 pp. (P)

Brennan, Alice. *Hollywood Nurse*. New York: Avon, 1966. 143 pp. (P)

Brennan, Alice. *Mary Adams, Student Nurse*. Derby, CT: Monarch, 1964. 128 pp. (P)

Brennan, Alice. *Nurse Keane's Affair*. New York: Belmont, 1963. 141 pp. (P)

Brennan, Alice. *Nurse's Dormitory*. New York: Lancer, 1962. 128 pp. (P)

Brennan, Alice. *Visiting Nurse*. New York: Berkley, 1962. 127 pp. (P)

Brenner, Dorothy. *Nurse at Playland Park*. New York: Avalon, 1976. 232 pp. (P)

Brenner, Dorothy. *Nurse in the Caribbean*. New York: Avalon, 1974. 192 pp.

Brinkley, William. *Don't Go Near the Water*. New York: Random House, 1956. 373 pp.

Brock, Stuart. *Bring Back Her Body*. New York: Ace, 1953. 142 pp. (P)

Bromfield, Louis. *The Rains Came*. New York: Harper and Brothers, 1937. 597 pp.

Brown, Marion Marsh. *Nurse Abroad*. New York: Avalon, 1963, 261 pp.

Bryan, Michael. *Intent to Kill*. New York: Dell, 1956. 191 pp. (P)

Buckingham, Callie. *Nurse at Orchard Hill*. New York: Avalon, 1978, 222 pp.

Burchell, Mary. *Hospital Corridors*. New York: Harlequin, 1958. 192 pp. (P)

Burchell, Mary. *Loyal in All*. New York: Harlequin, 1957. 192 pp. (P)

Burchell, Mary. *Surgeon of Distinction*. New York: Harlequin, 1959. 191 pp. (P)

Burnett, Ruth. *Nurse and the Talisman*. New York: Avalon, 1974. 192 pp.

Burnett, Ruth. *Nurse of Mount Juliet*. New York: Avalon, 1975. 192 pp.

Bush, Christine. *Nurse at Deer Hollow*. New York: Airmont, 1977. 186 pp. (P)

Cabot, Isabel. *Come Summer, Come Love*. New York: Airmont, 1977. 186 pp. (P)

Cabot, Isabel. *The Lost Inheritance*. New York: Dell, 1971. 187 pp. (P)

Cabot, Isabel. *Nurse at Sea Lair*. New York: Avalon, 1975. 186 pp.

Cabot, Isabel. *Nurse Audrey's Mission*. New York: Dell, 1969. 155 pp. (P)

Cabot, Isabel. *Nurse Craig*. New York: Ace, 1957. 128 pp. (P)

Cabot, Isabel. *Nurse Janice Calling*. New York: Avalon, 1964. 191 pp.

Cabot, Isabel. *Private Duty Nurse*. New York: Bantam, 1958. 121 pp. (P)

Caine, Hall. *The Christian*. New York: D. Appleton, 1897. 540 pp.

Caine, Mitchell. *Creole Surgeon.* New York: Fawcett, 1977. 446 pp. (P)

Capeto, Isabel. *Nurse in Doubt.* New York: Arcadia House, 1968. 189 pp. (P)

Cardwell, Ann. *Crazy to Kill.* New York: Arcadia House, 1941. 144 pp. (P)

Carew, Jean. *Doctor Lochinvar.* New York: Arcadia House, 1969. 176 pp. (P)

Carew, Jean. *Nurse's Masquerade.* New York: Pyramid, 1964. 126 pp. (P)

Carew, Jean. *Run, Nurse, Run.* New York: Pyramid, 1965. 126 pp. (P)

Carr, Patti. *A Nurse to Marry.* New York: Arcadia House, 1967. 160 pp. (P)

Carr, Patti. *Pam Green: Rehabilitation Nurse.* New York: Signet, 1966. 128 pp. (P)

Carr, Patti. *TV Nurse.* New York: New American Library, 1965. 126 pp. (P)

Carr, William H. A. *Medical Examiner.* New York: Prestige, 1963. 143 pp. (P)

Cassiday, Bruce. *General Hospital: In the Name of Love.* New York: Award, 1974. 155 pp. (P)

Cassiday, Bruce. *General Hospital: Surgeon's Crisis.* New York: Award, 1972. 157 pp. (P)

Cassiday, Bruce. *Marcus Welby, M.D.: The Acid Test.* New York: Ace, 1970. 189 pp. (P)

Cassiday, Bruce. *Marcus Welby, M.D.: The Fire's Center.* New York: Ace, 1971. 187 pp. (P)

Cassiday, Bruce. *Marcus Welby, M.D.: Rock a Cradle Empty.* New York: Ace, 1970. 189 pp. (P)

Cassill, R. V. *Nurses' Quarters.* New York: Fawcett, 1961. 176 pp. (P)

Castle, Helen B. *Emergency Ward Nurse.* New York: Paperback Library, 1963. 127 pp. (P)

Chace, Isobel. *The Flamboyant Tree.* New York: Harlequin, 1973. 192 pp. (P)

Chace, Isobel. *Home Is Goodbye.* New York: Harlequin, 1971. 192 pp. (P)

Chace, Isobel. *The Hospital of Fatima.* New York: Harlequin, 1963. 189 pp. (P)

Chambers, Helene. *Nurse in Research.* New York: Avalon, 1974. 192 pp.

Christie, Agatha. *Murder on the Orient Express.* New York: Dodd, Mead, 1933. 213 pp.

Christopher, Louis. *Robin West: Nurse's Aide.* New York: Dell, 1963. 119 pp. (P)

Claire, Marvin. *The Drowning Wire.* New York: Ace, 1953, 156 pp. (P)

Cleary, Jon. *Back of Sunset.* New York: Fawcett, 1959. 224 pp. (P)

Cleaver, Vera. *The Nurse's Dilemma.* New York: Pyramid, 1966. 141 pp. (P)

Clemence, Ruth. *A Cure with Kindness.* New York: Harlequin, 1970. 188 pp. (P)

Cole, Dorothy. *Country Club Nurse.* New York: Arcadia House, 1967. 192 pp. (P)

Cole, Dorothy. *Nurse at the Fair.* New York: Lenox Hill, 1971. 172 pp. (P)

Coleman, Mitchell. *Ward Nurse.* New York: Publication House, 1957. 130 pp. (P)

Collins, Lynne. *Doctor in Pursuit.* London: Mills and Boon, 1982. 188 pp. (P)

Connor, Ralph. *The Doctor.* Old Tappan, NJ: Fleming H. Revell, 1906. 399 pp.

Connor, Ralph. *The Sky Pilot in No Man's Land.* New York: George H. Doran, 1919. 349 pp.

Converse, Jane. *Accused Nurse.* New York: New American Library, 1974. 128 pp. (P)

Converse, Jane. *Alias Miss Saunders, R.N.* New York: New American Library, 1962. 127 pp. (P)

Converse, Jane. *Art Colony Nurse.* New York: New American Library, 1969. 175 pp. (P)

Converse, Jane. *Backstage Nurse.* New York: New American Library, 1969. 144 pp. (P)

Converse, Jane. *Beth Lloyd, Surgical Nurse.* New York: New American Library, 1970. 128 pp. (P)

Converse, Jane. *Cinderella Nurse.* New York: New American Library, 1967. 128 pp. (P)

Converse, Jane. *Condemned Nurse.* New York: New American Library, 1971. 126 pp. (P)

Converse, Jane. *Crusading Nurse.* New York: New American Library, 1968. 128 pp. (P)

Converse, Jane. *Dr. Holland's Nurse.* New York: New American Library, 1963. 128 pp. (P)

Converse, Jane. *Emergency Nurse.* New York: New American Library, 1962. 128 pp. (P)

Converse, Jane. *Expedition Nurse.* New York: New American Library, 1968. 127 pp. (P)

Converse, Jane. *Heartbreak Nurse.* New York: New American Library, 1968. 127 pp. (P)

Converse, Jane. *Hometown Nurse.* New York: New American Library, 1968. 143 pp. (P)

Converse, Jane. *Hostage Nurse.* New York: New American Library, 1973. 159 pp. (P)

Converse, Jane. *Ice Show Nurse.* New York: New American Library, 1970. 128 pp. (P)

Converse, Jane. *Jet Set Nurse.* New York: New American Library, 1970. 128 pp. (P)

Converse, Jane. *Masquerade Nurse.* New York: New American Library, 1963. 126 pp. (P)

Converse, Jane. *Nurse Against the Town.* New York: New American Library, 1966. 126 pp. (P)

Converse, Jane. *Nurse Forrester's Secret.* New York: New American Library, 1965. 191 pp. (P)

Converse, Jane. *Nurse in Acapulco.* New York: New American Library, 1964. 126 pp. (P)

Converse, Jane. *Nurse in Charge.* New York: New American Library, 1969. 159 pp. (P)

Converse, Jane. *Nurse in Crisis.* New York: New American Library, 1966. 128 pp. (P)

Converse, Jane. *Nurse in Danger.* New York: New American Library, 1962. 128 pp. (P)

Converse, Jane. *Nurse in Hollywood.* New York: New American Library, 1965. 128 pp. (P)

Converse, Jane. *Nurse in Las Vegas.* New York: New American Library, 1975. 144 pp. (P)

Converse, Jane. *Nurse in London.* New York: New American Library, 1970. 176 pp. (P)

Converse, Jane. *Nurse in Panic.* New York: New American Library, 1971. 128 pp. (P)

Converse, Jane. *Nurse in Rome.* New York: New American Library, 1967. 128 pp. (P)

Converse, Jane. *Nurse in Turmoil.* New York: New American Library, 1974. 128 pp. (P)

Converse, Jane. *Nurse on the Riviera.* New York: New American Library, 1968. 127 pp. (P)

Converse, Jane. *Nurse on Trial.* New York: New American Library, 1966. 128 pp. (P)

Converse, Jane. *Obstetrical Nurse.* New York: New American Library, 1972. 175 pp. (P)

Converse, Jane. *The Party Nurses.* New York: New American Library, 1974. 143 pp. (P)

Converse, Jane. *Penthouse Nurse.* New York: New American Library, 1974. 127 pp. (P)

Converse, Jane. *Pleasure Cruise Nurse.* New York: New American Library, 1966. 126 pp. (P)

Converse, Jane. *Psychiatric Nurse.* New York: New American Library, 1963. 127 pp. (P)

Converse, Jane. *Recruiting Nurse.* New York: New American Library, 1968. 128 pp. (P)

Converse, Jane. *Second-Chance Nurse.* New York: New American Library, 1961. 143 pp. (P)

Converse, Jane. *Settlement-House Nurse.* New York: New American Library, 1965. 126 pp. (P)

Converse, Jane. *Society Nurse.* New York: New American Library, 1975. 154 pp. (P)

Converse, Jane. *Surf Safari Nurse.* New York: New American Library, 1966. 127 pp. (P)

Converse, Jane. *Terry Allen, Nurse in Love.* New York: New American Library, 1970. 126 pp. (P)

Converse, Jane. *Undercover Nurse.* New York: New American Library, 1972. 173 pp. (P)

Converse, Jane. *Winter Resort Nurse.* New York: New American Library, 1973. 175 pp. (P)

Converse, Jane. *The Young Nurses.* New York: New American Library, 1969. 128 pp. (P)

Conway, Celine. *White Doctor.* New York: Harlequin, 1957. 222 pp. (P)

Cook, Robin. *Coma.* New York: New American Library, 1977. 308 pp. (P)

Cook, Robin. *Year of the Intern.* New York: New American Library/Signet, 1972. 210 pp. (P)

Corby, Jane. *Nurse Liza Hale.* New York: Modern Promotions, 1965. 126 pp. (P)

Corby, Jane. *Nurse of Greenmeadow.* New York: Modern Promotions, 1964. 143 pp. (P)

Corby, Jane. *Nurse's Alibi.* New York: Arcadia House, 1966. 190 pp. (P)

Corby, Jane. *Nurse's Choice.* New York: Arcadia House, 1965. 126 pp. (P)

Corby, Jane. *Nurse with the Red-Gold Hair.* New York: Macfadden, 1964. 128 pp. (P)

Corby, Jane. *Staff Nurse.* New York: Dell, 1962. 156 pp. (P)

Corby, Jane. *Traveling Nurse.* New York: Arcadia House, 1964. 223 pp. (P)

Cosgrove, Rachel. *The Candystripers.* New York: Dell, 1964, 156 pp. (P)

Cotler, Gordon. *The Bottletop Affair.* New York: Paperback Library, 1968. 176 pp. (P)

Covert, Alice Lent. *Woman Doctor.* New York: Popular Library, 1952. 128 pp. (P)

Cozzens, James Gould. *The Last Adam.* New York: Harcourt, Brace, 1933. 301 pp.

Craig, Dolores. *Scalpel of Honor.* New York: Lancer, 1969. 189 pp. (P)

Craig, Georgia. *Grass Roots Nurse.* New York: Arcadia House, 1958. 224 pp.

Craig, Georgia. *Nurse at Guale Farms.* New York: Arcadia House, 1964. 128 pp. (P)

Craig, Georgia. *A Nurse Comes Home.* New York: Arcadia House, 1963. 219 pp.

Craig, Georgia. *Nurse Lucie.* New York: Macfadden, 1964. 128 pp. (P)

Craig, Georgia. *Nurse with Wings.* New York: Avon, 1945. 128 pp. (P)

Craig, Georgia. *Reach for Tomorrow.* New York: Avon, 1960. 128 pp. (P)

Craig, Georgia. *Society Nurse.* New York: Arcadia House, 1962. 128 pp. (P)

Craig, Vera. *Glen Hall.* New York: Dell, 1970. 151 pp. (P)

Craig, Vera. *Land of Enchantment.* New York: Dell, 1969. 192 pp.

Craig, Vera. *The Love Barrier.* New York: Dell, 1970. 192 pp. (P)

Craig, Vera. *Now and Forever.* New York: Dell, 1969. 191 pp. (P)

Craig, Vera. *Path of Peril.* New York: Dell, 1969. 191 pp. (P)

Crawford, F. Marion. *The White Sister.* New York: Macmillan, 1909. 335 pp.

Creese, Bethea. *Glorious Haven.* New York: Harlequin, 1958. 191 pp. (P)

Cronin, A. J. *Shannon's Way.* New York: Bantam, 1956. 312 pp. (P)

Cronin, A. J. *The Citadel.* Boston: Little, Brown, 1937. 401 pp.

Cullen, Carter. *The Deadly Chase.* New York: Fawcett, 1957. 144 pp. (P)

Curtiss, Ursula. *Danger: Hospital Zone.* New York: Dodd, Mead, 1966. 184 pp.

Dale, Nancy. *Army Nurse.* Racine, WI: Whitman, 1944. 248 pp.

Dana, Rose. *Arctic Nurse.* New York: Modern Promotions, 1966. 127 pp. (P)

Dana, Rose. *Bermuda Nurse.* New York: Macfadden-Bartell, 1965. 128 pp. (P)

Dana, Rose. *Construction Camp Nurse.* New York: Arcadia House, 1968. 176 pp. (P)

Dana, Rose. *Cruise Ship Nurse.* New York: Arcadia House, 1969. 192 pp.

Dana, Rose. *Department Store Nurse.* New York: Lenox Hill, 1970. 192 pp.

Dana, Rose. *Down East Nurse.* New York: Macfadden-Bartell, 1968. 128 pp. (P)

Dana, Rose. *Homecoming Nurse.* New York: Lancer, 1968. 205 pp.

Dana, Rose. *Labrador Nurse.* New York: Arcadia House, 1968. 192 pp.

Dana, Rose. *Network Nurse.* New York: Magnum, 1968. 160 pp. (P)

Dana, Rose. *Night Club Nurse.* New York: Macfadden-Bartell, 1967. 127 pp. (P)

Dana, Rose. *Nurse Freda.* New York: Macfadden-Bartell, 1950. 126 pp. (P)

Dana, Rose. *Nurse in Danger.* New York: Belmont Productions, 1967. 73 pp. (P)

Dana, Rose. *Nurse in Jeopardy.* New York: Macfadden-Bartell, 1968. 128 pp. (P)

Dana, Rose. *Operating Room Nurse.* New York: Macfadden-Bartell, 1965. 128 pp. (P)

Dana, Rose. *Resort Nurse.* New York: Lancer, 1969. 189 pp. (P)

Daniels, Dorothy. *Cruise Ship Nurse.* New York: Paperback Library, 1963. 128 pp. (P)

Daniels, Dorothy. *Island Nurse.* New York: Paperback Library, 1964. 128 pp. (P)

Daniels, Dorothy. *Nurse at Danger Mansion.* New York: Paperback Library, 1971. (P)

Daniels, Dorothy. *World's Fair Nurse.* New York: Paperback Library, 1964. 128 pp. (P)

Daniels, Norman. *County Hospital.* New York: Fawcett, 1963. 143 pp. (P)

Daniels, Norman. *Dr. Kildare's Finest Hour.* New York: Lancer, 1963. 143 pp. (P)

Daniels, Norman. *Dr. Kildare's Secret Romance.* New York: Lancer, 1962. 144 pp. (P)

Daniels, Norman. *Jennifer James, R.N.* New York: Fawcett, 1961. 160 pp. (P)

Daniels, Norman. *Stanton Bishop, M.D.* New York: Lancer, 1969. 192 pp. (P)

Daniels, Norman. *The Surgeon.* New York: Lancer, 1967. 174 pp. (P)

Davis, J. R. *The Right to Die.* Tower, 1976. 215 pp. (P)

Dean, Nell Marr. *Circus Nurse.* New York: Lancer, 1965. 206 pp. (P)

Dean, Nell Marr. *Flight Nurse.* New York: Julian Messner, 1963. 192 pp.

Dean, Nell Marr. *Nurse Kelly's Crusade.* New York: Dell, 1969. 185 pp. (P)

Dean, Nell Marr. *Nurse on Paradise Isle.* New York: Belmont, 1964. 156 pp. (P)

Dean, Nell Marr. *Nurse on Skis.* New York: Avalon, 1960. 221 pp.

Dean, Nell Marr. *Society Doctor.* New York: Airmont, 1961. 128 pp. (P)

Dean, Nell Marr. *A Time for Strength.* New York: Modern Promotions, 1964. 157 pp. (P)

Deiss, Jay. *The Blue Chips.* New York: Bantam, 1957. 243 pp. (P)

De Leeuw, Adele. *Doctor Ellen.* New York: Ace, 1944. 175 pp. (P)

De Leeuw, Cateau, and De Leeuw, Adele. *Nurses Who Led the Way.* Racine, WI: Whitman, 1961. 210 pp.

Deming, Dorothy. *Ginger Lee: War Nurse.* New York: Dodd, Mead, 1942. 212 pp.

Deming, Dorothy. *Hilda Baker: School Nurse.* New York: Dodd, Mead, 1955. 244 pp.

Deming, Dorothy. *Linda Kent, Student Nurse.* New York: Dodd, Mead, 1959. 274 pp.

Deming, Dorothy. *Mysterious Discovery in Ward K.* New York: Dodd, Mead, 1959. 210 pp.

Deming, Dorothy. *Nurse's Dilemma in the Private Corridor.* New York: Dodd, Mead, 1957. 213 pp.

Deming, Dorothy. *Pam Wilson, Registered Nurse.* New York: Dodd, Mead, 1946. 247 pp.

Deming, Dorothy. *Penny Marsh Finds Adventure.* New York: Dodd, Mead, 1957. 236 pp.

Deming, Dorothy. *Penny Marsh, R.N., Director of Nurses.* New York: Dodd, Mead, 1961. 247 pp.

Deming, Dorothy. *Strange Disappearance from Ward B.* New York: Dodd, Mead, 1955. 243 pp.

Deming, Dorothy. *Sue Morris, Sky Nurse.* New York: Dodd, Mead, 1960. 247 pp.

Deming, Dorothy. *Trudy Wells, R.N.: Pediatric Nurse.* New York: Dodd, Mead, 1957, 244 pp.

De Morgan, William. *Alice-for-Short.* New York: Henry Holt, 1907. 563 pp.

Denzer, Peter W. *Episode.* New York: Popular Library, 1954. 224 pp. (P)

Dern, Peggy. *Country Nurse.* New York: Macfadden-Bartell, 1956. 127 pp. (P)

Dern, Peggy. *County Doctor.* New York: Arcadia House, 1945. 198 pp.

Dern, Peggy. *County Nurse.* New York: Arcadia House, 1956. 216 pp.

Dern, Peggy. *The Doctor's Wife.* New York: Arcadia House, 1966. 190 pp. (P)

Dern, Peggy. *Florida Nurse.* New York: Arcadia House, 1961. 192 pp. (P)

Dern, Peggy. *Holiday Nurse.* New York: Arcadia House, 1963. 224 pp.

Dern, Peggy. *Leona Gregory, R.N.* New York: Arcadia House, 1961. 221 pp.

Dern, Peggy. *Nurse Angela.* New York: Arcadia House, 1965. 190 pp.

Dern, Peggy. *Nurse at Burford's Landing.* New York: Arcadia House, 1966. 128 pp. (P)

Dern, Peggy. *A Nurse Called Hope.* New York: Ace, 1963. 127 pp. (P)

Dern, Peggy. *Nurse Ellen.* New York: Macfadden, 1956. 128 pp. (P)

Dern, Peggy. *Nurse Felicity.* New York: Macfadden-Bartell, 1966. 128 pp. (P)

Dern, Peggy. *Nurse in the Tropics.* New York: Macfadden, 1963. 127 pp. (P)

Dern, Peggy. *Nurse's Dilemma.* New York: Arcadia House, 1966. 128 pp. (P)

Dern, Peggy. *Nurse with a Dream.* New York: Arcadia House, 1963. 127 pp. (P)

Dern, Peggy. *Orchids for a Nurse.* New York: Arcadia House, 1962. 144 pp. (P)

Dern, Peggy. *Understand, My Love.* New York: Arcadia House, 1966. 128 pp. (P)

Dickens, Charles. *The Life and Adventures of Martin Chuzzlewit.* Boston: Dana Estes, 1849. 1,257 pp.

Didion, Joan. *Play It as It Lays: A Novel.* New York: Farrar, Straus and Giroux, 1970. 266 pp.

Dingwell, Joyce. *Australian Hospital.* New York: Harlequin, 1960. 160 pp. (P)

Dingwell, Joyce. *Nurse Smith, Cook.* New York: Harlequin, 1968. 187 pp. (P)

Donarico, Elnora. *Nurse Jessica's Cruise.* New York: Avalon, 1980. 263 pp.

Donarico, Elnora. *Nurse Vicky's Love.* New York: Avalon, 1979. 236 pp.

Dooley, Thomas A., M.D. *Deliver Us from Evil.* New York: New American Library, 1956. 142 pp. (P)

Dorien, Ray. *The Heart of Dr. Hilary.* New York: Ace, 1962. 159 pp. (P)

Dorien, Ray. *Meet Nurse Lucinda.* New York: Ace, 1969. 158 pp. (P)

Dorien, Ray. *Noonday Nurse.* New York: Arcadia House, 1957. 192 pp. (P)

Dorien, Ray. *The Odds Against Nurse Pat.* New York: Ace, 1958. 159 pp. (P)

Dormandy, Clara. *The Doctors.* New York: Thomas Boureghy, 1959. 128 pp. (P)

Dorset, Ruth. *Behind Hospital Walls.* New York: Lenox Hill, 1970. 192 pp.

Dorset, Ruth. *Front Office Nurse.* New York: Manor, 1968. 206 pp. (P)

Dorset, Ruth. *Head Nurse.* New York: Lancer, 1970. 198 pp. (P)

Dorset, Ruth. *Nurse in Waiting.* New York: Arcadia House, 1967. 192 pp.

Dorset, Ruth. *Nurse Paula.* New York: Arcadia House, 1968. 192 pp.

Dorset, Ruth. *The Nurse Takes a Chance.* New York: Lancer, 1970. 205 pp. (P)

Dorset, Ruth. *Surgical Nurse.* New York: Arcadia House, 1970. 205 pp. (P)

Douglas, Colin. *Bleeders Come First.* New York: Taplinger, 1979. 171 pp.

Douglas, Diana. *Apollo Nurse.* New York: New American Library, 1970. 128 pp. (P)

Douglas, Diana. *Beauty Contest Nurse.* New York: New American Library, 1973. 125 pp. (P)

Douglas, Diana. *Caribbean Nurse.* New York: New American Library, 1972. 156 pp. (P)

Douglas, Diana. *Casino Nurse.* New York: New American Library, 1974. 127 pp. (P)

Douglas, Diana. *Doctor in Shadow.* New York: New American Library, 1967. 127 pp. (P)

Douglas, Diana. *Dude Ranch Nurse.* New York: New American Library, 1970. 127 pp. (P)

Douglas, Diana. *Duty Nurse.* New York: New American Library, 1968. 221 pp. (P)

Douglas, Diana. *The Fledgling Nurses.* New York: New American Library, 1971. 125 pp. (P)

Douglas, Diana. *Hockey Star Nurse.* New York: New American Library, 1972. 158 pp. (P)

Douglas, Diana. *Mystery Nurse.* New York: New American Library, 1968. 126 pp. (P)

Douglas, Diana. *New Orleans Nurse.* New York: New American Library, 1974. 157 pp. (P)

Douglas, Diana. *Nurse Chadwick's Sorrow.* New York: New American Library, 1967. 125 pp. (P)

Douglas, Diana. *Nurse Deceived.* New York: New American Library, 1973. 175 pp. (P)

Douglas, Diana. *Nurse in Spain.* New York: New American Library, 1975. 172 pp. (P)

Douglas, Diana. *Nurse Lambert's Conflict.* New York: New American Library, 1969. 125 pp. (P)

Douglas, Diana. *Nurse on Location.* New York: New American Library, 1968. 125 pp. (P)

Douglas, Diana. *Resort Nurse.* New York: New American Library, 1969. 160 pp. (P)

Douglas, Diana. *Sea Nurse.* New York: New American Library, 1970. 204 pp. (P)

Douglas, Diana. *Ski Lodge Nurse.* New York: New American Library, 1970. 207 pp. (P)

Douglas, Diana. *Surfing Nurse.* New York: New American Library, 1971. 128 pp. (P)

Douglas, Lloyd C. *Disputed Passage.* New York: P. F. Collier, 1938. 432 pp.

Douglas, Lloyd C. *Doctor Hudson's Secret Journal.* New York: P. F. Collier, 1939. 295 pp.

Douglas, Lloyd C. *Green Light.* Boston: Houghton Mifflin, 1934. 236 pp.

Douglas, Lloyd C. *Magnificent Obsession.* New York: P. F. Collier, 1929. 330 pp.

Douglas, Shane. *Air Surgeon.* New York: New American Library, 1962. 128 pp. (P)

Douglas, Shane. *Assistant Surgeon.* New York: New American Library, 1962. 128 pp. (P)

Douglas, Shane. *Doctor at Fault.* New York: New American Library, 1962. 126 pp. (P)

Douglas, Shane. *Doctor in Action.* New York: New American Library, 1966. 125 pp. (P)

Douglas, Shane. *Doctor in the Dark.* New York: New American Library, 1964. 127 pp. (P)

Douglas, Shane. *The Doctor's Past.* New York: New American Library, 1962. 127 pp. (P)

Douglas, Shane. *The Doctor's Pledge.* New York: New American Library, 1962. 127 pp. (P)

Douglas, Shane. *Emergency Surgeon.* New York: New American Library, 1962. 125 pp. (P)

Douglas, Shane. *The Mercy Heroes.* New York: New American Library, 1962. 126 pp. (P)

Douglas, Shane. *Sea Nurse.* New York: New American Library, 1970. 204 pp. (P)

Douglas, Shane. *Sky Doctor.* New York: New American Library, 1962. 125 pp. (P)

Douglas, Shane. *Surgeon on Call.* New York: New American Library, 1963. 126 pp. (P)

Douglas, Shane. *Surgeon Suspect.* New York: New American Library, 1967. 127 pp. (P)

Douglas, Sheila. *The Young Doctor.* New York: Harlequin, 1973. 190 pp. (P)

Dowd, Emma. *Polly of the Hospital Staff.* New York: Grosset and Dunlap, 1912. 290 pp.

Dowdell, Dorothy. *Arctic Nurse.* New York: Dell, 1966, 156 pp. (P)

Dowdell, Dorothy. *Border Nurse.* New York: Ace, 1963. 144 pp. (P)

Dunbar, Jean. *The Summer Nights.* New York: Harlequin, 1969. 190 pp. (P)

Dunn, Bob. *Hospital Happy.* New York: Avon, 1949. 126 pp. (P)

Dunne, Mary Collins. *Nurse of the Crystalline Valley.* New York: Avalon, 1971. 196 pp.

Dunne, Mary Collins. *Nurse of the Midnight Sun.* New York: Airmont, 1973. 192 pp. (P)

Dunne, Mary Collins. *Nurse of the Vineyards.* New York: Avalon, 1975. 246 pp.

Durham, Anne. *Mann of the Medical Wing.* New York: Harlequin, 1968. 192 pp. (P)

Durham, Anne. *Nurse Sally's Last Chance.* New York: Harlequin, 1967. 188 pp. (P)

Durham, Anne. *The Romantic Doctor Rydon.* New York: Harlequin, 1967. 190 pp. (P)

Durham, Anne. *The Youngest Night Nurse.* New York: Harlequin, 1966. 192 pp. (P)

Eberhart, Mignon G. *Eberhart's Mystery Omnibus.* New York: Grosset and Dunlap, 1929. 310 pp.

Eberhart, Mignon G. *From this Dark Stairway.* New York: Doubleday, 1931. 312 pp.

Eberhart, Mignon G. *Man Missing.* New York: Random House, 1953. 189 pp.

Eberhart, Mignon G. *Murder by an Aristocrat.* New York: Doubleday, 1932. 310 pp.

Eberhart, Mignon G. *The Mystery of Hunting's End.* New York: Doubleday, 1930. 341 pp.

Eberhart, Mignon G. *While the Patient Slept.* New York: Doubleday, 1930. 224 pp.

Eberhart, Mignon G. *Wolf in Man's Clothing.* New York: Random House, 1942. 221 pp.

Edwards, Monica. *Airport Nurse.* New York: Ace, 1964, 127 pp. (P)

Elias, Michael, and Eustis, Rich. *Young Doctors in Love.* New York: Avon, 1982. 172 pp. (P)

Elliott, Ellen. *High Flight Nurse.* New York: Arcadia House, 1968. 192 pp.

Elliott, Ellen. *Hong Kong Nurse.* New York: Dell, 1968. 141 pp. (P)

Ellis, Louise. *Nurse Sandra's Second Summer.* New York: Harlequin, 1969. 188 pp. (P)

Ellis, Louise. *Three Nurses.* New York: Harlequin, 1968. 192 pp. (P)

Elting, Mary. *Nurses.* New York: Scholastic, 1963. 64 pp. (P)

Emerson, Alice B. *Ruth Fielding at the War Front.* New York: Cupples and Leon, 1918. 204 pp.

Emerson, Alice B. *Ruth Fielding in the Red Cross.* New York: Cupples and Leon, 1918. 204 pp.

Erskine, Sylvia. *Nurses' Quarters.* New York: Detective House, 1953. 128 pp. (P)

Everett, Gail. *Journey for a Nurse.* New York: Ace, 1966. 127 pp. (P)

Felson, Henry Gregor. *Davey Logan, Interne.* New York: Berkley Medallion, 1965. 127 pp. (P)

Fenn, George Manville. *Nurse Elisia.* New York: Cassell, 1894. 364 pp.

Ferrari, Ivy. *Nurse Kate at Fallowfield.* New York: Harlequin, 1967. 189 pp. (P)

Ferrari, Ivy. *Surgery in the Hills.* New York: Harlequin, 1966. 192 pp. (P)

Field, Della. *Vietnam Nurse.* New York: Avon, 1966. 126 pp. (P)

Finley, Glenna. *Nurse Pro Tem.* New York: Dell, 1967. 156 pp. (P)

Fitzgerald, Arlene J. *Daredevil Nurse.* New York: Pyramid, 1964. 125 pp. (P)

Fitzgerald, Arlene J. *Double Duty Nurse.* New York: Belmont, 1968. 157 pp. (P)

Fitzgerald, Arlene J. *Log Camp Nurse.* New York: Avon, 1966. 160 pp. (P)

Fitzgerald, Arlene J. *Northwest Nurse.* New York: Ace, 1964. 144 pp. (P)

Fitzgerald, Arlene J. *Volunteer Nurse.* New York: Avon, 1967. 128 pp. (P)

Fitzgerald, Arlene J. *Young Nurse Rayburn.* New York: Pyramid, 1964. 144 pp. (P)

Fletcher, Dorothy. *House of Hate.* New York: Arcadia House, 1967, 123 pp. (P)

Fletcher, Dorothy. *New Yorker Nurse.* New York: Ace, 1969. 126 pp. (P)

Fletcher, Mary Mann. *Danger—Nurse at Work.* New York: Ace, 1966. 127 pp. (P)

Fletcher, Mary Mann. *Girl Intern.* New York: Lancer, 1970. 191 pp. (P)

Fletcher, Mary Mann. *Nurse Julie.* New York: Dell, 1967. 156 pp. (P)

Fletcher, Mary Mann. *Psychiatric Nurse.* New York: Ace, 1962. 127 pp. (P)

Ford, Marcia. *Dixie Doctor.* New York: Monarch, 1955. 142 pp. (P)

Ford, Marcia. *Flying Nurse.* New York: Avalon, 1971. 192 pp.

Ford, Marcia. *Island Nurse.* New York: Monarch, 1959. 142 pp. (P)

Ford, Marcia. *Nancy Craig, R.N.* New York: Harlequin, 1956. 152 pp. (P)

Ford, Marcia. *Nurse Craig.* New York: Berkley Medallion, 1953. 127 pp. (P)

Ford, Norrey. *Nurse with a Dream.* New York: Harlequin, 1959. 189 pp. (P)

Fox, Paula. *Desperate Characters.* New York: Harcourt, Brace and World, 1970.

Francis, Dorothy Brenner. *Nurse of Spirit Lake.* New York: Avalon, 1975. 192 pp.

Francis, Dorothy Brenner. *Nurse of the Keys.* New York: Avalon, 1974. 192 pp.

Francis, Dorothy Brenner. *Nurse on Assignment.* New York: Avalon, 1973. 196 pp.

Francis, Dorothy Brenner. *Nurse Under Fire.* New York: Avalon, 1973. 192 pp.

Francis, Jean. *The Doctor in Ward B.* New York: Prestige, 1969. 192 pp.

Francis, William. *Kill or Cure.* New York: Green, 1942. 128 pp. (P)

Franklin, Frieda K. *Combat Nurse.* New York: Pocket Books, 1955. 230 pp. (P)

Franklin, Irwin R. *Flight.* New York: Grosset and Dunlap, 1929. 245 pp.

Frazer, Diane. *An American Nurse in London.* New York: Pocket Books, 1968. 160 pp. (P)

Frazer, Diane. *An American Nurse in Paris*. New York: Pocket Books, 1963. 138 pp. (P)

Frazer, Diane. *An American Nurse in Vienna*. New York: Pocket Books, 1966. 174 pp. (P)

Frazer, Diane. *Confidential Nurse*. New York: Pocket Books, 1962. 150 pp. (P)

Frazer, Diane. *The Dilemma of Geraldine Addams*. New York: Pocket Books, 1965. 157 pp. (P)

Frazer, Diane. *First Year Nurse*. New York: Pocket Books, 1964. 158 pp. (P)

Frazer, Diane. *I, Theresa, Registered Nurse*. New York: Pocket Books, 1965. 156 pp. (P)

Frazer, Diane. *Nurse Lily and Mister X*. New York: Permabooks, 1961. 153 pp. (P)

Frazer, Diane. *Nurse Turner Runs Away*. New York: Permabooks, 1962. 151 pp. (P)

Frazer, Diane. *Nurse with a Past*. New York: Pocket Books, 1964. 138 pp. (P)

Frazer, Diane. *A Special Case for Peggy Bruce, R.N.* New York: Pocket Books, 1963. 152 pp. (P)

Frazer, Diane. *Starring Suzanne Carteret, R.N.* New York: Pocket Books, 1966. 156 pp. (P)

Frede, Richard. *The Interns*. New York: Bantam, 1960. 341 pp. (P)

Fredericks, Vic. *More for Doctors Only*. New York: Pocket Books, 1961. 164 pp. (P)

Freeman, Jean Todd. *Diagnosis Positive*. New York: Pocket Books, 1971. 298 pp. (P)

Fullbrook, Gladys. *Bush Hospital*. New York: Harlequin, 1968. 187 pp. (P)

Fullbrook, Gladys. *Hospital in the Tropics*. New York: Harlequin, 1966. 159 pp. (P)

Fullbrook, Gladys. *Nurse Prue in Ceylon*. New York: Harlequin, 1963. 190 pp. (P)

Fullbrook, Gladys. *Nurses of the Tourist Service*. New York: Harlequin, 1962. 191 pp. (P)

Furman, A. L. *Private Practice*. New York: Caxton House, 1939. 251 pp.

Gaddis, Peggy. *Bayou Nurse*. New York: Macfadden-Bartell, 1964. 128 pp. (P)

Gaddis, Peggy. *Betsy Moran, R.N.* New York: Macfadden-Bartell, 1964. 128 pp. (P)

Gaddis, Peggy. *Big City Nurse*. New York: Modern Promotions, 1956. 128 pp. (P)

Gaddis, Peggy. *Cadet Nurse*. New York: Arcadia House, 1945. 226 pp.

Gaddis, Peggy. *Challenges for Nurse Genie*. New York: Arcadia House, 1960. 128 pp. (P)

Gaddis, Peggy. *City Nurse*. New York: Harlequin, 1957. 157 pp. (P)

Gaddis, Peggy. *Clinic Nurse*. New York: Macfadden-Bartell, 1964. 126 pp. (P)

Gaddis, Peggy. *The Courtship of Nurse Genie Hayes*. New York: Macfadden, 1960. 128 pp. (P)

Gaddis, Peggy. *Doctor Jerry*. New York: Arcadia House, 1951. 128 pp. (P)

Gaddis, Peggy. *Doctor Merry's Husband*. New York: Macfadden-Bartell, 1947. 128 pp. (P)

Gaddis, Peggy. *Doctor Sara*. New York: Macfadden, 1963. 127 pp. (P)

Gaddis, Peggy. *Emergency Nurse*. New York: Modern Promotions, 1963. 128 pp. (P)

Gaddis, Peggy. *Everglades Nurse*. New York: Macfadden-Bartell, 1964. 127 pp. (P)

Gaddis, Peggy. *Flight Nurse*. New York: Arcadia House, 1945. 232 pp.

Gaddis, Peggy. *Future Nurse*. New York: Arcadia House, 1962. 223 pp.

Gaddis, Peggy. *Future Nurse/Student Nurse*. New York: Manor, 1962. 256 pp. (P)

Gaddis, Peggy. *Heiress Nurse*. New York: Lancer, 1959. 221 pp. (P)

Gaddis, Peggy. *Hill-Top Nurse*. New York: Modern Promotions, 1964. 128 pp. (P)

Gaddis, Peggy. *Island Nurse*. New York: Arcadia House, 1960. 222 pp.

Gaddis, Peggy. *Lady Doctor*. New York: Modern Promotions, 1956. 128 pp. (P)

Gaddis, Peggy. *Leota Foreman, R.N.* New York: Arcadia House, 1957. 128 pp. (P)

Gaddis, Peggy. *The Listening Nurse*. New York: Arcadia House, 1965. 128 pp. (P)

Gaddis, Peggy. *Luxury Nurse*. New York: Macfadden, 1956. 127 pp. (P)

Gaddis, Peggy. *Miss Doc*. New York: Arcadia House, 1959. 127 pp. (P)

Gaddis, Peggy. *Mountain Nurse*. New York: Arcadia House, 1959. 223 pp.

Gaddis, Peggy. *Nora Was a Nurse*. New York: Macfadden, 1953. 128 pp. (P)

Gaddis, Peggy. *The Nurse and the Pirate*. New York: Ace, 1961. 127 pp. (P)

Gaddis, Peggy. *The Nurse and the Star*. New York: Macfadden-Bartell, 1963. 126 pp. (P)

Gaddis, Peggy. *Nurse Angela*. New York: Macfadden-Bartell, 1965. 128 pp. (P)

Gaddis, Peggy. *Nurse at Spanish Cay*. New York: Arcadia House, 1962. 127 pp. (P)

Gaddis, Peggy. *Nurse at Sundown*. New York: Macfadden-Bartell, 1958. 128 pp. (P)

Gaddis, Peggy. *Nurse at the Cedars*. New York: Macfadden, 1963. 127 pp. (P)

Gaddis, Peggy. *A Nurse Called Happy*. New York: Macfadden, 1963. 126 pp. (P)

Gaddis, Peggy. *Nurse Christine*. New York: Macfadden, 1962. 128 pp. (P)

Gaddis, Peggy. *A Nurse Comes Home*. New York: Arcadia House, 1963. 219 pp.

Gaddis, Peggy. *Nurse Durand's Affair*. New York: Belmont, 1961. 141 pp. (P)

Gaddis, Peggy. *A Nurse for Apple Valley*. New York: Macfadden, 1964. 127 pp. (P)

Gaddis, Peggy. *Nurse in Flight*. New York: Arcadia House, 1965. 128 pp. (P)

Gaddis, Peggy. *Nurse in the Shadows*. New York: Modern Promotions, 1956. 128 pp. (P)

Gaddis, Peggy. *Nurse Melinda*. New York: Berkley Medallion, 1960. 128 pp. (P)

Gaddis, Peggy. *Nurse's Choice*. New York: Macfadden-Bartell, 1957. 126 pp. (P)

Gaddis, Peggy. *Nurse's Secret*. New York: Lancer, 1968. 226 pp.

Gaddis, Peggy. *The Nurse Was Juliet*. New York: Arcadia House, 1965. 128 pp. (P)

Gaddis, Peggy. *The Old Doctor*. New York: Arcadia House, 1943. 231 pp.

Gaddis, Peggy. *Palm Beach Nurse*. New York: Berkley Medallion, 1953. 142 pp. (P)

Gaddis, Peggy. *Piney Woods Nurse*. New York: Arcadia House, 1961. 224 pp.

Gaddis, Peggy. *Second Chance at Love*. New York: Arcadia House, 1965. 191 pp. (P)

Gaddis, Peggy. *Settlement Nurse*. New York: Arcadia House, 1959. 220 pp.

Gaddis, Peggy. *Strange Shadows of Love*. New York: Arcadia House, 1964. 128 pp. (P)

Gaddis, Peggy. *Student Nurse*. New York: Macfadden, 1959. 128 pp. (P)

Gaddis, Peggy. *Young Doctor Merry*. New York: Arcadia House, 1944. 228 pp.

Gaddis, Peggy. *Young Doctor Talbot*. New York: Berkley Medallion, 1961. 125 pp. (P)

Gaddis, Peggy, and Stuart, Florence. *Nurse Hilary*. New York: Manor Books, 1959. 132 pp. (P)

Gale, Adela. *Goddess of Terror*. New York: New American Library, 1967. 128 pp. (P)

Gardner, Erle Stanley. *The Case of the Fugitive Nurse*. New York: Pocket Books, 1954. 196 pp. (P)

Garrison, Joan. *Nurse Greer.* New York: Avon, 1954. 127 pp. (P)

Gelsthorpe, Annie L. *Dr. Lesley's Triumph.* New York: Dell, 1968. 187 pp. (P)

Gelsthorpe, Annie L. *Nurse Andrea Takes a Flier.* New York: Avalon, 1973. 192 pp.

Gibson, William. *The Cobweb.* New York: Bantam, 1955. 328 pp. (P)

Gillen, Lucy. *Good Morning, Doctor Houston.* New York: Harlequin, 1970. 192 pp. (P)

Gillen, Lucy. *Nurse Helen.* New York: Harlequin, 1971. 187 pp. (P)

Gilmer, Ann. *Kate Wilder, R.N.* New York: Macfadden-Bartell, 1964. 128 pp. (P)

Gilmer, Ann. *Nurse at Breakwater Hotel.* New York: Avalon, 1982. 221 pp.

Gilmer, Ann. *Nurse Crane . . . Emergency.* New York: Valentine, 1964. 222 pp. (P)

Gilmer, Ann. *Nurse in the Tropics.* New York: Lancer, 1967. 198 pp.

Gilmer, Ann. *Nurse on Call.* New York: Valentine, 1968. 192 pp. (P)

Gilmer, Ann. *Private Nurse.* New York: Thomas Bouregy, 1969. 191 pp.

Gilmer, Ann. *Surgeon's Nurse.* New York: Thomas Bouregy, 1969. 189 pp.

Gilmer, Ann. *Young Dr. Leinster.* New York: Avalon, 1964. 189 pp. (P)

Gilzean, Elizabeth. *Doctor in Corsica.* New York: Harlequin, 1965. 190 pp. (P)

Gilzean, Elizabeth. *Next Patient, Doctor Anne.* New York: Harlequin, 1958. 192 pp. (P)

Gino, Carol. *Nurse's Story.* New York: Linden, 1982. 352 pp. (P)

Gladson, Leslie. *Dr. Weiland's Treatment.* New York: Lancer, 1968. 192 pp. (P)

Glenn, Isa. *Transport.* New York: Knopf, 1929. 387 pp.

Golden, Dr. Francis Leo. *Just What the Doctor Ordered.* New York: Pocket Books, 1949. 223 pp. (P)

Gordon, Noah. *Bamboo Ward.* New York: New American Library, 1962. 126 pp. (P)

Gordon, Noah. *Night Ward.* New American Library, 1959. 128 pp. (P)

Gordon, Richard. *The Private Life of Florence Nightingale.* New York: Atheneum, 1978. 231 pp.

Gould, Lois. *Such Good Friends.* New York: Dell, 1971. 306 pp. (P)

Gray, Adrian. *Doctors' Desires.* New York: New American Library, 1973. 125 pp.

Gray, Adrian. *Doctors' Passions.* New York: New American Library, 1975. 188 pp. (P)

Gray, Adrian. *The Young Doctors.* New York: New American Library, 1971. 128 pp. (P)

Green, Gerald. *The Healers.* New York: Berkley, 1979. 516 pp. (P)

Green, Gerald. *The Last Angry Man.* New York: Scribner's, 1955. 494 pp.

Green, Hannah. *I Never Promised You a Rose Garden.* New York: New American Library, 1964. 256 pp. (P)

Green, Pam. *Rehabilitation Nurse.* New York: New American Library, 1966. 128 pp. (P)

Greer, Germaine. *The Female Eunuch.* New York: McGraw-Hill, 1971. 432 pp.

Greig, Maysie. *Doctor on Wings.* New York: Beagle, 1966. 157 pp. (P)

Greig, Maysie. *Doctor's Wife.* New York: Triangle, 1937. 278 pp.

Gunn, Betty R. *Nurse Whitney's Paradise.* New York: Avalon, 1981. 246 pp.

Hailey, Arthur. *The Final Diagnosis.* Garden City, NY: Doubleday, 1959. 319 pp.

Hale, Arlene. *Camp Nurse.* New York: Ace, 1966. 155 pp. (P)

Hale, Arlene. *Chicago Nurse.* New York: Ace, 1965. 127 pp. (P)

Hale, Arlene. *Community Nurse.* New York: Ace, 1967. 142 pp. (P)

Hale, Arlene. *Crossroads for Nurse Cathy.* New York: Ace, 1969. 171 pp. (P)

Hale, Arlene. *Disaster Area Nurse.* New York: Ace, 1965. 126 pp. (P)

Hale, Arlene. *The Disobedient Nurse.* New York: Ace, 1975. 157 pp. (P)

Hale, Arlene. *Dr. Barry's Nurse.* New York: Ace, 1968. 158 pp. (P)

Hale, Arlene. *Doctor Myra Comes Home.* New York: Airmont, 1962. 126 pp. (P)

Hale, Arlene. *Doctor's Daughter.* New York: Ace, 1967. 139 pp. (P)

Hale, Arlene. *Dude Ranch Nurse.* New York: Ace, 1963. 128 pp. (P)

Hale, Arlene. *Emergency Call.* New York: Ace, 1968. 158 pp. (P)

Hale, Arlene. *Emergency for Nurse Selena.* New York: Ace, 1966. 125 pp. (P)

Hale, Arlene. *Executive Nurse.* New York: Ace, 1971. 169 pp. (P)

Hale, Arlene. *Frightened Nurse.* New York: Ace, 1976. 147 pp.

Hale, Arlene. *Journey for a Nurse.* New York: Ace, 1966. 125 pp. (P)

Hale, Arlene. *The Lady Is a Nurse.* New York: Arcadia House, 1967. 190 pp. (P)

Hale, Arlene. *Lake Resort Nurse.* New York: Ace, 1966. 136 pp. (P)

Hale, Arlene. *Leave It to Nurse Kathy.* New York: Ace, 1963. 128 pp. (P)

Hale, Arlene. *Mountain Nurse.* New York: Ace, 1966. 126 pp. (P)

Hale, Arlene. *My Favorite Nurse.* New York: Ace, 1968. 153 pp. (P)

Hale, Arlene. *New Nurse at Crest View.* New York: Ace, 1966. 125 pp. (P)

Hale, Arlene. *The New Nurses.* New York: Ace, 1970. 159 pp. (P)

Hale, Arlene. *Nurse Connor Comes Home.* New York: Ace, 1964. 127 pp. (P)

Hale, Arlene. *A Nurse for Sand Castle.* New York: Dell, 1969. 159 pp. (P)

Hale, Arlene. *Nurse from the Shadows.* New York: Ace, 1975. 158 pp. (P)

Hale, Arlene. *Nurse in Residence.* New York: Dell, 1968. 160 pp. (P)

Hale, Arlene. *Nurse Jean's Strange Case.* New York: Ace, 1970. 159 pp. (P)

Hale, Arlene. *Nurse Julia's Tangled Loves.* New York: Ace, 1976. 185 pp. (P)

Hale, Arlene. *Nurse Lora's Love.* New York: Ace, 1967. 136 pp.

Hale, Arlene. *Nurse Marcie's Island.* New York: Ace, 1964. 126 pp. (P)

Hale, Arlene. *Nurse Nicole's Decision.* New York: Ace, 1965. 125 pp. (P)

Hale, Arlene. *Nurse on Leave.* New York: Ace, 1965. 124 pp. (P)

Hale, Arlene. *Nurse on the Beach.* New York: Ace, 1967. 143 pp. (P)

Hale, Arlene. *Nurse on the Run.* New York: Ace, 1965. 125 pp. (P)

Hale, Arlene. *Nurse Shelley Decides.* New York: Pyramid, 1964. 126 pp. (P)

Hale, Arlene. *A Nurse's Strange Romance.* New York: Ace, 1964. 128 pp. (P)

Hale, Arlene. *Nurse Sue's Romance.* New York: Ace, 1964. 127 pp. (P)

Hale, Arlene. *Orphanage Nurse.* New York: Dell, 1970. 155 pp. (P)

Hale, Arlene. *Private Duty for Nurse Scott.* New York: Ace, 1965. 125 pp. (P)

Hale, Arlene. *Private Hospital.* New York: Dell, 1969. 156 pp. (P)

Hale, Arlene. *Private Nurse.* New York: Belmont, 1968. 141 pp. (P)

Hale, Arlene. *School Nurse.* New York: Ace, 1960. 180 pp. (P)

Hale, Arlene. *The Secret Longing.* New York: Dell, 1971. 184 pp. (P)

Hale, Arlene. *Special Duty.* New York: Dell, 1970. 156 pp. (P)

Hale, Arlene. *Symptoms of Love.* New York: Ace, 1964. 128 pp. (P)

Hale, Arlene. *University Nurse.* New York: Ace, 1967. 128 pp. (P)

Hale, Arlene. *Walk Softly, Doctor.* New York: Ace, 1971. 158 pp. (P)

Hale, Arlene. *When Dreams Come True.* New York: Dell, 1969. 176 pp. (P)

Hale, Arlene. *Whistle Stop Nurse.* New York: Lancer, 1968. 192 pp.

Hall, Bennie C. *No Escape from Love.* New York: Arcadia House, 1968. 192 pp. (P)

Hall, Bennie C. *Redheaded Nurse.* New York: Dell, 1960. 191 pp. (P)

Hamill, Ethel. *Aloha Nurse.* New York: Thomas Bouregy, 1961. 222 pp.

Hamill, Ethel. *Bluegrass Doctor.* New York: Airmont, 1953. 128 pp. (P)

Hamill, Ethel. *Candy Frost: Emergency Nurse.* New York: Hillman, 1952. 144 pp. (P)

Hamill, Ethel. *A Nurse Comes Home.* New York: Dell, 1954. 157 pp. (P)

Hamill, Ethel. *A Nurse for Galleon Key.* New York: Bantam, 1957. 120 pp. (P)

Hamill, Ethel. *Runaway Nurse.* New York: Ace, 1955. 143 pp. (P)

Hamilton, Robert W. *Belinda of the Red Cross.* New York: World Syndicate, 1916. 342 pp.

Hancock, Frances Dean. *Resident Nurse.* New York: Thomas Bouregy, 1966. 192 pp.

Hancock, Lucy Agnes. *Calling Nurse Blair.* New York: Harlequin, 1954. 160 pp. (P)

Hancock, Lucy Agnes. *Community Nurse.* Philadelphia: Blakiston, 1944. 250 pp.

Hancock, Lucy Agnes. *Graduate Nurse.* New York: Bantam, 1947. 151 pp. (P)

Hancock, Lucy Agnes. *North Side Nurse.* New York: Triangle, 1940. 285 pp.

Hancock, Lucy Agnes. *The Nurse at Whittle's.* Philadelphia: Blakiston, 1945. 256 pp.

Hancock, Lucy Agnes. *Nurse Barlow.* Philadelphia: Macrae-Smith, 1946. 255 pp.

Hancock, Lucy Agnes. *Nurse in White.* New York: Penn, 1939. 251 pp.

Hancock, Lucy Agnes. *Nurse Kathy Decides.* New York: Macrae-Smith, 1951. 268 pp.

Hancock, Lucy Agnes. *Nurse's Aide.* New York: Triangle, 1943. 249 pp.

Hancock, Lucy Agnes. *Nurses Are People.* New York: Triangle, 1942. 279 pp.

Hancock, Lucy Agnes. *Pat Whitney, R.N.* New York: Sun Dial, 1942. 288 pp.

Hancock, Lucy Agnes. *Special Nurse.* New York: Pocket Books, 1948. 211 pp. (P)

Hancock, Lucy Agnes. *Staff Nurse.* New York: Triangle, 1942. 288 pp.

Hancock, Lucy Agnes. *Student Nurse.* Philadelphia: Blakiston, 1944. 250 pp.

Hancock, Lucy Agnes. *West End Nurse.* Philadelphia: Triangle, 1944. 272 pp.

Harding, Matt. *Nurse or Woman.* New York: Softcover Library, 1967. 155 pp. (P)

Harpole, James. *A Surgeon's Heritage.* London: Pan, 1956. 191 pp. (P)

Harris, Kathleen. *Camp Nurse.* New York: Berkley Medallion, 1961. 127 pp. (P)

Harris, Kathleen. *Flight Nurse.* New York: Thomas Bouregy, 1960. 220 pp.

Harris, Kathleen. *Jane Arden: Head Nurse.* New York: Popular Library, 1959. 128 pp. (P)

Harris, Kathleen. *Jane Arden: Space Nurse.* New York: Popular Library, 1963. 126 pp. (P)

Harris, Kathleen. *Jane Arden: Student Nurse.* New York: Avalon, 1955. 256 pp.

Harris, Kathleen. *Jane Arden: Surgery Nurse.* New York: Popular Library, 1961. 128 pp. (P)

Harris, Kathleen. *Nurse on Holiday.* New York: Dell, 1964. 159 pp. (P)

Harris, Kathleen. *Nurse on the Run.* New York: Arcadia House, 1965. 176 pp. (P)

Harrison, Barbara. *The Gorlin Clinic.* New York: Avon, 1975. 345 pp. (P)

Harrison, Elizabeth. *Ambulance Call.* New York: Pocket Books, 1974. 144 pp. (P)

Harrison, Elizabeth. *Emergency Call.* New York: Pocket Books, 1970. 143 pp. (P)

Harrison, Elizabeth. *Surgeon's Call.* New York: Pocket Books, 1973. 159 pp. (P)

Hart, Helen. *The Campfire Girls: Red Cross Work.* Racine, WI: Whitman, 1915. 117 pp.

Harte, Majorie. *Strange Journey.* New York: Lenox Hill, 1971. 189 pp. (P)

Hartman, Shirley, and Ellerbeck, Walter. *The Surgeons.* New York: Pyramid, 1974. 381 pp. (P)

Harvey, Gene. *Doctor's Nurse.* New York: Pyramid, 1951. 143 pp. (P)

Haskell, Frank. *Young Doctor Masters.* New York: Belmont, 1953. 125 pp. (P)

Hayes, Ralph E. *Ellen Matthews, Mission Nurse.* New York: Dell, 1966. 156 pp. (P)

Hayes, Ralph E. *Nurse in Istanbul.* New York: Thomas Bouregy, 1970. 189 pp.

Hayle, Felicity. *A Promise Is for Keeping.* New York: Harlequin, 1967. 190 pp. (P)

Heath, Sharon. *Jungle Nurse.* New York: Ace, 1965. 126 pp. (P)

Heath, Sharon. *Nurse at Cliff End.* New York: Ace, 1970. 126 pp. (P)

Heath, Sharon. *Nurse at Moorcroft Manor.* New York: Ace, 1967. 157 pp. (P)

Heath, Sharon. *Nurse at Shadow Manor.* New York: Ace, 1966. 126 pp. (P)

Heath, Sharon. *Nurse Elaine and the Sapphire Star.* New York: Ace, 1973. 157 pp. (P)

Heath, Sharon. *Nurse on Castle Island.* New York: Ace, 1968. 127 pp. (P)

Heath, Sharon. *The Sunshine Nurse.* New York: Ace, 1969. 157 pp. (P)

Heath, Sharon. *A Vacation for Nurse Dean.* New York: Ace, 1966. 159 pp. (P)

Heinrich, Willi. *The Cross of Iron.* New York: Bantam, 1957. 437 pp. (P)

Heinz, W. C. *Emergency.* Greenwich, CT: Fawcett, 1975. 304 pp. (P)

Hejinian, John. *Extreme Remedies.* New York: Bantam, 1974. 280 pp. (P)

Heller, Joseph. *Catch-22.* New York: Simon and Schuster, 1955. 472 pp.

Hemingway, Ernest. *A Farewell to Arms.* New York: Scribner's, 1929. 332 pp.

Hendron, Grace Muirhead. *Nurse in Alaska.* New York: Dell, 1965. 156 pp. (P)

Highmore, Jane. *Big City Nurse.* New York: Permabooks, 1961. 188 pp. (P)

Hilton, James. *The Story of Dr. Wassell.* Boston: Little, Brown, 1943. 158 pp.

Hirschfeld, Burt. *General Hospital.* New York: Lancer, 1965. 143 pp. (P)

Hobart, Lois. *Elaine Forrest: Visiting Nurse.* New York: Paperback Library, 1959. 157 pp. (P)

Hoke, Helen. *Nurses, Nurses, Nurses.* New York: F. Watts, 1961. 217 pp.

Holden, Joanne. *Holiday for a Nurse.* New York: Pyramid, 1965. 143 pp. (P)

Holden, Joanne. *Nurse at the Castle.* New York: Arcadia House, 1965. 158 pp. (P)

Holden, Joanne. *Nurse Gina.* New York: Macfadden-Bartell, 1964. 127 pp. (P)

Holden, Joanne. *Village Nurse.* New York: Macfadden-Bartell, 1963. 126 pp. (P)

Holloway, Teresa. *Nurse Farley's Decision.* New York: Avalon, 1959. 219 pp.

Holloway, Teresa. *Nurse for the Fishermen.* New York: Avalon, 1974. 221 pp.

Holloway, Teresa. *Nurse Karen's Secret.* New York: Ace, 1971. 220 pp. (P)

Holloway, Teresa. *The Nurse on Dark Island.* New York: Ace, 1969. 125 pp. (P)

Holloway, Teresa. *Nurse Paige's Triumph.* New York: Thomas Bouregy, 1972. 192 pp.

Holloway, Teresa. *Nurse to Remember.* New York: Ace, 1970. 125 pp. (P)

Holloway, Teresa. *River Nurse.* New York: Arcadia House, 1969. 192 pp. (P)

Holmes, David. *Night Nurse.* New York: Pyramid, 1951. 143 pp. (P)

Holmgren, Virginia C. *Nurse Kilmer's Vow*. New York: Dell, 1963. 157 pp. (P)

Hooker, Richard. *M*A*S*H*. New York: Pocket Books, 1969. 180 pp. (P)

Hooker, Richard. *M*A*S*H Goes to Maine*. New York: Pocket Books, 1971. 192 pp. (P)

Hooker, Richard, and Butterworth, William E. *M*A*S*H Goes to Hollywood*. New York: Pocket Books, 1976. 206 pp. (P)

Hooker, Richard, and Butterworth, William E. *M*A*S*H Goes to Las Vegas*. New York: Pocket Books, 1976. 239 pp. (P)

Hooker, Richard, and Butterworth, William E. *M*A*S*H Goes to Moscow*. New York: Pocket Books, 1977, 1975. 217 pp. (P)

Houghton, Elizabeth. *Island Hospital*. New York: Harlequin, 1959. 189 pp. (P)

Houghton, Elizabeth. *New Surgeon at St. Lucian's*. New York: Harlequin, 1967. 191 pp. (P)

Howe, Margaret. *Calling Dr. Merryman*. New York: Ace, 1954. 131 pp. (P)

Howe, Margaret. *Debutante Nurse*. New York: Thomas Bouregy, 1958. 220 pp.

Howe, Margaret. *The Girl in the White Cap*. New York: Ace, 1957. 144 pp. (P)

Howe, Margaret. *Special Nurse*. New York: Bantam, 1958. 121 pp. (P)

Howe, Margaret. *Visiting Nurse*. New York: Pocket Books, 1956. 122 pp. (P)

Hoy, Elizabeth. *Nurse Tenant*. New York: Harlequin, 1959. 189 pp. (P)

Hoy, Elizabeth. *You Took My Heart*. New York: Harlequin, 1957. 189 pp. (P)

Hughes, Rupert. *The Patent Leather Kid*. New York: Grosset and Dunlap, 1917. 240 pp.

Hughes, Rupert. *She Goes to War*. New York: Grosset and Dunlap, 1918. 302 pp.

Hulme, Kathryn. *The Nun's Story*. New York: Pocket Books, 1956. 314 pp. (P)

Humphries, Adelaide. *Ann Star, Nurse*. New York: Arcadia House, 1944. 241 pp.

Humphries, Adelaide. *Ann Star, Senior Nurse*. New York: Arcadia House, 1945. 245 pp.

Humphries, Adelaide. *Ann Star, Staff Nurse*. New York: Arcadia House, 1946. 267 pp.

Humphries, Adelaide. *A Case for Nurse Marian*. New York: Bantam, 1957. 119 pp. (P)

Humphries, Adelaide. *Clinic Nurse*. New York: Airmont, 1958. 128 pp. (P)

Humphries, Adelaide. *Danger for Nurse Vivian*. New York: Avalon, 1979. 231 pp.

Humphries, Adelaide. *A Feather in Her Cap*. New York: Dell, 1964. 159 pp. (P)

Humphries, Adelaide. *Flight Nurse*. New York: Thomas Bouregy, 1960. 220 pp.

Humphries, Adelaide. *Glamour Nurse*. New York: Arcadia House, 1950. 221 pp.

Humphries, Adelaide. *Home Front Nurse*. New York: Bouregy and Curl, 1952. 210 pp.

Humphries, Adelaide. *Jane Arden, Staff Nurse*. New York: Avalon, 1957. 197 pp.

Humphries, Adelaide. *Jane Arden, Student Nurse*. New York: Avalon, 1956. 221 pp.

Humphries, Adelaide. *Jane Arden, Surgery Nurse*. New York: Avalon, 1958. 206 pp.

Humphries, Adelaide. *Love Has No Logic*. New York: Dell, 1967. 157 pp. (P)

Humphries, Adelaide. *Luxury Nurse*. New York: Thomas Bouregy, 1966. 192 pp.

Humphries, Adelaide. *Miracle for Nurse Louisa*. New York: Avalon, 1978. 226 pp.

Humphries, Adelaide. *Mission Nurse*. New York: Bantam, 1960. 119 pp. (P)

Humphries, Adelaide. *Navy Nurse*. New York: Airmont, 1954. 126 pp. (P)

Humphries, Adelaide. *New England Nurse*. New York: Avon, 1956. 144 pp. (P)

Humphries, Adelaide. *Nurse Barclay's Dilemma*. New York: Avalon, 1954. 230 pp.

Humphries, Adelaide. *The Nurse Had a Secret*. New York: Bantam, 1960. 149 pp. (P)

Humphries, Adelaide. *Nurse Had Red Hair*. New York: Avalon, 1957. 227 pp.

Humphries, Adelaide. *Nurse in a Nightmare*. New York: Lancer, 1971. 189 pp. (P)

Humphries, Adelaide. *Nurse in Flight*. New York: Lancer, 1968. 224 pp. (P)

Humphries, Adelaide. *The Nurse Knows Best*. New York: Monarch, 1953. 140 pp. (P)

Humphries, Adelaide. *Nurse Lady*. New York: Bouregy and Curl, 1953. 162 pp.

Humphries, Adelaide. *Nurse Landon's Challenge*. New York: Bantam, 1952. 120 pp. (P)

Humphries, Adelaide. *Nurse Laurie's Cruise*. New York: Airmont, 1956. 126 pp. (P)

Humphries, Adelaide. *The Nurse Made Headlines*. New York: Dell, 1962. 156 pp. (P)

Humphries, Adelaide. *Nurse on Holiday*. New York: Avalon, 1964. 226 pp.

Humphries, Adelaide. *A Nurse on Horseback*. New York: Bantam, 1959. 120 pp. (P)

Humphries, Adelaide. *Nurses Are People*. New York: Bouregy and Curl, 1951. 231 pp.

Humphries, Adelaide. *Nurse Was Kidnapped*. New York: Avalon, 1976. 227 pp.

Humphries, Adelaide. *Nurse with Wings*. New York: Avalon, 1955. 223 pp.

Humphries, Adelaide. *Orchids for the Nurse*. New York: Airmont, 1955. 126 pp. (P)

Humphries, Adelaide. *Park Avenue Nurse*. New York: Avalon, 1956. 222 pp.

Humphries, Adelaide. *Substitute Nurse*. New York: Arcadia House, 1944. 236 pp.

Humphries, Adelaide. *A Test for Nurse Barbi*. New York: Avalon, 1975. 192 pp.

Humphries, Adelaide. *Visiting Nurse*. New York: Arcadia House, 1944. 221 pp.

Humphries, Adelaide. *Young Dr. Bob*. New York: Arcadia House, 1945. 251 pp.

Hunt, Rosamund. *Nurse Martin's Dilemma*. New York: Thomas Bouregy, 1961. 222 pp.

Hunt, Rosamund. *Nurse Martin's Secret*. New York: Paperback Library, 1961. 128 pp. (P)

Hunt, Rosamund. *Night Nurse*. New York: Dell, 1962, 157 pp. (P)

Hunt, Rosamund. *Settlement Nurse*. New York: Thomas Bouregy, 1966. 192 pp.

Hunter, Elizabeth. *Cherry-Blossom Clinic*. New York: Harlequin, 1962. 160 pp. (P)

Ibanez, Vicente Blasco. *The Four Horsemen of the Apocalypse*. New York: Dell, 1961, 415 pp. (P)

Irving, John. *The World According to Garp*. New York: Pocket Books, 1976. 609 pp. (P)

Irving, Luella. *Nurse Patsy's Last Chance*. New York: Avalon, 1980. 230 pp.

Ives, Ruth. *Congo Nurse*. New York: Modern Promotions, 1963. 143 pp. (P)

Ives, Ruth. *Navy Nurse*. New York: New American Library, 1968. 96 pp. (P)

Ives, Ruth. *Surgical Nurse*. New York: Berkeley Medallion, 1962. 144 pp. (P)

Jackson, Charles. *The Lost Weekend*. New York: Farrar and Rinehart, 1944. 244 pp.

Jackson, Kathryn. *Nurse Nancy*. New York: Golden, 1958. 22 pp.

Jaffe, Susanne. *Cruise Ship M.D.* New York: Ace, 1975. 223 pp. (P)

Jaffe, Susanne. *Group Therapy M.D.* New York: Ace, 1975. 201 pp. (P)

James, Florence Alice Price. *Nurse Revel's Mistake*. New York: G. Munro, 1890. 306 pp.

James, Josephine. *An Affair of the Heart*. New York: Golden, 1965. 186 pp. (P)

James, Josephine. *The Patient in 202*. New York: Golden, 1961. 186 pp.

James, Josephine. *Peace Corps Nurse*. New York: Golden, 1965. 187 pp. (P)

James, Josephine. *Private Nurse*. New York: Golden, 1962. 223 pp. (P)

James, Josephine. *Senior Nurse*. New York: Golden, 1960. 186 pp. (P)

James, Norah C. *Nurse Adriane: A Novel*. New York: Covici, Friede, 1933. 281 pp.

James, Rian. *The White Parade*. New York: Alfred H. King, 1934. 316 pp.

Johnson, Martha. *Ann Bartlett, Navy Nurse*. New York: Thomas Y. Crowell, 1941. 321 pp.

Johnston, William. *Ben Casey*. New York: Lancer, 1962. 144 pp. (P)

Johnston, William. *Dr. Starr in Crisis*. New York: Monarch, 1964. 128 pp. (P)

Johnston, William. *Emergency for Dr. Starr*. New York: Monarch, 1963. 144 pp. (P)

Johnston, William. *The New Interns*. New York: Bantam, 1964. 346 pp. (P)

Johnston, William. *Nurses*. New York: Bantam, 1963. 123 pp.

Johnston, William. *Surgeon's Oath*. New York: Arcadia House, 1968. 224 pp. (P)

Johnston, William. *Two Loves Has Nurse Powell*. Las Vegas: Medical Fiction, 1963. 176 pp. (P)

Jones, Irene Heywood. *Sister*. London: W. H. Allen, 1982. 220 pp. (P)

Jordan, Gail. *Student Nurse*. New York: Universal, 1950. 124 pp. (P)

Josephs, Michelle. *Cruise Ship Nurse*. New York: Belmont, 1969. 123 pp. (P)

Judson, Jeanne. *City Nurse*. New York: Bantam, 1959. 121 pp. (P)

Judson, Jeanne. *A Doctor for the Nurse*. New York: Avalon, 1954. 255 pp.

Judson, Jeanne. *John Keith, Intern*. New York: Dell, 1963. 159 pp. (P)

Judson, Jeanne. *A Strange Case for Dr. Rolland*. New York: Thomas Bouregy, 1962. 125 pp. (P)

Judson, Jeanne. *Visiting Nurse*. New York: Bantam, 1954. 119 pp. (P)

Kafka, Franz. *The Trial*. New York: Modern Library, 1937. 341 pp.

Karp, Marvin Allen, ed. *Men in White*. New York: Popular Library, 1966. 128 pp. (P)

Karson, Arlene. *Walk Out of Darkness*. New York: Monarch, 1963. 126 pp. (P)

Katzman, Lawrence. *Nurse Nellie's Naughties*. New York: Dell, 1964. 127 pp. (P)

Kaus, Gina. *Luxury Liner*. New York: Ray Long and Richard R. Smith, 1932. 316 pp.

Kellier, Elizabeth. *The Patient at Tonesbury Manor*. New York: Ace, 1964. 175 pp. (P)

Kellier, Elizabeth. *Wayneston Hospital*. New York: Ace, 1963. 159 pp. (P)

Kesey, Ken. *One Flew over the Cuckoo's Nest*. New York: New American Library, 1962. 272 pp. (P)

Ketchum, Philip. *The Quartet in White*. Las Vegas: Medical Fiction, 1963. 176 pp. (P)

Kirby, Jean. *Nurses Three: A Career for Kelly*. Racine, WI: Whitman, 1963. 216 pp. (P)

Kirby, Jean. *Nurses Three: First Assignment*. Racine, WI: Whitman, 1963. 216 pp.

Kirby, Jean. *Nurses Three: Tracy's Little People*. Racine, WI: Whitman, 1965. 211 pp.

Kirby, Jean. *Nurses Three: A Very Special Girl*. Racine, WI: Whitman, 1963. 216 pp.

Knickerbocker, Charles. *The Dynasty*. New York: Dell, 1969. 352 pp. (P)

Knickerbocker, Charles. *Summer Doctor*. New York: Macfadden-Bartell, 1964. 256 pp. (P)

Knight, Doris. *Nurse on Terror Island*. New York: Modern Promotions, 1967. 141 pp. (P)

Knight, Doris. *Runaway Nurse*. New York: Belmont, 1968. 124 pp. (P)

Kramer, Charles. *The Negligent Doctor*. New York: Popular Library, 1968. 204 pp. (P)

Kramm, Joseph. *The Shrike*. New York: Random House, 1952. 198 pp.

Kyne, Peter B. *Lord of Lonely Valley*. New York: H. C. Kinsey, 1932. 294 pp.

Laklan, Carli. *Nancy Kimball, Nurse's Aide*. Garden City, NY: Doubleday, 1962. 142 pp.

Laklan, Carli. *Nurse in Training*. Garden City, NY: Doubleday, 1965. 144 pp.

Laklan, Carli. *Second Year Nurse: Nancy Kimball at City Hospital*. Garden City, NY: Doubleday, 1967. 144 pp.

Lambert, Alice Eleanor. *Hospital Nocturne*. New York: Dell, 1932. 239 pp. (P)

Lane, Roumelia. *Nurse at Noongwalla*. New York: Harlequin, 1974. 190 pp. (P)

Lees, Marguerite. *A Case for Nurse Clare*. New York: Harlequin, 1955. 191 pp. (P)

Levin, Beatrice. *Safari Smith*. New York: Nova, 1965. 156 pp. (P)

Lewis, Colleen. *Nurse at Lookout Rock*. New York: Avalon, 1982. 202 pp.

Lewis, Sinclair. *Arrowsmith*. New York: Harcourt, Brace and World, 1924. 464 pp.

Lewis, Sinclair. *Babbitt*. New York: Grosset and Dunlap, 1924. 536 pp.

Libby, Patricia. *Cover Girl Nurse*. New York: Ace, 1963. 141 pp. (P)

Libby, Patricia. *Hollywood Nurse*. New York: Ace, 1962. 128 pp. (P)

Libby, Patricia. *Winged Victory for Nurse Kerry*. New York: Ace, 1965. 128 pp. (P)

Littleton, Kay. *Jean Craig, Nurse*. Cleveland: World, 1949. 216 pp.

Lloyd, Sylvia. *Dr. Walker's People*. New York: Thomas Bouregy, 1965. 190 pp.

Lloyd, Sylvia. *Down East Nurse*. New York: Ace, 1965. 156 pp. (P)

Logan, Louise. *Nurse*. New York: Arcadia House, 1940. 221 pp.

Logan, Louise. *Nurse Merton: Army Spy*. New York: Arcadia House, 1942. 235 pp.

Logan, Louise. *Nurse Merton Comes Home*. New York: Arcadia House, 1946. 211 pp.

Logan, Louise. *Nurse Merton: Desert Captive*. New York: Arcadia House, 1943. 236 pp.

Logan, Louise. *Nurse Merton in the Pacific*. New York: Arcadia House, 1944. 217 pp.

Logan, Louise. *Nurse Merton on the Russian Front*. New York: Arcadia House, 1945. 239 pp.

Logsdon, Patricia. *Nurse of the Ozarks*. New York: Avalon, 1974. 192 pp.

Longfellow, Henry Wadsworth. *The Poetical Works of Longfellow*. Boston: Houghton Mifflin, 1878. 401 pp.

Lorraine, Anne. *Emergency Nurse*. New York: Harlequin, 1961. 191 pp. (P)

Lowry, Nan. *Crystal Manning, Maternity Nurse*. New York: Paperback Library, 1964. 128 pp. (P)

Luis, Earlene. *Listen, Lissa!* New York: Dodd, Mead, 1968. 144 pp.

Lynch, Miriam. *Dr. Garrett's Girl*. New York: Dell, 1970. 156 pp. (P)

McBain, Edward. *Death of a Nurse*. New York: New American Library, 1955. 160 pp. (P)

McCall, Virginia. *Navy Nurse*. New York: Julian Messner, 1968. 191 pp.

McCarthy, Jane. *Nurse April's Dilemma*. New York: Avalon, 1974. 177 pp.

McCarthy, Jane. *Nurse of Thorne Grotto*. New York: Avalon, 1977. 142 pp.

McCarthy, Justin Huntly, and Critchett, R. C. *Nurse Benson*. New York: John Lane, 1919. 163 pp.

McComb, Katherine. *Night-Duty Nurse*. New York: Avalon, 1970. 189 pp.

McComb, Katherine. *Nurse April*. New York: Arcadia House, 1967. 190 pp. (P)

McComb, Katherine. *Nurse on Trial*. New York: Avalon, 1973. 198 pp.

McComb, Katherine. *Princess of White Starch.* New York: Ace, 1963. 128 pp. (P)

McCoy, Horace. *Scalpel.* New York: Signet, 1953. 256 pp. (P)

McCulloch, Margaret. *Second Year Nurse.* New York: Scholastic, 1964. 222 pp. (P)

MacDonald, Zillah K. *A Cap for Corrine.* New York: Julian Messner, 1952. 184 pp.

MacDonald, Zillah K. *Roxanne, Company Nurse.* New York: Berkeley Medallion, 1957. 158 pp. (P)

MacDonald, Zillah K., and Ahl, Vivian J. *Nurse Todd's Strange Summer.* New York: Paperback Library, 1960. 144 pp. (P)

McDonnell, R. N., and McDonnell, Virginia B. *Annapolis Nurse.* New York: Macfadden, 1965. 126 pp. (P)

McDonnell, Virginia B. *The Nurse with the Silver Skates.* New York: Ace, 1964. 126 pp. (P)

McDonnell, Virginia B. *Trouble at Mercy Hospital.* Garden City, NY: Doubleday, 1968. 142 pp.

McElfresh, Adeline. *Ann and the Hoosier Doctor.* New York: Avalon, 1955. 169 pp.

McElfresh, Adeline. *Ann Foster, Lab Technician.* New York: Avalon, 1956. 176 pp.

McElfresh, Adeline. *Ann Kenyon: Surgeon.* New York: Dell, 1960. 192 pp. (P)

McElfresh, Adeline. *Calling Dr. Jane.* New York: Avalon, 1957. 224 pp.

McElfresh, Adeline. *Challenge for Dr. Jane.* New York: Avalon, 1957. 163 pp.

McElfresh, Adeline. *Doctor Barbara.* New York: Avalon, 1958. 182 pp.

McElfresh, Adeline. *Doctor for Blue Hollow.* New York: Dell, 1971. 165 pp. (P)

McElfresh, Adeline. *Doctor Jane.* New York: Bantam, 1956. 122 pp. (P)

McElfresh, Adeline. *Dr. Jane Comes Home.* New York: Thomas Bouregy, 1959. 220 pp.

McElfresh, Adeline. *Dr. Jane, Interne.* New York: Bantam, 1966. 137 pp. (P)

McElfresh, Adeline. *Dr. Jane's Choice.* New York: Thomas Bouregy, 1961. 221 pp.

McElfresh, Adeline. *Dr. Jane's Mission.* New York: Avalon, 1958. 224 pp.

McElfresh, Adeline. *Ellen Randolph, R.N.* New York: Dell, 1971. 144 pp. (P)

McElfresh, Adeline. *Flight Nurse.* New York: Dell, 1971. 152 pp. (P)

McElfresh, Adeline. *Jill Nolan, R.N.* New York: Dell, 1962. 160 pp. (P)

McElfresh, Adeline. *Jill Nolan, Surgical Nurse.* New York: Dell, 1962. 158 pp. (P)

McElfresh, Adeline. *Kay Manion, M.D.* New York: Dell, 1959. 160 pp. (P)

McElfresh, Adeline. *The Magic of Dr. Farrar.* New York: Belmont, 1965. 159 pp. (P)

McElfresh, Adeline. *New Nurse at Dorn Memorial.* New York: Ace, 1969. 190 pp. (P)

McElfresh, Adeline. *Night Call.* New York: Dell, 1961. 190 pp. (P)

McElfresh, Adeline. *Nurse Anne.* New York: Ace, 1971. 143 pp. (P)

McElfresh, Adeline. *Nurse for Mercy's Mission.* New York: Dell, 1969. 156 pp. (P)

McElfresh, Adeline. *A Nurse for Rebel's Run.* New York: Thomas Bouregy, 1960. 220 pp.

McElfresh, Adeline. *Nurse in Yucatan.* New York: Dell, 1971. 155 pp. (P)

McElfresh, Adeline. *Nurse Kathy.* New York: Permabooks, 1956. 153 pp. (P)

McElfresh, Adeline. *Nurse Nolan's Private Duty.* New York: Belmont, 1966. 157 pp. (P)

McElfresh, Adeline. *The Two Loves of Nurse Ellen.* New York: Ace, 1969. 156 pp. (P)

McElfresh, Adeline. *Wings for Nurse Bennett.* New York: Dell, 1960. 160 pp. (P)

McElfresh, Adeline. *Young Doctor Randall.* New York: Bantam, 1957. 122 pp. (P)

MacLeod, Jean S. *Air Ambulance.* New York: Harlequin, 1958. 192 pp. (P)

MacLeod, Ruth. *Born To Be a Nurse.* New York: Paperback Library, 1969. 128 pp. (P)

MacLeod, Ruth. *Nurse Ann in Surgery.* New York: Ace, 1965. 128 pp. (P)

MacLeod, Ruth. *A Nurse for Dr. Sterling.* New York: Ace, 1962. 126 pp. (P)

Macleod, Ruth. *Waikiki Nurse.* New York: Avon 1963. 160 pp. (P)

Macy, Dora. *Night Nurse.* New York: Grosset and Dunlap, 1931. 282 pp.

Maguire, Anne. *Nurse at Towpath Lodge.* New York: Avalon, 1976. 211 pp.

Maguire, Anne. *Nurse in Las Palmas.* New York: Avalon, 1980. 203 pp.

Malcolm, Margaret. *The Healing Touch.* New York: Harlequin, 1952. 192 pp. (P)

Malcolm, Margaret. *Village Hospital.* New York: Harlequin, 1961. 192 pp. (P)

Mallette, Gertrude E. *Probation Nurse.* New York: Paperback Library, 1951. 192 pp. (P)

Mann, Abby. *Medical Story.* New York: New American Library, 1975. 167 pp. (P)

Mann, Thomas. *The Magic Mountain.* New York: Knopf, 1924. 901 pp.

March, Kim. *Bachelor Nurse.* New York: Universal, 1962. 155 pp. (P)

Mark, Polly. *Nurse at Seaview.* New York: Avalon, 1977. 219 pp.

Marnay, Jane. *Nurse Afloat.* New York: Harlequin, 1965. 192 pp. (P)

Marsh, Ngaio, and Jellett, Dr. Henry. *The Nursing Home Murder.* Cleveland: World, 1943. 280 pp.

Marsh, Rebecca. *Nurse Annette.* New York: Arcadia, 1962. 224 pp.

Marsh, Rebecca. *Nurse of Ward B.* New York: Pyramid, 1963. 127 pp. (P)

Marsh, Rebecca. *Office Nurse.* New York: Macfadden, 1960. 128 pp. (P)

Marsh, Rebecca. *Recovery Room Nurse.* New York: Macfadden, 1965. 128 pp. (P)

Marshall, Douglas. *Doctor Ben.* New York: Thomas Bouregy, 1941. 256 pp.

Marshall, Marguerite Mooers. *Her Soul To Keep.* New York: Bantam, 1940. 152 pp. (P)

Marshall, Marguerite Mooers. *Nurse into Woman.* New York: Triangle, 1941. 307 pp.

Marshall, Marguerite Mooers. *Nurse with Wings.* New York: Bantam, 1952. 150 pp. (P)

Marshall, Marguerite Mooers. *Wilderness Nurse.* New York: Pocket Books, 1949. 230 pp.

Maugham, W. Somerset. *Trio.* Garden City, NY: Doubleday, 1950. 156 pp.

Maxwell, Portia. *Nurse's Training.* New York: Gramercy, 1951. 137 pp.

Mercer, Charles. *Rachel Cade.* New York: Putnam's, 1956. 318 pp.

Mergendahl, Charles. *The Bramble Bush.* New York: Putnam's, 1958. 382 pp.

Michener, James A. *Selected Writings.* New York: Random House, 1957. 425 pp.

Michener, James A. *Tales of the South Pacific.* New York: Pocket Books, 1947. 375 pp. (P)

Middleton, Jan. *Learn To Say Goodbye.* New York: Bantam, 1965. 120 pp. (P)

Miller, John J. *New Doctor at Tower General.* New York: Monarch, 1964. 125 pp. (P)

Miller, Marcia. *Nurse in Peril.* New York: Avalon, 1975. 201 pp.

Miller, Marcia. *Nurse Kris's Trust.* New York: Thomas Bouregy, 1973. 191 pp.

Miller, Marcia. *Nurse of the High Sierras.* New York: Avalon, 1973. 218 pp.

Mitchell, Edward. *The Captive Nurse.* New York: Publisher's Consultants, 1978. 159 pp. (P)

Mitchell, Kerry. *Crisis at Waite Memorial.* New York: Dell, 1965. 156 pp. (P)

Mitchell, Kerry. *Doctor on Approval: A Dr. Brian Temple Story.* New York: Dell, 1962. 157 pp. (P)

Mitchell, Kerry. *Doctor on Test.* New York: Dell, 1963. 156 pp. (P)

Mitchell, Kerry. *The Doctor's Challenge.* New York: Dell, 1961. 156 pp. (P)

Mitchell, Kerry. *The Doctor's Decision.* New York: Dell, 1963. 159 pp. (P)

Mitchell, Kerry. *Emergency Doctor.* New York: Dell, 1962. 159 pp. (P)

Mitchell, Kerry. *Security Surgeon.* New York: Dell, 1963. 155 pp. (P)

Mitchell, Kerry. *Wrong Diagnosis.* New York: Dell, 1962. 158 pp. (P)

Mitchell, Paige. *A Wilderness of Monkeys.* New York: Bantam, 1966. 378 pp. (P)

Moore, Marjorie. *Senior Surgeon.* New York: Harlequin, 1954. 192 pp. (P)

Moore, Marjorie. *To Please the Doctor.* New York: Harlequin, 1959. 192 pp. (P)

Morgan, Millicent. *Mollie Sloan: Special Nurse.* New York: Permabooks, 1962. 120 pp. (P)

Morris, Carol. *Nurse Said Yes.* New York: Arcadia House, 1947. 233 pp.

Mosler, Blanche Y. *Marie Warren, Night Nurse.* New York: Paperback Library, 1963. 128 pp. (P)

Mosler, Blanche Y. *Terror Stalks the Night Nurse.* New York: Paperback Library, 1963. 128 pp. (P)

Moura, Joni, and Sutherland, Jackie. *If It Moves, Kiss It!* Greenwich, CT: Fawcett, 1973. 254 pp. (P)

Moura, Joni, and Sutherland, Jackie. *Tender Loving Care.* Greenwich, CT: Fawcett, 1969. 287 pp. (P)

Munroe, Val. *Doctors and Wives.* New York: Softcover Library, 1968. 156 pp. (P)

Muskett, Netta. *Through Many Waters.* London: Arrow, 1961. 192 pp. (P)

Myers, Harriett Kathryn. *Prodigal Nurse.* New York: Ace, 1963. 127 pp. (P)

Naughton, Bill. *Alfie.* New York: Ballantine, 1966. 221 pp. (P)

Neal, Hilary. *Charge Nurse.* New York: Harlequin, 1965. 159 pp. (P)

Neal, Hilary. *Factory Nurse.* New York: Harlequin, 1961. 191 pp. (P)

Neels, Betty. *Cassandra by Chance.* New York: Harlequin, 1973. 191 pp. (P)

Neels, Betty. *Heaven Is Gentle.* New York: Harlequin, 1974. 187 pp. (P)

Neels, Betty. *The Magic of Living.* New York: Harlequin, 1974. 190 pp. (P)

Neels, Betty. *Nurse in Holland.* New York: Harlequin, 1970. 190 pp. (P)

Neels, Betty. *Surgeon from Holland.* New York: Harlequin, 1970. 192 pp. (P)

Neels, Betty. *Tabitha in Moonlight.* New York: Harlequin, 1975. 192 pp. (P)

Neels, Betty. *Three for a Wedding.* New York: Harlequin, 1973. 189 pp. (P)

Nelson, Marguerite. *Dr. Gail's Dilemma.* New York: Arcadia House, 1968. 173 pp. (P)

Nelson, Marguerite. *Hollywood Nurse.* New York: Macfadden, 1963. 128 pp. (P)

Nelson, Marguerite. *Tropics Nurse.* New York: Thomas Bouregy, 1969. 190 pp.

Nelson, Valerie K. *Nurse Ann Wood.* New York: Harlequin, 1963. 192 pp. (P)

Nelson, Valerie K. *Nurse Jan and Cousin Paul.* New York: Harlequin, 1964. 191 pp. (P)

Nelson, Valerie K. *Two Sisters.* New York: Harlequin, 1962. 192 pp. (P)

Nelson, Valerie K. *Verena Fayre, Probationer.* New York: Harlequin, 1963. 224 pp. (P)

Neubauer, William Arthur. *Nurse Anne's Emergency.* New York: Arcadia House, 1965. 176 pp.

Neubauer, William Arthur. *Nurse Greer.* New York: Arcadia House, 1954. 169 pp.

Neubauer, William Arthur. *Nurse March.* New York: Arcadia House, 1957. 171 pp.

Neubauer, William Arthur. *Nurse of Ward B.* New York: Arcadia House, 1961. 174 pp.

Neubauer, William Arthur. *Nurse To Marry.* New York: Arcadia House, 1959. 168 pp.

Neubauer, William Arthur. *Police Nurse.* New York: Macfadden-Bartell, 1964. 127 pp. (P)

Neubauer, William Arthur. *Prison Nurse.* New York: Arcadia House, 1962. 127 pp. (P)

Neubauer, William Arthur. *The Trouble in Ward J.* New York: Arcadia House, 1964. 191 pp.

Newcomb, Norma. *A Nurse To Marry.* New York: Arcadia House, 1967. 190 pp.

Newell, Hope. *A Cap for Mary Ellis.* New York: Harper and Brothers, 1953. 200 pp.

Newell, Hope. *Mary Ellis, Student Nurse.* New York: Berkley Medallion, 1958. 157 pp. (P)

Nichols, Sarah. *Amy Marsh in Copenhagen.* New York: Curtis, 1973. 157 pp. (P)

Nichols, Sarah. *Amy Marsh in London.* New York: Curtis, 1973. 158 pp. (P)

Nichols, Sarah. *Amy Marsh, TV Nurse.* New York: Curtis, 1972. 189 pp. (P)

Nickson, Hilda. *Nurse Adele.* New York: Harlequin, 1966. 192 pp. (P)

Nickson, Hilda. *Operation Love.* New York: Harlequin, 1962. 190 pp. (P)

Nickson, Hilda. *Surgeon at Witteringham.* New York: Harlequin, 1971. 190 pp. (P)

Nickson, Hilda. *The World of Nurse Mitchell.* New York: Harlequin, 1964. 191 pp. (P)

Nielsen, Virginia. *Marry Me Nurse.* New York: Lancer, 1969. 222 pp. (P)

Nielsen, Virginia. *Nurse in the Navy.* New York: Valentine, 1969. 222 pp. (P)

Norrell, Marjorie. *Change of Duty.* New York: Harlequin, 1970. 192 pp. (P)

Norrell, Marjorie. *Doctor Geyer's Project.* New York: Harlequin, 1967. 191 pp. (P)

Norrell, Marjorie. *Dr. Maitland's Secretary.* New York: Harlequin, 1971. 192 pp. (P)

Norrell, Marjorie. *More than Kind.* New York: Harlequin, 1969. 188 pp. (P)

Norrell, Marjorie. *Nurse Barlow's Jinx.* New York: Harlequin, 1968. 174 pp. (P)

Norrell, Marjorie. *Nurse Deborah.* New York: Harlequin, 1969. 188 pp. (P)

Norrell, Marjorie. *Nurse Kelsey Abroad.* New York: Harlequin, 1971. 188 pp. (P)

Norrell, Marjorie. *Nurse Lavinia's Mistake.* New York: Harlequin, 1968. 189 pp. (P)

Norrell, Marjorie. *Nurse Molly.* New York: Harlequin, 1964. 188 pp. (P)

Norrell, Marjorie. *Pride's Banner.* New York: Harlequin, 1971. 192 pp. (P)

Norrell, Marjorie. *Sister Darling.* New York: Harlequin, 1969. 189 pp. (P)

Norrell, Marjorie. *Staff Nurse Sally.* New York: Harlequin, 1965. 188 pp. (P)

Norrell, Marjorie. *Thank You, Nurse Conway.* New York: Harlequin, 1967. 189 pp. (P)

Norrell, Marjorie. *The Torpington Annexe.* New York: Harlequin, 1966. 190 pp. (P)

Norris, Kathleen. *Beauty's Daughter.* New York: Triangle, 1934. 354 pp.

Norton, Bess. *The Quiet One.* New York: Harlequin, 1959. 192 pp. (P)

Norway, Kate. *Dedication Jones.* New York: Harlequin, 1969. 158 pp. (P)

Norway, Kate. *Paper Halo.* New York: Harlequin, 1970. 158 pp. (P)

Nourse, Alan E. *Star Surgeon.* New York: Scholastic, 1964. 190 pp. (P)

Olivier, Stefan. *I Swear and Vow.* Greenwich, CT: Crest, 1962. 271 pp. (P)

O'More, Peggy. *Disaster Nurse.* New York: Arcadia House, 1965. 190 pp.

O'More, Peggy. *Doctor Angel.* New York: Arcadia House, 1952. 162 pp.

O'More, Peggy. *Door to Door Nurse*. New York: Arcadia House, 1967. 187 pp.

O'More, Peggy. *Emergency Calling Nurse Mallon*. New York: Arcadia House, 1964. 182 pp.

O'More, Peggy. *Harmony Hospital*. New York: Arcadia House, 1967. 159 pp.

O'More, Peggy. *I Love You but . . .* New York: Arcadia House, 1965. 128 pp. (P)

O'More, Peggy. *Love Needs a Nurse*. New York: Hillman, Curl, 1961. 164 pp.

O'More, Peggy. *Medicare Nurse*. New York: Arcadia House, 1967. 152 pp.

O'More, Peggy. *A Nurse Involved*. New York: Arcadia House, 1968. 192 pp. (P)

O'More, Peggy. *Nurse Kathryn*. New York: Arcadia House, 1965. 183 pp.

O'More, Peggy. *Nurse Kathryn and Disaster Nurse*. New York: Manor, 1972. 161 pp.

O'More, Peggy. *Seacliff Nurse*. New York: Arcadia House, 1966. 174 pp. (P)

O'More, Peggy. *Shoreline Nurse*. New York: Arcadia House, 1965. 137 pp.

O'More, Peggy. *Small Town Nurse*. New York: Arcadia House, 1959. 142 pp.

O'More, Peggy. *Stand-by Nurse*. New York: Arcadia House, 1968. 192 pp. (P)

O'More, Peggy. *Surgeon in Uniform*. New York: Grammercy, 1944. 179 pp.

O'More, Peggy. *When a Nurse Needs a Doctor*. New York: Arcadia House, 1961. 183 pp.

Osborne, O. O. *The Rise and Fall of Dr. Carey*. Greenwich, CT: Fawcett, 1958. 207 pp. (P)

Oursler, Will. *Departure Delayed*. New York: Ace, 1947. 164 pp. (P)

Overholtzer, Merle C. *Nurse Loreen's Nightmare*. New York: Avalon, 1981. 186 pp.

Palmer, Bernard, and Palmer, Marjorie. *Sandra Emerson, R.N.* Chicago: Moody, 1966. 127 pp. (P)

Palmer, Bernard, and Palmer, Marjorie. *Student Nurse*. Chicago: Moody, 1960. 125 pp. (P)

Palmer, Florence K. *Surgical Nurse*. New York: Monarch, 1963. 125 pp. (P)

Palmer, Frederick. *Invisible Wounds*. New York: Dodd, Mead, 1925. 432 pp.

Pasternak, Boris. *Doctor Zhivago*. New York: Pantheon, 1958. 559 pp.

Patterson, Norma. *Jenny*. New York: Grosset and Dunlap, 1928. 271 pp.

Patton, Frances Gray. *Good Morning, Miss Dove*. New York: Dodd, Mead, 1947. 218 pp.

Payes, Rachel C. *Peace Corps Nurse*. New York: Avalon, 1967. 189 pp.

Perkins, Barbara. *Dear Doctor Marcus*. New York: Harlequin, 1970. 189 pp. (P)

Perkins, Barbara. *My Sisters and Me*. New York: Harlequin, 1971. 187 pp. (P)

Phillips, Teresa Hyde. *The Prodigal Nurse*. New York: Triangle, 1936. 301 pp.

Pianka, Phyllis Taylor. *Sharon Garrison, Clinic Nurse*. New York: Airmont, 1977. 184 pp. (P)

Piercy, Marge. *Small Changes*. Garden City, NY: Doubleday, 1973. 178 pp.

Pinchot, Ann. *Calling Nurse Adams*. New York: Bantam, 1960. 121 pp. (P)

Pinchot, Ann. *Rival to My Heart*. New York: Bantam, 1943. 124 pp. (P)

Porter, Gene Stratton. *The Harvester*. New York: Grosset and Dunlap, 1911. 564 pp.

Presser, Hilda. *A Love of Her Own*. New York: Harlequin, 1968. 188 pp. (P)

Pressley, Hilda. *Night Superintendent*. New York: Harlequin, 1963. 192 pp. (P)

Pressley, Hilda. *Nurse's Dilemma*. New York: Harlequin, 1965. 192 pp. (P)

Pressley, Hilda. *Senior Staff Nurse*. New York: Harlequin, 1965. 192 pp. (P)

Pressley, Hilda. *Theatre Nurse*. New York: Harlequin, 1960. 160 pp. (P)

Preston, Hilary. *Nurse Angela*. New York: Harlequin, 1959. 159 pp. (P)

Quandt, Albert L. *Big City Nurse*. New York: Original Novels, 1953. 130 pp. (P)

Queen, Ellery. *The Dutch Shoe Mystery: A Problem in Deduction*. New York: New American Library, 1931. 214 pp. (P)

Quentin, Dorothy. *Nurse Sally Dean*. New York: Arcadia House, 1943. 217 pp.

Quintin, Conrad. *Young Doctor Mallory*. New York: Modern Promotions, 1967. 127 pp. (P)

Radford, Ruby L. *Doctor Diane's Decision*. New York: Airmont, 1961. 127 pp. (P)

Radford, Ruby L. *Nancy Dale: Army Nurse*. Racine, WI: Whitman, 1944. 248 pp.

Radford, Ruby L. *Once upon a Spring*. New York: Thomas Bouregy, 1961. 224 pp.

Rae, Patricia. *Charge Nurse*. New York: Zebra, 1980. 365 pp. (P)

Rae, Patricia. *Student Nurse*. New York: Zebra, 1982. 361 pp. (P)

Rae, Patricia. *Trauma Nurse*. New York: Zebra, 1982. 350 pp. (P)

Raef, Laura C. *Nurse in Fashion*. New York: Avalon, 1972. 190 pp.

Raef, Laura C. *Nurse Jan and the Legacy*. New York: Avalon, 1972. 192 pp.

Randall, Rona. *Lab Nurse*. New York: Berkley Medallion, 1958. 128 pp. (P)

Randall, Rona. *Leap in the Dark*. New York: Ace, 1956. 173 pp. (P)

Randall, Rona. *Nurse Stacey Comes Aboard*. New York: Ace, 1958. 158 pp. (P)

Randolph, Ellen. *The Haunting of Nurse Jean*. New York: Valentine, 1968. 221 pp. (P)

Randolph, Ellen. *Nurse of the North Woods*. New York: Macfadden, 1966. 127 pp. (P)

Ravin, Neil. *M.D.* New York: Delacorte, 1981. 372 pp.

Reece, Colleen L. *Nurse Autumn's Secret Love*. New York: Avalon, 1979. 189 pp.

Reece, Colleen L. *Nurse Camilla's Love*. New York: Avalon, 1978. 191 pp.

Reece, Colleen L. *Nurse Julie's Sacrifice*. New York: Avalon, 1980. 188 pp.

Reece, Colleen L. *Nurse of the Crossroads*. New York: Airmont, 1977. 186 pp. (P)

Reed, Barry. *The Verdict*. New York: Bantam, 1981. 246 pp. (P)

Remarque, Erich Maria. *All Quiet on the Western Front*. Boston: Little, Brown, 1929. 291 pp.

Rembo, Kent. *Visiting Hours*. New York: Pinnacle, 1982. 218 pp. (P)

Renault, Mary. *North Face*. New York: William Morrow, 1948. 280 pp.

Renault, Mary. *Promise of Love*. New York: Dell, 1939. 336 pp. (P)

Rey, Margaret, and Rey, H. A. *Curious George Goes to the Hospital*. New York: Scholastic, 1966. 161 pp. (P)

Rinehart, Mary Roberts. *The Doctor*. New York: Farrar and Rinehart, 1936. 386 pp.

Rinehart, Mary Roberts. *K.* Boston: Houghton Mifflin, 1915. 410 pp.

Rinehart, Mary Roberts. *Miss Pinkerton: Adventures of a Nurse Detective*. New York: Farrar and Rinehart, 1932. 382 pp.

Roberts, Mary D. *Get with It, Joan*. New York: Ives Washburn, 1961. 179 pp.

Roberts, Suzanne. *Celebrity Suite Nurse*. New York: Ace, 1965. 127 pp. (P)

Roberts, Suzanne. *Co-Ed in White*. New York: Ace, 1964. 127 pp. (P)

Roberts, Suzanne. *Cross Country Nurse*. New York: Ace, 1967. 159 pp. (P)

Roberts, Suzanne. *Emergency Nurse*. New York: Ace, 1962. 127 pp. (P)

Roberts, Suzanne. *Holly Andrews, Nurse in Alaska*. New York: Dell, 1967. 189 pp. (P)

Roberts, Suzanne. *Hootenanny Nurse*. New York: Ace, 1964. 127 pp. (P)

Roberts, Suzanne. *Hope Farrell's Crusading Nurse*. New York: Arcadia House, 1968. 190 pp. (P)

Roberts, Suzanne. *Julie Jones, Cape Canaveral Nurse*. New York: Ace, 1963. 127 pp. (P)

Roberts, Suzanne. *Nurse Penny*. New York: Thomas Bouregy, 1968. 191 pp.

Roberts, Suzanne. *A Prize for Nurse Darci*. New York: Ace, 1965. 126 pp. (P)

Roberts, Suzanne. *Rangeland Nurse*. New York: Ace, 1967. 127 pp. (P)

Roberts, Suzanne. *Sisters in White*. New York: Ace, 1965. 126 pp. (P)

Roberts, Suzanne. *The Two Dr. Barlowes*. New York: Ace, 1965. 128 pp. (P)

Roberts, Suzanne. *Vietnam Nurse*. New York: Ace, 1966. 142 pp. (P)

Roberts, Virginia. *Nurse Howard's Assignment*. New York: Bantam, 1959. 122 pp. (P)

Roberts, Virginia. *Studio Nurse*. New York: Airmont, 1961. 127 pp. (P)

Roberts, Virginia. *Terry Randolph: Registered Nurse*. New York: Berkley Medallion, 1959. 144 pp. (P)

Roberts, Willo Davis. *Nurse at Mystery Villa*. New York: Ace, 1967. 126 pp. (P)

Roberts, Willo Davis. *Nurse in Danger*. New York: Ace, 1972. 159 pp. (P)

Roberts, Willo Davis. *Nurse Kay's Conquest*. New York: Ace, 1966. 143 pp. (P)

Roberts, Willo Davis. *Nurse Robin*. New York: Lenox Hill, 1973. 167 pp.

Roberts, Willo Davis. *The Nurses*. New York: Ace, 1972. 288 pp. (P)

Roberts, Willo Davis. *Once a Nurse*. New York: Ace, 1966. 190 pp. (P)

Ross, Ann B. *The Murder Cure*. New York: Avon, 1978. 158 pp. (P)

Ross, Dan. *Nurse's Choice*. New York: Avalon, 1972. 183 pp.

Ross, Helaine. *No Tears Tomorrow*. New York: Popular Library, 1964. 126 pp. (P)

Ross, Marilyn. *Decision for Nurse Baldwin*. New York: Paperback Library, 1965. 128 pp. (P)

Ross, Marilyn. *Tread Softly, Nurse Scott*. New York: Paperback Library, 1966. 126 pp. (P)

Ross, Phyllis. *Headline Nurse*. New York: Pocket Books, 1965. 187 pp. (P)

Ross, Phyllis. *Sybil Larson, Hospital Nurse*. New York: Pocket Books, 1963. 167 pp. (P)

Ross, Walter. *The Man with the Miracle Cure*. New York: Macfadden-Bartell, 1965. 240 pp. (P)

Ross, Willim Edward Daniel. *Beauty Doctor's Nurse*. New York: New American Library, 1971. 160 pp. (P)

Ross, William Edward Daniel. *Nurse Ann's Secret*. New York: Avalon, 1981. 159 pp.

Ross, William Edward Daniel. *Nurse Grace's Dilemma*. New York: Avalon, 1982. 174 pp. (P)

Ross, William Edward Daniel. *Nurse in Jeopardy*. New York: Arcadia House, 1967. 161 pp.

Ross, William Edward Daniel. *Nurse in Waiting*. New York: Arcadia House, 1967. 143 pp.

Rossiter, Jane. *Backstage Nurse*. New York: Macfadden, 1963. 128 pp. (P)

Rosten, Leo. *Captain Newman, M.D.* Greenwich, CT: Fawcett, 1956. 272 pp. (P)

Rush, Ann. *Nell Shannon, R.N.* New York: Ace, 1963. 126 pp. (P)

Rush, Ann. *Special Duty Nurse*. New York: Berkley Medallion, 1960. 143 pp. (P)

Rush, Ann. *White Cap of Courage*. New York: Bantam, 1960. 122 pp. (P)

Russell, Sheila MacKay. *A Lamp Is Heavy*. Philadelphia: J. B. Lippincott, 1950. 257 pp.

Ryder, Sabin. *Dr. Stephanie's Decision*. New York: Berkley Medallion, 1959. 140 pp. (P)

Sale, Richard. *Passing Strange*. New York: Ace, 1942. 176 pp. (P)

Sanderson, Nora. *The Taming of Nurse Conway*. New York: Harlequin, 1965. 189 pp. (P)

Sanderson, Nora. *The Two Faces of Nurse Roberts*. New York: Harlequin, 1963. 188 pp. (P)

Sandstrom, Flora. *The Midwife of Pont Clery*. New York: Permabooks, 1958. 217 pp. (P)

Sangster, Margaret E. *Surgical Call*. New York: Sun Dial, 1937. 254 pp.

Sargent, Joan. *Cruise Nurse*. New York: Ace, 1960. 125 pp. (P)

Sargent, Joan. *My Love an Altar*. New York: Ace, 1963. 126 pp. (P)

Sault, Madeline. *Private Duty for Nurse Peggy*. New York: Pyramid, 1965. 157 pp. (P)

Saunders, John Monk. *Wings*. New York: Grosset and Dunlap, 1927. 249 pp.

Saunders, Rubie. *Marilyn Morgan, Cruise Nurse*. New York: New American Library, 1971. 128 pp. (P)

Saunders, Rubie. *Marilyn Morgan, R.N.* New York: New American Library, 1969. 160 pp. (P)

Saunders, Rubie. *Nurse Morgan Sees It Through*. New York: New American Library, 1971. 142 pp. (P)

Saunders, Rubie. *Nurse Morgan's Triumph*. New York: New American Library, 1970. 144 pp. (P)

Schellenberg, Helene Chambers. *Beth Adams, Private Duty Nurse*. New York: Arcadia House, 1964. 190 pp.

Schellenberg, Helene Chambers. *Breath of Life*. New York: Arcadia House, 1968. 192 pp.

Shellenberg, Helene Chambers. *Nurse in Research*. New York: Thomas Bouregy, 1974. 191 pp.

Schellenberg, Helene Chambers. *Nurse's Journey*. New York: Dell, 1967. 155 pp. (P)

Scher, Bertha. *The Torch of Life*. New York: Gem, 1926. 358 pp.

Schulman, Alix Kates. *Memoirs of an Ex-Prom Queen: A Novel*. New York: Knopf, 1972. 389 pp.

Scott, Jane. *A Nurse for Rebel's Run*. New York: Thomas Bouregy, 1960. 220 pp.

Scott, Jane. *Nurse Nancy*. New York: Bantam, 1959. 120 pp. (P)

Sears, Jane L. *Las Vegas Nurse*. New York: Avon, 1963. 143 pp. (P)

Sears, Jane L. *Television Nurse*. New York: Avon, 1963. 144 pp. (P)

Sears, Ruth McCarthy. *Circus Nurse*. New York: Lenox Hill, 1972. 192 pp.

Sears, Ruth McCarthy. *Jolie Benoit, R.N.* New York: Dell, 1970. 157 pp. (P)

Sears, Ruth McCarthy. *Nurse in Acapulco*. New York: Dell, 1971. 156 pp. (P)

Sears, Ruth McCarthy. *Nurse Nora's Folly*. New York: Avalon, 1979. 183 pp.

Sears, Ruth McCarthy. *Nurse of Glen Lock*. New York: Lenox Hill, 1973. 169 pp.

Sears, Ruth McCarthy. *A Nurse's Quest*. New York: Airmont, 1971. 191 pp.

Sears, Ruth McCarthy. *Timberline Nurse*. New York: Dell, 1965. 157 pp. (P)

Seifert, Elizabeth. *Army Doctor*. New York: Aeonian, 1973. 201 pp.

Seifert, Elizabeth. *Bachelor Doctor*. New York: Dodd, Mead, 1969. 257 pp.

Seifert, Elizabeth. *Bright Scalpel*. New York: Popular Library, 1941. 255 pp.

Seifert, Elizabeth. *A Call for Doctor Barton*. New York: Dell, 1956. 221 pp. (P)

Seifert, Elizabeth. *A Certain Doctor French*. New York: Aeonian, 1973. 216 pp.

Seifert, Elizabeth. *Challenge for Dr. Mays*. New York: Dodd, Mead, 1955. 279 pp.

Seifert, Elizabeth. *Doctor at the Crossroads*. New York: Dell, 1954. 224 pp. (P)

Seifert, Elizabeth. *A Doctor Comes to Bayard*. New York: Dell, 1965. 192 pp. (P)

Seifert, Elizabeth. *The Doctor Disagrees*. New York: Dodd, Mead, 1953. 205 pp.

Seifert, Elizabeth. *Doctor Ellison's Decision*. New York: Aeonian, 1973. 188 pp.

Seifert, Elizabeth. *A Doctor for Blue Jay Cove*. New York: Dodd, Mead, 1956. 179 pp.

Seifert, Elizabeth. *A Doctor in Judgement*. New York: Beagle, 1972. 211 pp.

Seifert, Elizabeth. *Doctor in Love*. New York: G. K. Hall, 1975. 182 pp.

Seifert, Elizabeth. *A Doctor in the Family*. New York: Dodd, Mead, 1955. 189 pp.

Seifert, Elizabeth. *Dr. Jeremy's Wife*. New York: Aeonian, 1974. 173 pp.

Seifert, Elizabeth. *The Doctor Makes a Choice*. New York: Dodd, Mead, 1961. 186 pp.

Seifert, Elizabeth. *Doctor of Mercy*. New York: Dodd, Mead, 1951. 240 pp.

Seifert, Elizabeth. *Doctor on Trial*. New York: Dell, 1959. 288 pp. (P)

Seifert, Elizabeth. *Doctor Samaritan*. New York: Dell, 1965. 222 pp. (P)

Seifert, Elizabeth. *The Doctor's Affair*. New York: Dodd, Mead, 1975. 198 pp.

Seifert, Elizabeth. *The Doctor's Bride*. New York: Dodd, Mead, 1960. 186 pp.

Seifert, Elizabeth. *The Doctor's Confession*. New York: Dodd, Mead, 1968. 206 pp.

Seifert, Elizabeth. *Dr. Scott, Surgeon on Call*. New York: Dell, 1963. 189 pp. (P)

Seifert, Elizabeth. *The Doctor's Daughter*. New York: Dodd, Mead, 1974. 224 pp.

Seifert, Elizabeth. *The Doctor's Desperate Hour*. New York: Dodd, Mead, 1959. 231 pp.

Seifert, Elizabeth. *Doctor's Destiny*. New York: Beagle, 1972. 187 pp. (P)

Seifert, Elizabeth. *The Doctor's Husband*. New York: Dodd, Mead, 1957. 183 pp.

Seifert, Elizabeth. *Doctor's Kingdom*. New York: New American Library, 1970. 191 pp. (P)

Seifert, Elizabeth. *The Doctors on Eden Place*. New York: Dodd, Mead, 1959. 196 pp.

Seifert, Elizabeth. *Doctors on Parade*. New York: Dodd, Mead, 1960. 189 pp.

Seifert, Elizabeth. *The Doctor's Private Life*. New York: Dodd, Mead, 1973. 231 pp.

Seifert, Elizabeth. *The Doctor's Promise*. New York: Dodd, Mead, 1972. 227 pp.

Seifert, Elizabeth. *The Doctor's Reputation*. New York: New American Library, 1974. 207 pp. (P)

Seifert, Elizabeth. *The Doctor's Second Love*. New York: Dodd, Mead, 1971. 217 pp.

Seifert, Elizabeth. *The Doctor's Strange Secret*. New York: Dodd, Mead, 1962. 221 pp.

Seifert, Elizabeth. *The Doctor's Two Lives*. New York: J. Curley, 1976. 196 pp.

Seifert, Elizabeth. *The Doctors Were Brothers*. New York: Dodd, Mead, 1978. 231 pp.

Seifert, Elizabeth. *The Doctor Takes a Wife*. New York: Pocket Books, 1962. 233 pp. (P)

Seifert, Elizabeth. *Doctor Tuck*. New York: Dodd, Mead, 1977. 212 pp.

Seifert, Elizabeth. *Doctor with a Mission*. New York: Dodd, Mead, 1967. 192 pp.

Seifert, Elizabeth. *Dr. Woodward's Ambition*. New York: Bantam, 1945. 209 pp. (P)

Seifert, Elizabeth. *For Love of a Doctor*. New York: J. Curley, 1976. 189 pp.

Seifert, Elizabeth. *Four Doctors, Four Wives*. New York: Dodd, Mead, 1975. 203 pp.

Seifert, Elizabeth. *Girl Intern*. New York: Aeonian, 1973. 226 pp.

Seifert, Elizabeth. *Hegerty, M.D.* New York: Pocket Books, 1966. 201 pp. (P)

Seifert, Elizabeth. *Hillbilly Doctor*. New York: Aeonian, 1973. 194 pp.

Seifert, Elizabeth. *Home-Town Doctor*. New York: Dodd, Mead, 1959. 215 pp.

Seifert, Elizabeth. *The Honor of Dr. Shelton*. New York: Dell, 1962. 223 pp. (P)

Seifert, Elizabeth. *Hospital Zone*. New York: Aeonian, 1973. 184 pp.

Seifert, Elizabeth. *Katie's Young Doctor*. New York: Dell, 1964. 192 pp. (P)

Seifert, Elizabeth. *Legacy for a Doctor*. New York: Dell, 1963. 221 pp. (P)

Seifert, Elizabeth. *Love Calls the Doctor*. New York: Dodd, Mead, 1958. 216 pp.

Seifert, Elizabeth. *Lucinda Marries the Doctor*. New York: Dodd, Mead, 1953. 245 pp.

Seifert, Elizabeth. *Miss Doctor*. New York: Dodd, Mead, 1951. 240 pp.

Seifert, Elizabeth. *The New Doctor*. New York: Dodd, Mead, 1958. 306 pp.

Seifert, Elizabeth. *Old Doc*. New York: Aeonian, 1973. 217 pp.

Seifert, Elizabeth. *Ordeal of Three Doctors*. New York: Dodd, Mead, 1969. 265 pp.

Seifert, Elizabeth. *The Problems of Dr. A*. New York: Dodd, Mead, 1963. 231 pp.

Seifert, Elizabeth. *Rebel Doctor*. New York: Dodd, Mead, 1967. 241 pp.

Seifert, Elizabeth. *The Rival Doctors*. New York: Dodd, Mead, 1967. 241 pp.

Seifert, Elizabeth. *The Story of Andrea Fields: Woman and Doctor*. Greenwich, CT: Fawcett, 1950. 256 pp. (P)

Seifert, Elizabeth. *The Strange Loyalty of Dr. Carlisle*. New York: Aeonian, 1973. 196 pp.

Seifert, Elizabeth. *Substitute Doctor*. New York: Dodd, Mead, 1957. 307 pp.

Seifert, Elizabeth. *Surgeon in Charge*. New York: Dodd, Mead, 1942. 256 pp.

Seifert, Elizabeth. *Take Three Doctors*. New York: Aeonian, 1973. 230 pp.

Seifert, Elizabeth. *Thus Doctor Mallory*. New York: Aeonian, 1973. 227 pp.

Seifert, Elizabeth. *To Wed a Doctor*. New York: Dodd, Mead, 1968. 269 pp.

Seifert, Elizabeth. *Two Doctors and a Girl*. New York: Dodd, Mead, 1976. 232 pp.

Seifert, Elizabeth. *Two Doctors, Two Loves*. New York: Dodd, Mead, 1982. 239 pp.

Seifert, Elizabeth. *The Two Faces of Dr. Collier*. New York: Dodd, Mead, 1973. 241 pp.

Seifert, Elizabeth. *When Doctors Marry*. New York: Dodd, Mead, 1960. 226 pp.

Seifert, Elizabeth. *Young Doctor Galahad*. New York: Pocket Books, 1938. 290 pp. (P)

Seifert, Shirley. *The Medicine Man*. New York: J. B. Lippincott, 1971. 243 pp.

Seigel, Benjamin. *Doctors and Wives*. New York: Dell, 1977. 218 pp. (P)

Shann, Renee. *Nurse in Paris*. New York: Lancer, 1968. 253 pp. (P)

Shann, Renee. *Ring for the Nurse*. New York: Berkley Medallion, 1959. 128 pp. (P)

Shann, Renee. *Student Nurse*. New York: Carlton House, 1941. 296 pp.

Shem, Samuel. *The House of God*. New York: Dell, 1978. 419 pp. (P)

Shepard, Fern. *College Nurse*. New York: Arcadia House, 1965. 192 pp. (P)

Shepard, Fern. *Courtroom Nurse*. New York: Arcadia House, 1968. 192 pp.

Shepard, Fern. *Graveyard Nurse*. New York: Arcadia House, 1967. 192 pp.

Shepard, Fern. *Night Nurse*. New York: Avon, 1962. 124 pp. (P)

Shepard, Fern. *Nurse in Danger*. New York: Macfadden, 1963. 128 pp. (P)

Shepard, Fern. *A Nurse's Longing*. New York: Arcadia House, 1965. 127 pp. (P)

Shepard, Fern. *Nurse Under Fire*. New York: Arcadia House, 1964. 189 pp.

Shepard, Fern. *Psychiatric Nurse*. New York: Arcadia House, 1967. 188 pp.

Shepard, Fern. *Sacrifice for Love*. New York: Arcadia House, 1963. 128 pp. (P)

Shiff, Nathan A. *Ambulance Call*. New York: Lancer, 1967. 223 pp. (P)

Shore, Juliet. *Hospital of Bamboo*. New York: Harlequin, 1972. 192 pp. (P)

Shore, Juliet. *The Palm-Thatched Hospital*. New York: Harlequin, 1963. 191 pp. (P)

Slaughter, Frank G. *Battle Surgeon*. New York: Pocket Books, 1944. 263 pp. (P)

Slaughter, Frank G. *Code Five*. New York: Pocket Books, 1971. 287 pp. (P)

Slaughter, Frank G. *Daybreak*. New York: Doubleday, 1958. 320 pp.

Slaughter, Frank G. *Doctors' Wives*. New York: Pocket Books, 1967. 330 pp. (P)

Slaughter, Frank G. *East Side General*. Garden City, NY: Doubleday, 1952. 311 pp.

Slaughter, Frank G. *The Healer*. Garden City, NY: Doubleday, 1955. 316 pp.

Slaughter, Frank G. *A Savage Place*. New York: Pocket Books, 1965. 264 pp. (P)

Slaughter, Frank G. *Spencer Brade, M.D.* New York: Pocket Books, 1942. 316 pp. (P)

Slaughter, Frank G. *Surgeon's Choice*. New York: Popular Library, 1969. 350 pp. (P)

Slaughter, Frank G. *Surgeon, U.S.A.* New York: Pocket Books, 1966. 327 pp. (P)

Slaughter, Frank G. *Sword and Scalpel*. New York: Pocket Books, 1957. 231 pp. (P)

Slaughter, Frank G. *That None Should Die*. New York: Pocket Books, 1941. 390 pp. (P)

Slaughter, Frank G. *Women in White*. New York: Pocket Books, 1974. 377 pp. (P)

Sloan, Gladys. *Professional Passion*. Cleveland: World, 1947. 190 pp.

Smiley, Virginia Kester. *High Country Nurse*. New York: Dell, 1970. 179 pp. (P)

Smiley, Virginia Kester. *Mansion of Mystery*. New York: Dell, 1973. 176 pp. (P)

Smiley, Virginia Kester. *Nurse Delia's Choice*. New York: Avalon, 1967. 192 pp.

Smiley, Virginia Kester. *Nurse for the Civic Center*. New York: Avalon, 1974. 196 pp.

Smiley, Virginia Kester. *Nurse Kate's Mercy Flight*. New York: Ace, 1968. 126 pp. (P)

Smiley, Virginia Kester. *Nurse of the Grand Canyon*. Greenwich, CT: Fawcett, 1973. 128 pp. (P)

Sobel, Irwin Philip. *The Hospital Makers*. Greenwich, CT: Fawcett, 1973. 352 pp. (P)

Somkin, Arnold. *The Crazy World of Julius Vrooder*. New York: Dell, 1974. 173 pp. (P)

Sorrell, Phillip. *Doctors' Women*. New York: Beacon, 1962. 155 pp. (P)

Soubiran, Andre, M.D. *The Doctors*. New York: Popular Library, 1953. 380 pp. (P)

Southam, Gertrude, and Southam, Ethel A. *Hors de Combat, or Three Weeks in a Hospital*. London: Cassell, 1891. 456 pp.

Sparkia, Roy. *Doctors and Lovers*. New York: Pyramid, 1960. 159 pp. (P)

Sparkia, Roy. *Operating Room 4*. New York: Pyramid, 1973. 203 pp. (P)

Sparks, Christine. *The Elephant Man*. New York: Ballantine, 1980. 281 pp. (P)

Starr, Kate. *Wrong Doctor John*. New York: Harlequin, 1966. 192 pp. (P)

Starrett, William. *Nurse Blake at the Front*. New York: Gramercy, 1944.

Starret, William. *Nurse Blake Overseas*. New York: Gramercy, 1943. 210 pp.

Starret, William. *Nurse Blake, U.S.A.* New York: Gramercy, 1942.

Stewart, Donald. *Sanatorium*. London: Chatto and Windus, 1930. 306 pp.

Stinetorf, Louise A. *White Witch Doctor*. New York: Pocket Books, 1950. 261 pp. (P)

Stolz, Mary. *Hospital Zone*. New York: Harper and Row, 1956. 250 pp.

Stolz, Mary. *The Organdy Cupcakes*. New York: Harper and Row, 1951. 213 pp.

Stolz, Mary. *Student Nurse*. New York: Berkley Highland, 1951. 173 pp. (P)

Stone, Fay. *Challenge for Nurse Laurel*. New York: Arcadia House, 1970. 208 pp. (P)

Stone, Fay. *Nurse on Call*. New York: Lenox Hill, 1970. 192 pp.

Stone, Patti. *Beyond the Storm*. New York: Bantam, 1970. 172 pp. (P)

Stone, Patti. *Calling Nurse Linda*. New York: Ace, 1961. 115 pp. (P)

Stone, Patti. *Nina Grant: Pediatric Nurse*. New York: Hillman, 1960. 160 pp. (P)

Stone, Patti. *Sandra: Surgical Nurse*. New York: Bantam, 1961. 122 pp. (P)

Stonebraker, Florence. *Nurse from Alaska*. New York: Arcadia House, 1964. 190 pp.

Stonebraker, Florence. *Nurse Under Fire*. New York: Arcadia House, 1964. 192 pp.

Stonebraker, Florence. *Young Doctor Elliot*. New York: Modern Promotions, 1946. 141 pp. (P)

Stratton, Chris. *Emergency!* New York: Popular Library, 1972. 159 pp. (P)

Stratton, Chris. *Medical Center*. New York: Popular Library, 1970. 192 pp. (P)

Stratton-Porter, Gene. *The Harvester*. New York: Grosset and Dunlap, 1911. 564 pp.

Strong, Charles Stanley. *Nurses' Home*. New York: Phoenix, 1956. 128 pp.

Stuart, Alex. *Spencer's Hospital*. New York: Harlequin, 1962. 224 pp. (P)

Stuart, Florence. *Believe in Miracles*. New York: Arcadia House, 1968. 141 pp. (P)

Stuart, Florence. *Her Doctor's Past*. New York: Arcadia House, 1963. 127 pp. (P)

Stuart, Florence. *Highway Nurse*. New York: Macfadden-Bartell, 1966. 128 pp. (P)

Stuart, Florence. *Hope Wears White*. New York: Ace, 1961. 128 pp. (P)

Stuart, Florence. *The New Nurse*. New York: Arcadia House, 1947. 126 pp. (P)

Stuart, Florence. *The Nurse and the Crystal Ball*. New York: Arcadia House, 1969. 173 pp. (P)

Stuart, Florence. *The Nurse and the Orderly*. New York: Arcadia House, 1964. 224 pp.

Stuart, Florence. *A Nurse Named Courage*. New York: Pyramid, 1967. 127 pp. (P)

Stuart, Florence. *A Nurse's Nightmare*. New York: Arcadia House, 1967. 128 pp. (P)

Stuart, Florence. *Nurse Under Fire*. New York: Modern Promotions, 1964. 126 pp. (P)

Stuart, Florence. *Research Nurse*. New York: Macfadden, 1967. 128 pp. (P)

Stuart, Florence. *Runaway Nurse*. New York: Macfadden, 1963. 126 pp. (P)

Stuart, Florence. *Strange Triangle*. New York: Arcadia House, 1964. 128 pp. (P)

Stuart, Vivian. *Nurse in Malaya*. New York: Harlequin, 1960. 192 pp. (P)

Taber, Gladys. *Nurse in Blue*. Philadelphia: Blakiston, 1944. 250 pp.

Tatham, Julie. *Cherry Ames at Spencer*. New York: Grossett and Dunlap, 1949. 213 pp.

Tatham, Julie. *Cherry Ames, Clinic Nurse*. New York: Grossett and Dunlap, 1952. 208 pp.

Tatham, Julie. *Cherry Ames, Country Doctor's Nurse*. New York: Grossett and Dunlap, 1955. 214 pp.

Tatham, Julie. *Cherry Ames, Dude Ranch Nurse*. New York: Grossett and Dunlap, 1953. 210 pp.

Tatham, Julie. *Cherry Ames, Mountaineer Nurse*. New York: Grossett and Dunlap, 1951. 212 pp.

Tatham, Julie. *Cherry Ames, Night Supervisor*. New York: Grossett and Dunlap, 1950. 209 pp.

Tatham, Julie. *Cherry Ames, Rest Home Nurse.* New York: Grossett and Dunlap, 1954. 214 pp.

Tennyson, Alfred. *Poems.* Boston: Ginn and Company, 1903. 221 pp.

Thompson, Jim. *The Alcoholics.* New York: Zenith, 1953. 127 pp. (P)

Thompson, Morton. *Not as a Stranger.* New York: New American Library, 1954. 790 pp. (P)

Thompson, Sydney. *Dr. Parrish, Resident.* Philadelphia: Blakiston, 1944. 250 pp.

Thorne, Emily. *Small Town Nurse.* New York: Avon, 1956. 126 pp. (P)

Treibich, S. J. *Burwyck's Wander.* New York: Lancer, 1967. 221 pp. (P)

Trench, Caroline. *Nurse Warding Takes Charge.* New York: Harlequin, 1957. 191 pp. (P)

Truax, Rhoda. *Hospital.* New York: E. P. Dutton, 1932. 312 pp.

Trumbo, Dalton. *Johnny Got His Gun.* New York: Bantam, 1939. 243 pp.

Ullman, James Ramsey. *Windom's Way.* New York: J. B. Lippincott, 1952. 286 pp.

Uren, Rhona. *Nurse Foster.* London: Mills and Boon, 1980. 160 pp. (P)

Uris, Leon. *Exodus.* Garden City, NY: Doubleday, 1958. 626 pp.

Van Atta, Winfred. *Shock Treatment.* Greenwich, CT: Fawcett, 1961. 160 pp. (P)

Vandercook, Margaret. *The Red Cross Girls with the Russian Army.* Philadelphia: John C. Winston, 1917. 265 pp.

van der Meersch, Maxence. *The Strange Diagnosis.* New York: Hillman, 1960. 191 pp. (P)

Van Dine, S. S. *The Garden Murder Case.* New York: Scribner's, 1935. 332 pp.

Van Hoosen, Bertha. *Petticoat Surgeon.* Chicago: Pellegrini and Cudahy, 1947. 324 pp.

Van Zandt, Eleanor, ed. *Hit Parade of Nurse Stories.* New York: Scholastic, 1964. 156 pp. (P)

Vinton, Anne. *Nurse to the Cruise.* New York: Harlequin, 1960. 189 pp. (P)

Voss, Carroll. *White Cap for Rechinda.* New York: Ives Washburn, 1966. 171 pp.

Vroman, Mary Elizabeth. *Esther.* New York: Bantam, 1963. 154 pp. (P)

Wagnalls, Mabel. *The Rose-Bush of a Thousand Years.* New York: Funk and Wagnalls, 1919. 77 pp.

Walsh, Patricia L. *Forever Sad the Hearts.* New York: Avon, 1982. 385 pp. (P)

Ward, Mary Jane. *The Snake Pit.* New York: Random House, 1946. 277 pp.

Ward, Mrs. Humphry. *Marcella.* Boston: Houghton Mifflin, 1911. 942 pp.

Warner, Anne. *The Rejuvenation of Aunt Mary.* Boston: Little, Brown, 1911. 323 pp.

Warren, Beatrice. *Nurse in Yosemite.* New York: Avalon, 1982. 192 pp. (P)

Warren, Beatrice. *Nurse Paula's New Look.* New York: Avalon, 1982. 189 pp. (P)

Warren, Maude Radford. *The House of Youth.* Indianapolis: Bobbs-Merrill, 1923. 376 pp.

Warren, Paulette. *Nurse of Brooding Mansion.* New York: Lancer, 1967. 176 pp. (P)

Way, Isabel Stewart. *Calling Nurse Lorrie.* New York: Thomas Bouregy, 1972. 192 pp.

Way, Isabel Stewart. *Dr. Jenny of Timberland.* New York: Avon, 1964. 143 pp. (P)

Way, Isabel Stewart. *Fighting Dr. Diana.* New York: Airmont, 1973. 192 pp. (P)

Way, Isabel Stewart. *Nurse Christy.* New York: Thomas Bouregy, 1968. 192 pp.

Way, Isabel Stewart. *Nurse in Love.* New York: Avon, 1963. 128 pp. (P)

Webb, Jean Francis. *Nurse from Hawaii.* New York: Avalon, 1964. 192 pp.

Webb, Jean Francis. *Nurse on Horseback.* New York: Bouregy and Curl, 1952.

Weiner, Gina Ingoglio. *Pepper Plays Nurse.* New York: Golden, 1964. 22 pp. (P)

Weinstein, Alfred A. *The Scalpel's Edge.* New York: Lancer, 1964. 399 pp. (P)

Welch, Maud McCurdy. *Country Nurse.* New York: Lancer, 1959. 128 pp. (P)

Welch, Maud McCurdy. *Nurse Carol.* New York: Avalon, 1955. 131 pp.

Welch, Maud McCurdy. *Nurses Marry Doctors.* New York: Airmont, 1956. 126 pp. (P)

Welch, Maud McCurdy. *Special Nurse.* New York: Lancer, 1967. 128 pp. (P)

Wells, Helen. *Cherry Ames, Army Nurse.* New York: Grosset and Dunlap, 1944. 214 pp.

Wells, Helen. *Cherry Ames at Hilton Hospital.* New York: Grosset and Dunlap, 1959. 180 pp.

Wells, Helen. *Cherry Ames, Boarding School Nurse.* New York: Grosset and Dunlap, 1955. 212 pp.

Wells, Helen. *Cherry Ames, Camp Nurse.* New York: Grosset and Dunlap, 1957. 182 pp.

Wells, Helen. *Cherry Ames, Chief Nurse.* New York: Grosset and Dunlap, 1944. 213 pp.

Wells, Helen. *Cherry Ames, Companion Nurse.* New York: Grosset and Dunlap, 1964. 178 pp.

Wells, Helen. *Cherry Ames, Cruise Nurse.* New York: Grosset and Dunlap, 1948. 216 pp.

Wells, Helen. *Cherry Ames, Department Store Nurse.* New York: Grosset and Dunlap, 1956. 212 pp.

Wells, Helen. *Cherry Ames, Flight Nurse.* New York: Grosset and Dunlap, 1945. 215 pp.

Wells, Helen. *Cherry Ames, Island Nurse.* New York: Grosset and Dunlap, 1960. 184 pp.

Wells, Helen. *Cherry Ames, Private Duty Nurse.* New York: Grosset and Dunlap, 1946. 216 pp.

Wells, Helen. *Cherry Ames, Senior Nurse.* New York: Grosset and Dunlap, 1944. 217 pp.

Wells, Helen. *Cherry Ames, Staff Nurse.* New York: Grosset and Dunlap, 1962. 177 pp.

Wells, Helen. *Cherry Ames, Student Nurse.* New York: Grosset and Dunlap, 1943. 213 pp.

Wells, Helen. *Cherry Ames, Veterans' Nurse.* New York: Grosset and Dunlap, 1946. 216 pp.

Wells, Helen. *Cherry Ames, Visiting Nurse.* New York: Grosset and Dunlap, 1947. 216 pp.

Wellsley, Julie. *The Fateful Tide.* New York: Modern Promotions, 1967. 128 pp. (P)

Wesley, Elizabeth. *Doctor Dee.* New York: Bantam, 1960. 120 pp. (P)

Wesley, Elizabeth. *The Patient in 711.* New York: Dell, 1972. 146 pp. (P)

West, Rebecca. *War Nurse.* New York: A. L. Burt, 1930. 265 pp.

Westbrook, Robert. *The Magic Garden of Stanley Sweetheart.* New York: Bantam, 1969. 214 pp. (P)

Weverka, Robert. *I Love My Wife.* New York: Bantam, 1971. 152 pp. (P)

Wharton, Edith. *Ethan Frome.* New York: Scribner's, 1911. 489 pp.

Wharton, Edith. *The Fruit of the Tree.* New York: Scribner's, 1907. 633 pp.

White, W. L. *They Were Expendable.* New York: Harcourt, Brace, 1942. 205 pp.

Whitten, Kathryn Marion. *The Horses of the Sun.* Boston: Meador, 1942. 314 pp.

Whittington, Harry. *The Young Nurses.* New York: Pyramid, 1961. 157 pp. (P)

Williams, Rose. *Airport Nurse.* New York: Valentine, 1968. 190 pp. (P)

Williams, Rose. *Department Store Nurse.* New York: Belmont, 1967. 86 pp. (P)

Williams, Rose. *Five Nurses.* New York: Pyramid, 1964. 128 pp. (P)

Williams, Rose. *Nurse in Doubt.* New York: Pyramid, 1965. 144 pp. (P)

Williams, Rose. *Nurse in Jeopardy.* New York: Lancet, 1966. 144 pp. (P)

Williams, Rose. *Nurse in Nassau.* New York: Arcadia House, 1967. 206 pp. (P)

Wilmont, Robert Patrick. *Blood in Your Eye.* New York: Pocket Books, 1953. 213 pp. (P)

Wilson, Harry Leon. *Oh, Doctor!* New York: Grosset and Dunlap, 1929. 261 pp.

Wood, Nancy. *The New Adventures of the Nurses.* New York: Ace, 1973. 282 pp. (P)

Wood, Nancy. *The Nurses.* New York: Ace, 1973. 282 pp. (P)

Worley, Dorothy. *Cinderella Nurse.* New York: Lancer, 1962. 237 pp. (P)

Worley, Dorothy. *Dr. Jeffrey's Awakening.* New York: Thomas Bouregy, 1961. 221 pp.

Worley, Dorothy. *Dr. John's Decision.* New York: Bantam, 1958. 122 pp. (P)

Worley, Dorothy. *Dr. Kilbourne Comes Home.* New York: Ace, 1954. 108 pp. (P)

Worley, Dorothy. *Dr. Michael's Challenge.* New York: Berkley Medallion, 1960. 144 pp. (P)

Worley, Dorothy. *Doctor's Nurse.* New York: Popular Library, 1961. 125 pp. (P)

Worley, Dorothy. *The High Road.* New York: Dell, 1962. 157 pp. (P)

Worthy, Judith. *Nurse at Sea.* London: Mills and Boon, 1981. 189 pp. (P)

Wyndham, Lee. *Candy Stripers.* New York: Julian Messner, 1958. 191 pp.

Wyndham, Lee. *The Lady with the Lamp.* New York: Scholastic, 1970. 191 pp. (P)

Yoder, Marie A. *The Nurse's Victory.* Grand Rapids, MI: Zondervan, 1962. 158 pp.

Young, Agatha. *The Town and Dr. Moore.* Greenwich, CT: Fawcett, 1963. 351 pp. (P)

Young, Edward. *Hospital Doctor.* New York: Pyramid, 1938. 190 pp.

MAGAZINE ARTICLES

Abbott, L.F. "Hospital Impressions." *Outlook* 139 (April 8, 1925): 525–26.

"America's Health: Supply of Nurses." *Today's Health* 28 (November 1950): 46.

Ames, M. "Fifty Ways to Use the Hourly Nurse." *Hygeia* 9 (December 1931): 115–17.

"Angel: Nurse on Duty During Construction of Union Carbide Skyscraper."

New Yorker 35 (November 28, 1959): 41–42.

"Angel with the Thermometer." *Saturday Evening Post* 197 (February 7, 1925): 39.

"Angry Women in White." *Newsweek* 29 (May 26, 1947): 62.

"Army's First Man Nurse." *Scholastic* 67 (October 20, 1955): 15.

Aynes, E.A., and Stuart, N.G. "Coming Scandal in Nursing." *McCalls* 91 (March 1964): 100–101.

Balcome, M. "Modern Nursing in the Home." *Harper's Bazaar* 35 (July 1901): 244–47.

Banfield, M. "Bathing the Sick." *Ladies' Home Journal* 20 (March 1903): 24.

Banfield, M. "Giving of Medicines." *Ladies' Home Journal* 20 (April 1903): 24.

Banfield, M. "Ventilation and Disinfection of Sick-Room." *Ladies' Home Journal* 20 (January 1903): 22.

Barrett, G. "Making the Rounds with a Nurse." *New York Times Magazine*, 108 (November 15, 1959): 17.

Barry, J. "Bedside Manners." *Ladies' Home Journal* 63 (February 1946): 187.

Bauer, W.W. "Knocking at Your Door." *Hygeia* 8 (December 1930): 145–51.

Bax, E. "Are Nurses Overpaid?" *Hygeia* 9 (August 1931): 727–31.

Baylee, J.T. "Army Nursing Reform and Men Nurses." *Westminster Review* 155 (March 1901): 235–37.

Beatty, J. "She Never Gave Up: Lifesaver Lillian Wald." *Forum* 96 (August 1936):70–73.

"Behind the Masks: Head Nurses Who Played Key Roles in the World's First Transplants of Human Hearts." *Time* 91 (March 1, 1968): 36.

Berg, R.H. "Where Did All the Nurses Go?" *Look* 32 (January 23, 1968): 26.

"Blonde Curls and Stern Tasks: Story of the Army Nurse." *Newsweek* 37 (March 12, 1951): 50–52.

Blue, R. "Lookout on the Mountain." *Ladies' Home Journal* 37 (April 1920): 45.

Blumer, G.A. "Nursing the Wounded Civilian." *Nation* 106 (January 24, 1918): 89.

"Bootleg Nurses." *Time* 31 (January 24, 1938): 33.

"Boys Jeered Her, V. Jaspers." *Newsweek* 48 (September 10, 1956): 90.

Breckinridge, M. "Maternity in the Mountains." *North American Review* 226 (December 1928): 765.

Breckinridge, M. "Nurse on Horseback." *Woman's Journal* 13 (February 1928): 5–7.

Bromley, D.D. "Career for College Girls." *Harper's* 195 (June 1942): 76–82.

Bromley, D.D. "Crisis in Nursing." *Harper's* 161 (July 1930): 159–71.

Bromley, D.D. "Do You Want To Be a Nurse?" *Good Housekeeping* 114 (March 1942): 42–43.

Bruce, H.A. "When Illness Is in the Home." *Good Housekeeping* 80 (June 1925): 51.

Bruere, M.B. "Impossible Profession: Nurse, the Doctor and the Third Partner." *Century* 113 (September 1926): 584–92.

Butts, M.F. "Concerning Care-Taking." *Outlook* 48 (September 2, 1983): 435–36.

"Call for Women To Volunteer." *Literary Digest* 57 (June 22, 1918): 30.

Candau, M.G. "World Needs Nurses." *Rotarian* 84 (May 1954): 8.

"Careers in Brief: Nursing." *Scholastic* 34 (April 29, 1939): 4.

"Careers in Nursing." *Changing Times* 16 (December 1962): 29–30.

Carter, G. "Medicine's Forgotten Women." *Reporter* 26 (March 1, 1962): 35–37.

Case, V. "Good Morning, I'm the County Nurse." *Saturday Evening Post* 213 (May 7, 1941): 36.

Casey, C.M. "Uncle Sam Needs Nurses!" *Scholastic* 39 (December 8, 1941): 29.

Chamberlain, M.E. "Obligation of Empire." *North American Review* 170 (April 1900): 498–503.

Chow, M. "Nurses for China's Army." *Independent Woman* 23 (December 1944): 366–67.

Clift, E. "New Family Doctor Is a Nurse." *McCalls* 103 (October 1975): 35.

Cole, A.M.F. "French Red Cross Nurses." *Catholic World* 87 (July 1908): 522–30.

"Compulsory Training in Nursing." *Literary Digest* 60 (February 8, 1919): 26–27.

Comstock, S. "Home Nurse Militant." *Good Housekeeping* 61 (September, October, November 1915): 280–88, 421–29, 588–96.

Connolly, V. "Angels in Blue Gingham: Household Nursing Association, Boston." *Good Housekeeping* 103 (November 1936): 62–63.

Coolidge, E.L. "What To Do When the Baby Is Sick." *Ladies' Home Journal* 20 (April, May 1903): 38, 37.

Coppage, N. "It's Supernurse to the Rescue: The Pediatric Nurse Associate." *Parents Magazine* 47 (July 1972): 54.

"Correspondence School Nurses." *Hygeia* 5 (May 1927): 254.

Coser, R.L., and Lewis, L. "Hospitals Can Give Patients a Break." *Look* 23 (July 7, 1959): 23–25.

Courtney, W.B. "Angel in Furs: M. Keaton, Sweetheart of Alaska." *Collier's* 100 (November 20, 1937): 67.

Cutting, M.S. "Amateur Nurse and Patient." *Harper's Bazaar* 44 (July 1910): 446–47.

Dagett, M.P. "Our Lady with the Lamp." *Good Housekeeping* 63 (November 1916): 34–35.

Davis, M.L. "Grendel Walks Again: Amateur Nurse in an Epidemic." *Atlantic Monthly* 144 (August 1929): 173–85.

Davis, R.H. "Trained Nurse." *Independent* 63 (October 3, 1907): 814–16.

Delano, J.A. "Red Cross Nursing as a Career for Girls." *St. Nicholas Magazine* 44 (August 1917): 880–81.

Deming, D. "Hilltop Benny." *Hygeia* 9 (February 1931): 116–51.

Deming, D. "Practical Nursing, Career for Women Under Fifty." *Today's Health* 30 (December 1952): 32–33.

De Pledge, J.L. "History and Progress of Nursing in Poor-Law Infirmaries." *Westminster Review* 142 (August 1894): 173–82.

"Diary of Captivity, by a Polish Nurse: Seizure of a Front-Line Polish Hospital by the Bolsheviks." *Atlantic Monthly* 165 (February, March 1940): 347–60.

Dix, R.D. "Night Nurse on Duty." *Hygeia* 14 (January 1936): 57.

Drake, K. "Our Flying Nightingales in Vietnam." *Reader's Digest* 91 (December 1967): 73–79.

Earl, H.G. "Your Next Nurse May Be a Man." *Today's Health* 44 (February 1966): 38–39.

"Eight-Year Survey Finds Hospitals Train Too Many Nurses." *Newsweek* 4 (October 6, 1934): 28.

"Elizabeth Caps Some 'Nurses' Among Schoolgirls." *Rotarian* 78 (April 1951): 37.

Ellison, J.C. "I've Had a Thousand Babies." *Saturday Evening Post* 225 (June 6, 1953): 22–23.

Ely, H. "The Most Wounded, the Most Sick, the Most Tired." *Reader's Digest* 58 (June 1951): 9–10.

"Emergency Angel." *Look* 21 (April 2, 1957): 105–9.

"Everybody's Favorite Nurse: Barbara Lloyd." *Look* 24 (March 15, 1960): 100–104.

Favel, W. "Professional Nurse." *Scholastic* 52 (April 26, 1948): 23.

Faville, K. "So She Wants To Be a Nurse." *Survey* 68 (April 1, 1932): 35–37.

Fenwick, E.G. "Evolution of the Trained Nurse." *Outlook* 64 (January 6, 1900): 56–57.

Fenwick, E.G. "State Registration of Trained Nurses." *Nineteenth Century* 67 (June 1910): 1049–60.

Ferguson, H.M. "State Registration of Nurses." *Nineteenth Century* 55 (February 1904): 310–17.

Fischl, I. "Why Are Nurses Shook-up over Abortion." *Look* 35 (February 9, 1971): 66.

Fishbein, M. "Nursing as a Career." *Hygeia* 25 (December 1947): 915.

"Flight Angel, Charlotte Cooley." *Cosmopolitan* 134 (May 1953): 112–21.

Foley, M. "Her Lamp Still Shines: Florence Nightingale." *Good Housekeeping* 117 (July 1943): 34–35.

Folks, H.J. "Be a Nurse and See the World." *Independent Woman* 20 (October 1941): 300–302.

Fox, E.G. "Professional Nursing as a Career." *Woman's Home Companion* 49 (April 1922): 20.

France, B. "If Illness Comes Which Type of Nurse Should You Engage?" *Good Housekeeping* 106 (April 1938): 235–38.

"Frontier Nurse." *Literary Digest* 124 (August 28, 1937): 12.

Fulton, S. "Home Care of the Sick." *Cosmopolitan* 28 (January 1900): 283–89.

Furnas, J.C. "House that Saves Lives in Liberia." *Saturday Evening Post* 225 (May 16, 1953): 22–23.

Gilkey, H.H. "Does Higher Education Have an Obligation for Nursing Education?" *School & Society* 77 (February 14, 1953): 101–3.

"Good Voyage Home: Flight Nurse." *Woman's Home Companion* 78 (July 1951): 21–25.

Gordon, E. "Needed: 50,000 Nurses." *New York Times Magazine* 91 (April 12, 1942): 10–11.

Gordon, H.P. "Nursing: A Changing Profession." *School & Society* 69 (April 9, 1949): 265–68.

Grafton, S. "Too Busy for Back Rubs: Today's Nurse is an Executive!" *McCalls* 86 (September 1959): 52–53.

Gross, L. "Introducing: The Supernurse." *McCalls* 98 (March 1971): 75.

Haldane, E.S. "Nursing as a Profession." *Nineteenth Century* 92 (September 1922): 442–48.

Hale, T. "What's Wrong with American Hospitals? A Doctor's Opinion: Nursing Shortage." *Saturday Review* 50 (February 4, 1967): 62–65.

Harger, M. "What's the Matter with Farm Health?" *Outlook* 130 (March 29, 1922): 507–8.

Harrison, E. "Home Nursing of Today." *Harper's Bazaar* 39 (July 1905): 659–61.

Hassenplug, L.W. "Nurse's Cap for You?" *National Parent-Teacher* 50 (June 1956): 7–8.

Hawes, E. "There's a Career in Nursing." *Woman's Home Companion* 70 (January 1943): 66–67.

"Help Wanted." *Commonweal* 62 (August 26, 1955): 510.

Herrick, C.T. "How To Care for a Sick Child." *Harper's Bazaar* 33 (January 27, 1900): 67.

Hewlett, L.A. "Home Nursing." *Woman's Home Companion* 47 (May 1920): 64–66.

Hickey, M. "Nurses: A Major National Need." *Ladies' Home Journal* 72 (June 1955): 29.

Hirschowitz, R.G. "Psychiatric Nurse: Fox or Hedgehog?" *Mental Hygiene* 54 (January 1970): 123–28.

Hoffman, B.H. "Junior Home Nurses: Teensters in Princeton, NJ." *Ladies' Home Journal* 60 (May 1943): 26–29.

Hoffman, R. "Angel of Mercy Is Dead." *Mademoiselle* 66 (December 1967): 134–35.

Holland, S. "State Registration of Nurses." *Nineteenth Century* 68 (July 1910): 143–47.

Horn, F.H. "Nurses for Our New World." *School & Society* 69 (April 9, 1949): 257–60.

Hosokawa, B. "Angel of the Hills: Teller County, Colorado." *Saturday Evening Post* 228 (May 26, 1956): 44–45.

Howard, M. "Nursing the Poor in Their Homes." *Nineteenth Century* 44 (November 1898): 834–39.

Hunt, M. "Have the New Nurses Come to Your Town?" *Woman's Home Companion* 79 (September 1952): 36–37.

Hunter, H.R. "Training Black Mammies." *Hygeia* 6 (July 1928): 395–97.

Hunter, Mrs. "Hospital Nursing." *Review of Reviews* 3 (June 1891): 505–6.

"If Boss Hires Nurse." *Business Week* 23 (March 20, 1937): 45.

Ingells, D.J. and Whitman, H. "Don't Curse the Nurse." *Collier's* 119 (May 31, 1947): 26.

"Interested in Being a Licensed Practical Nurse?" *Good Housekeeping* 149 (July 1959): 115.

Irwin, H.A. "Profession of Nursing." *Woman's Home Companion* 41 (October 1914): 34.

Jackson, E.M. "Future of District Nursing." *Nineteenth Century* 102 (October 1927): 494–99.

Jacobsen, R.S. "Why I Went Back to Nursing." *Saturday Evening Post* 230 (August 3, 1957): 26–27.

James, P. "Men as Nurses and the Hamilton Association for Providing Trained Male Nurses." *Westminster Review* 147 (March 1897): 309–10.

"Jobscope: Nonhospital Nursing Opportunities." *Mademoiselle* 66 (December 1967): 144–45.

Johnson, C. "Life, Death and Miracles: Student Nurse in Her First Year." *Seventeen* 22 (December 1963): 80–81.

Johnston, M.F. "Case Against Hospital Nurses." *Nineteenth Century* 51 (April 1902): 596–603.

Johnston, M.F., et al. "Questions of the Modern Trained Nurses." *Nineteenth Century* 51 (June 1902): 966–79.

Jones, M.C.R. "Training of a Nurse." *Scribner's Monthly* 8 (November 1890): 613–24.

Kane, H. "Nurse and Her Patient." *American Mercury* 19 (February 1930): 189–92.

Kearney, C. "Nurses Are Human." *Scribner's Monthly* 96 (July 1934): 46–48.

"Keep the Patient Comfortable." *Popular Mechanics* 79 (April 1943): 14–15.

Klein, H.H. "Rural Nursing Association." *Good Housekeeping* 49 (August 1909): 223–24.

Krueger, C. "Do Bad Girls Become Good Nurses?" *Trans-Action* 5 (July 1968): 31–36.

Kruger, D.H. "Bargaining and the Nursing Profession." *Monthly Labor Review* 84 (July 1961): 699–705.

"Lady in GI White." *Newsweek* 28 (November 11, 1946): 71.

Lake, A. "Andrea: A Nurse Who Cares." *Ladies' Home Journal* 82 (August 1965): 74–75.

Lewis, L., and Coser, R.L. "Hospitals Can Give Patients a Break." *Look* 23 (July 7, 1959): 23–25.

Liickes, E.C.E. "State Registration of Nurses." *Nineteenth Century* 55 (May 1904): 827–39.

Lin, T. "Nurse Training for China." *Independent Woman* 20 (December 1941): 363.

McCaul, E. "Army Nursing." *Nineteenth Century* 49 (April 1901): 580–87.

McCracken, E. "Nursing the Wounded Civilian." *Nation* 105 (December 13, 1917): 663–64.

MacCracken, N. "Girls Who Want To Go to France: Vassar College Training Camp for Nurses." *Independent* 94 (May 11, 1918): 248.

McGee, A.N. "Nurses and Nursing: American Nurses in Japan." *Century* 69 (April 1905): 895–906.

McLaughlin, K. "Needed: More Nurses." *New York Times Magazine* 90 (March 9, 1941): 9.

McMurdy, R. "Chicago Training School for Nurses." *Outlook* 69 (November 9, 1901): 662.

"Making Nurses in Eight Weeks." *Literary Digest* 68 (March 5, 1921): 22–23.

Mansfield, R. "If You Hire a Baby Nurse." *McCalls* 88 (March 1961): 180C–180D.

Marley, F. "Training Nurses for War." *Hygeia* 21 (November 1943): 788–89.

Martin, J. "Hospitals Without Nurses." *National* 201 (October 18, 1965): 245–46.

Martin. L.G. "Angels of Viet Nam: U. S. Military Nurses." *Today's Health* 45 (August 1967): 16–23.

Maxwell, A. "Girl With a Future." *Woman's Home Companion* 71 (September 1944): 88–89.

"Men as Nurses." *America* 94 (October 22, 1955): 89.

Merrick, E. "Cross Section: People Encountered by a District Nurse During the Course of a Snowy Day." *Scribner's Monthly* 96 (September 1934): 175–79.

Merrick, E. "Northern Nurse." *Scholastic* 41 (January 10, 1944): 25–26.

"Mike the Cop Studies to be Mike the Nurse." *Life* 70 (May 14, 1971): 47–48.

Miles, D. "Heroines on Horseback." *Collier's* 118 (August 31, 1946): 24–26.

Miller, F. "Celebration for Mary Donnelly, Block Island's Public Health Nurse." *Reader's Digest* 103 (October 1973): 122–27.

"Ministering Blue Angel of Mercy." *Literary Digest* 123 (June 12, 1937): 16.

"Misuse of Nursing Talent." *Science Digest* 67 (January 1970): 56.

"Mobilizing Women as Nurses." *Literary Digest* 57 (April 27, 1918): 33.

"More Glamour, Pay, Glory Needed To Attract Nurses." *Science Newsletter* 88 (August 7, 1965): 89.

Moss, M. "Evolution of the Trained Nurse." *Atlantic Monthly* 91 (May 1903): 587–99.

Murphy, M. "My Most Sweetest Smile: Interview with A. Bry, Nurse on Dutch Transports." *New Yorker* 18 (October 24, 1942): 53–60.

Murray, F. "For Services Rendered." *Collier's* 155 (May 19, 1945): 33.

Murray, G.H. "Home Nursing Helps: Vital Things You Should Know How To Do." *Parents Magazine* 14 (April 1930): 25.

Myers, P. "Mountain Mothers of Kentucky." *Hygeia* 7 (April 1929): 353–56.

"Need for Nurses." *Time* 38 (October 12, 1941): 81.

Nelson, J. "Calling All Nurses." *Independent Woman* 22 (May 1943): 138–40.

Nelson, J. "Nurses for Our Fighting Men: Nation's Womanpower Shortage." *Independent Woman* 24 (February 1945): 34–35.

"New Measure of Devotion." *Scribner's Monthly* 66 (August 1919): 251–52.

"New Mother's Best Friend: The Visiting Nurse." *Ladies' Home Journal* 71 (June 1954): 23.

"Next Advance in Public Health." *New Republic* 31 (July 12, 1922): 175–76.

Nightingale, F. "Trained Nurses." *Century* 81 (November 1910): 159–60.

"Nightingale Needed." *Time* 40 (December 28, 1942): 55.

Noyes, C.D. "Message to American Girls." *St. Nicholas Magazine* 45 (August 1918): 879–81.

"Nurse Betty." *Time* 43 (October 7, 1946): 50.

"Nurse! Nurse!" *Time* 63 (April 12, 1954): 79.

"Nurses." *Outlook* 52 (August 3, 1895): 190.

"Nurse's Aid Society." *Harper's Bazaar* 33 (January 13, 1900): 33.

"Nurses Are Being Shortchanged." *Life* 61 (January 23, 1966): 6.

"Nurses Have Not Lagged Behind." *Saturday Evening Post* 217 (April 28, 1945): 108.

"Nurse Shortage." *Survey* 83 (September 1947): 256–57.

"Nurses in Los Angeles: Concurrent Conventions of Three National Nurses' Associations." *Time* 28 (July 1936): 41–43.

"Nurses Needed." *Outlook* 119 (July 17, 1918): 439.

"Nurses of Five Wars." *New York Times Magazine* 91 (June 21, 1942): 18–19.

"Nurse's Voice." *Literary Digest* 55 (November 10, 1917): 27.

"Nurses with Gloves." *Literary Digest* 68 (March 26, 1921): 69.

"Nursing as a Calling." *Spectator* 79 (September 4, 1897): 305–6.

"Nursing as a Career for Both Girls and Men." *School & Society* 69 (April 9, 1949): 261–62.

"Nursing Is Emerging as a Profession." *Literary Digest* 118 (November 10, 1934): 17.

"Nursing Service by the Hour." *Hygeia* 4 (September 1926): 533.

Nye, A., and Smith, L. "Feminine Enough To Mother You, Tough Enough To Bark." *Today's Health* 50 (May 1972): 22–25.

Oldfield, J. "Nurse of the Future." *Westminster Review* 164 (December 1905): 655–62.

Olds, B., and Herr, D. "Where's That Nurse?" *Saturday Evening Post* 219 (January 4, 1947): 17.

Palmer, G. "What Happens When Trained Nurses Won't Nurse the Sick?" *Ladies' Home Journal* 64 (December 1947): 50.

"Parachute-Jumping Nurses Bring First Aid from the Sky: French Corps." *Popular Science* 132 (April 1938): 58.

Penny, L. "County Hires a Nurse." *Hygeia* 9 (August 1931): 712–14.

Perry, G.S. "Angels in Blue: Visiting Nurses." *Saturday Evening Post* 226 (May 15, 1954): 28–29.

Perry, G.S. "Nurses Are Lucky Girls!" *Saturday Evening Post* 226 (February 20, 1954): 24–25.

Phillips, W. "Rx for Hospitals, R.N." *New York Times Magazine* 106 (August 25, 1957): 25.

Piggott, M.W. "You Would Hardly Believe It." *Nineteenth Century* 68 (July 1910): 148–54.

Pigrebin, L.C. "Why Do Women In White See Red?" *Ladies' Home Journal* 89 (August 1972): 40.

Poole, E. "Nurse on Horseback: Frontier Nursing Service." *Good Housekeeping* 94 (January 1930): 38–39.

Poore, A. "You Can Help the War Effort by Conserving Medical and Nursing Care!" *American Home* 29 (January 1943): 31.

"Position of Organized Nursing." *Saturday Review* 50 (February 4, Mar. 4, 1967): 61–62, 60–62.

"Preventive Nursing." *Independent* 74 (February 26, 1913): 481–82.

Priestley, E.C. "Nurses à la Mode." *Nineteenth Century* 41 (January 1897): 28–37.

"Private Duty Nurse." *Hygeia* 9 (February 1931): 158.

"Private-Practice Nurses." *Time* 101 (March 12, 1973): 70.

"Privileged Profession." *Westminster Review* 135 (January 1891): 6–10.

"Public Health Nurse." *Nation* 108 (March 22, 1919): 418.

Purwin, L., and Block, R. "Nurses for China." *Independent Woman* 23 (March 1944): 66–67.

Ralston, L.B. "Is There a Nurse in the House?" *Woman's Home Companion* 70 (March 1943): 40.

Rawlings, B.B. "Nurses in Hospitals." *Nineteenth Century* 64 (November 1908): 824–36.

Reynolds, Q. "Young Women in White: Louise Jaissle." *Reader's Digest* 69 (November 1956): 79–83.

Richmond, C. "Nursing in Group Medical Practice." *American Journal of Public Health* 41 (October 1951): 1268–74.

Rood, M.J. "How We Support Our District Nurses." *Delineator* 88 (May 1916): 14.

Rose, D. "Genteel Art of Nursing." *North American Review* 229 (February 1930): 251–53.

"Rx for Sick Hospitals." *Newsweek* 68 (July 11, 1966): 57–61.

Safran, C. "Their Patients Call Them Supernurses: Nurse Practitioners." *Today's Health* 53 (July 1975): 20–23.

"St. Louis Rotarians Help Train More Nurses." *Rotarian* 61 (December 1942): 19–21.

Salter, L.C. "Epics of Courage: How American Nurses Are Serving Our Fighting Men, and America." *Hygeia* 22 (February 1944): 116–17.

"Samaritans on Wings: Nurses Fly Transoceanic Missions Evacuating Injured GIs from Vietnam." *Ebony* 25 (May 1970): 60–62.

Samuels, G. "With Army Nurses Somewhere in Korea." *New York Times Magazine* 100 (April 16, 1951): 14–15.

Sangster, M.E. "Care of a Convalescent." *Harper's Bazaar* 32 (November 17, 1900): 1860.

"Saving Lives on the Last Frontier." *Literary Digest* 119 (February 2, 1935): 22.

Schloss, M.H. "How I Nursed Some Invalids to Health." *Ladies' Home Journal* 25 (November 1908): 40.

Schultz, K. "If the Baby's Ill: Simple Rules of Nursing Care." *Parents Magazine* 15 (June 1940): 31.

Scott, A. "Case Number 10,000." *Hygeia* 11 (March 1933): 210–11.

Scott, R.B. "Problem of a Degree?" *National Business Woman* 36 (May 1957): 8–9.

"Sickness in the Hospitals: Resignation Threat by Public Health Nurses in New York City." *Newsweek* 67 (May 30, 1966): 78.

Silver, G.A. "Women in Medicine." *Nation* 220 (June 21, 1975): 741.

Simpson, D. "College Woman as Nurse." *Review of Reviews* 57 (May 1918): 527–28.

Simpson, H. "Public Health Nursing." *Review of Reviews* 61 (June 1920): 635–38.

Sissman, L.E. "Extreme Mercy." *Atlantic* 235 (January 1975): 16.

"Sisters of the Poor: Owners and Operators of St. Francis Hospital." *New Yorker* 42 (December 31, 1966): 24.

Sloan, R. "Short Course in Nursing: Red Cross Volunteer Nurse's Aide Course." *Parents Magazine* 17 (October 1942): 37.

Smith, W.R. "They Call Her Mrs. Doctor Man." *Sunset* 55 (November 1925): 50.

Star, J. "What Happened to the Nurses?" *Look* 26 (September 11, 1962): 22–28.

Stewart, I. "State Registration of Nurses." *Nineteenth Century* 55 (June 1904): 987–95.

Strong, A.H. "Need for Nurses." *Nation* 106 (June 1, 1918): 645–46.

Stuart, N.G., and Aynes, E.A. "Coming Scandal in Nursing." *McCalls* 91 (March 1964): 100–101.

"Superprofessionals Ride Again, or How To Perpetuate a Nursing Shortage." *Trans-Action* 7 (June 1970): 8

Swallow, W. "I Never Thought of That: Suggestions for the Home Nurse." *Woman's Home Companion* 69 (October 1942): 38.

"Team Nursing." *Newsweek* 41 (June 29, 1953): 78.

"Teen-Age Civil War Nurse Susie King Taylor." *Ebony* 25 (February 1970): 96–98.

"These Angels Must Eat." *Newsweek* 51 (June 23, 1958): 60.

Thruelsen, R. "Registered Nurse." *Saturday Evening Post* 220 (April 3, 1948): 34–35.

"Trained Nurse." *Outlook* 103 (April 19, 1913): 831.

"Trained Nurses and Reconstruction." *Outlook* 122 (June 11, 1919): 228.

"Trained Nurses in Industrial Plants." *World's Work* 22 (June 1911): 631–36.

"Training-Schools for Nurses." *Fraser's Magazine* 10 (December 1874): 706–13.

Trench, M. "Sick Nurses." *MacMillan's Magazine* 34 (September 1876): 423–29.

Trimble, A. "Nurses and Those They Serve." *Hygeia* 21 (May 1943): 335–37.

"Trojans of the Civil War." *Literary Digest* 44 (February 10, 1912): 307.

Tunley, R. "Career Where the Action Is." *Seventeen* 27 (March 1968): 140–41.

Tunley, R. "Why We Need More Nurses Now." *Redbook* 129 (July 1967): 68–69.

"Twin Nurses." *Look* 19 (May 3, 1955): 61–63.

Van Blarcom, C.C. "Trained Nurse and the Depression." *Nation* 137 (October 11, 1933): 406–7.

Villet, B. "More than Compassion: Head Nurse, Judy Strickland." *Life* 72 (April 7, 1972): 68–75.

Walburn, N. "Nursing Is a Woman's Job." *Independent Woman* 19 (July 1940): 208–10.

Wang, H. "China Needs Nurses!" *Independent Woman* 21 (November 1942): 341.

Washburn, H. "So You Want To Be a Nurse." *Good Housekeeping* 110 (April 1940): 39.

"We Are Trying To Find One Hundred Thousand Women." *Good Housekeeping* 115 (December 1942): 14.

Werminghaus, E.A. "Your Stake in Private Duty Nursing." *Today's Health* 33 (October 1955): 13

"What Is a Nurse?" *Literary Digest* 69 (May 21, 1921): 22.

"What Makes a Good Nurse for Babies: Nursing School of Babies' Hospital, NY." *Good Housekeeping* 112 (April 1941): 26–27.

Wheeler, C.T. "Trained Nurse in Turkey." *Outlook* 84 (September 1, 1906): 32–35.

"Who Has Heard the Nightingale?" *Ladies' Home Journal* 65 (May 1948): 11.

Winslow, A. "Public Health Nursing." *Forum* 78 (November 1972): 726–32.

Winterburn, F.H. "For the Home Nurse." *Harper's Bazaar* 46 (September 1912): 470.

"Women in White." *Coronet* 30 (May 1951): 71–86.

Woodbury, C. "Student Nurse, Could You Take It?" *Woman's Home Companion* 76 (June 1949): 36–38.

Worden, H. "She Nurses Her Patients for a Dollar a Year: Frontier Nursing Service." *American Magazine* 112 (December 1931): 69–70.

"You Need Public Health Nurses." *Ladies' Home Journal* 64 (April 1947): 11.

Young, L. "Unforgettable Sister Winifred." *Reader's Digest* 88 (March 1966): 173–74.

"Your Next Nurse May Be a Man." *Today's Health* 44 (February 1966): 38–39.

MOTION PICTURES

Abandon Ship! 100 min. B & W. Released: 5/57. Distributor: Columbia. Director: Richard Sale. Screenplay: Richard Sale.

Adele 6 reels. B & W. Released: 2/1/19. Distributor: United Pictures. Director: Wallace Worsley. Screenplay: Jack Cunningham, based on the novel by Adele Bleneau, *The Nurse's Story: In Which Reality Meets Romance* (Indianapolis: Bobbs-Merrill, 1915).

Against the Law 60 min. B & W. Reviewed: 11/21/34. Distributor: Colum-bia. Director: Lambert Hillyer. Screenplay: Harold Shumate.

Air Hostess 63 min. B & W. Released: 1/21/33. Distributor: Columbia. Director: Al Rogell. Screenplay: Keene Thompson, Milton Raison, adapted from a story by Grace Perkins.

Air Hostess 61 min. B & W. Released: 8/25/49. Distributor: Columbia. Director: Lew Landers. Screenplay: Robert Libott, Frank Burt, adapted from an original story by Louise Rousseau.

The Amazing Doctor Clitterhouse 87 min. B & W. Released: 7/30/38. Distributor: Warner Brothers. Director: Anatole Litvak. Screenplay: John Wexley, John Huston, from a three-act play by Barre Lyndon, *The Amazing Dr. Clitterhouse.*

And Soon the Darkness 98 min. Color. Released: 4/71. Distributor: Levitt-Pickman. Director: Robert Fuest. Screenplay/Story: Brian Clemens, Terry Nation.

Angel Face 90 min. B & W. Released: 12/11/52. Distributor: RKO. Director: Otto Preminger. Screenplay: Frank Nugent, Oscar Millard, from an original story by Chester Erskine.

Angel of Mercy 1 reel. B & W. Released: 5/20/39. Distributor: MGM. Director: Edward Cahn.

The Angel of the Battlefield 2 reels. B & W. Released: 1917. Director: Frederick W. Hornby.

Angels of Mercy 10 min. B & W. Released: 1/23/42. Distributor: Soundies Distributing Corp.

Army Surgeon 63 min. B & W. Released: 12/4/42. Distributor: RKO. Director: A. Edward Sutherland. Screenplay: Barry Trivers, Emmett Lavery, adapted from a screen story by John Twist.

Arrowsmith 108 min. B & W. Released: 12/13/31. Distributor: United Artists. Director: John Ford. Screenplay: Sidney Howard, adapted from the book by Sinclair Lewis, *Arrowsmith* (New York: Harcourt, 1925).

Atlantic Convoy 66 min. B & W. Released: 7/2/42. Distributor: Columbia. Director: Lew Landers. Screenplay: Robert Lee Johnson.

AW Nurse 10 min. B & W. Released: 3/24/34. Distributor: Screen Gems. Story: Sid Marcus.

Bad Boy's Joke on the Nurse 6 min. B & W. Released: 12/9/04. Distributor: Edison.

Bad For Each Other 83 min. B & W. Reviewed: 12/16/53. Distributor: Columbia. Director: Irving Rapper. Screenplay: Irving Wallace, from the book by Horace McCoy, *Scalpel* (New York: Appleton-Century-Crofts, 1952).

Battle Circus 90 min. B & W. Released: 3/6/53. Distributor: MGM. Director: Richard Brooks. Screenplay: Richard Brooks, adapted from a story by Allen Rivkin, Laura Kerr.

The Battle of Paris 62 min. B & W. Released: 11/30/29. Distributor: Paramount Famous-Lasky. Director: Robert Florey. Story/Dialoguer: Gene Markey.

Battle Flame 78 min. B & W. Released: 7/26/59. Distributor: Allied Artists. Director: R.G. Springsteen. Screenplay: Ellwood Ullman. Written by Lester A. Sansom, Ellwood Ullman.

Battle Zone 82 min. B & W. Released: 10/26/52. Distributor: Allied Artists. Director: Lesley Selander. Screenplay: Steve Fisher.

The Beast with Five Fingers 88 min. B & W. Released: 12/20/46. Distributor: Warner Brothers. Director: Robert Florey. Screenplay: Curt Siodmak, adapted from the novel by W. Fryer Harvey, *The Beast with Five Fingers: Twenty Tales of the Uncanny* (New York: Dutton, 1947).

Because of You 95 min. B & W. Released: 11/52. Distributor: Universal. Director: Joseph Pevney. Screenplay: Ketti Frings, from an original story by Thelma Robinson.

Bedside 65 min. B & W. Reviewed: 3/6/34. Distributor: Warner Brothers. Director: Robert Florey. Screenplay: Lillie Hayward, James Wharton, Rian James, from a story by Manuel Seff, Harvey Thew.

Bedside Manner 79 min. B & W. Released: 6/22/45. Distributor: United Artists. Director: Andrew Stone. Screenplay: Frederick Jackson, Malcolm Stuart Boylan, adapted from an original story by Robert Carson.

Beneath the Valley of the Ultravixens 96 min. Eastman Color. Released: 1978. Distributor: Signal. Director: Russ Meyer.

Between Two Women 95 min. B & W. Released: 7/9/37. Distributor: MGM. Director: George B. Seitz. Screenplay: Frederick Stephani, Marion Parsonnet, from an original story by Eric von Stroheim, "General Hospital."

Between Two Women 83 min. B & W. Reviewed: 12/18/44. Distributor: MGM. Director: Willis Goldbeck. Screenplay: Harry Ruskin, adapted from an original story by Erich von Stroheim, "General Hospital."

Beyond the Poseidon Adventure 122 min. Color. Released: 5/79. Distributor: Warner Brothers. Director: Irwin Allen. Screenplay: Nelson Gidding, based on the novel by Paul Gallico, *The Poseidon Adventure* (New York: Coward-McCann, 1969).

Billy's Nurse 14 min. B & W. Released: 8/12/15. Distributor: MinA. Director: Alice Buy Blache.

Birth Control 5 reels. B & W. Released: 4/21/17. Distributor: Message Photoplay.

The Black Butterfly 5 reels. B & W. Released: 12/21/16. Distributor: Metro. Director: Burton L. King. Screenplay: Wallace C. Clifton.

Born to Love 84 min. B & W. Released: 4/26/31. Distributor: Pathe. Director: Paul L. Stein. Screenplay: Ernest Pascal, from a story and screenplay by Ernest Pascal.

Bowery Boy 71 min. B & W. Released: 1/3/41. Distributor: Republic. Director: William Morgan. Screenplay: Robert Chapin, Harry Kronman, Eugene Solow, adapted from the original by Sam Fuller, Sidney Sutherland.

The Bramble Bush 105 min. Technicolor. Released: 2/13/60. Distributor: Warner Brothers. Director: Daniel Petrie. Screenplay: Milton Sperling, adapted from the novel by Charles H. Mergendahl, *The Bramble Bush* (New York: Putnam, 1958).

Brink of Life (Sweden) 82 min. B & W. Released: 1958 (U.S.: 11/7/59). Distributor: Ajay Film. Director: Ingmar Bergman. Screenplay: Ella Isaksson.

Bullet Scars 59 min. B & W. Released: 3/7/43. Distributor: Warner Brothers. Director: D. Ross Lederman. Screenplay: Robert E. Kent, from an idea by Charles Belden, Sy Bartlett.

Buried Alive 74 min. B & W. Reviewed: 1/23/40. Distributor: Producers Distributing. Director: Victor Halperin. Screenplay: George Bricker, from the book by Arnold Bennett, *Buried Alive* (London: Chapman and Hall, 1908).

Cactus Flower 103 min. Technicolor. Released: 12/16/69. Distributor: Columbia. Director: Gene Saks. Screenplay: I.A.L. Diamond, adapted from the play by Abe Burrows, *Cactus Flower.*

Calling Dr. Death 63 min. B & W. Released: 12/30/43. Distributor: Universal. Director: Reginald LeBorg. Screenplay: Edward Dein.

Calling Dr. Gillespie 82 min. B & W. Reviewed: 6/17/42. Distributor: MGM. Director: Harold S. Bucquet. Screenplay: Willis Goldbeck, Harry Ruskin, from an original screen story by Kubec Glasmon, based on the character created by Max Brand.

Calling Dr. Kildare 86 min. B & W. Released: 4/28/39. Distributor: MGM. Director: Harold S. Bucquet. Screenplay: Harry Ruskin, Willis Goldbeck, from the book by Max Brand, *Calling Dr. Kildare* (New York: Dodd, Mead, 1940).

The Call of the Soul 5 reels. B & W. Released: 1/19/19. Distributor: Fox. Director: Edward J. LeSaint. Screenplay: Denison Clift. Story: Julia Burnham.

Candy Stripe Nurses 80 min. Metrocolor. Released: 5/74. Distributor: New World. Director: Allan Holleb. Screenplay: Allan Holleb.

Captain Newman M.D. 126 min. Eastman Color. Released: 12/25/63. Distributor: Universal. Director: David Miller. Screenplay: Richard L. Breen, Phoebe Ephron, Henry Ephron, adapted from the novel by Leo Rosten, *Captain Newman M.D.* (New York: Harper, 1961).

The Caretakers 97 min. B & W. Released: 8/21/63. Distributor: United Artists. Director: Hall Bartlett. Screenplay: Henry F. Greenberg, adapted from the novel by Dariel Telfer, *The Caretakers* (New York: Simon and Schuster, 1959).

The Carey Treatment 101 min. Metrocolor. Released: 3/72. Distributor: MGM. Producer: William Belasco. Director: Blake Edwards. Screenplay: James P. Bonner, based on the novel by Jeffrey Hudson, *A Case of Need* (New York: New American Library, 1968).

Carnaby, M.D. (Great Britain; originally titled *Doctor in Clover*) 101 min. Eastman Color. Released: 3/66 (U.S.: 8/67). Distributor: Continental Distributing. Director: Ralph Thomas. Screenplay: Jack Davies, adapted from the novel by Richard Gordon, *Doctor in Clover* (London: Joseph, 1960).

Carry On Again, Doctor (Great Britain) 89 min. Eastman Color. Released: 5/69. Distributor: Rank. Director: Gerald Thomas. Story: Talbot Rothwell.

Carry On Doctor (Great Britain) 94 min. Eastman Color. Released: 11/67 (U.S.: 1973). Distributor: Rank. Producer: Peter Rogers. Director: Gerald Thomas. Story: Talbot Rothwell.

Carry On Matron (Great Britain) 89 min. Color. Released: 6/72 (U.S.: 1973). Distributor: Rank. Director: Gerald Thomas.

Carry On Nurse (Great Britain) 90 min. B & W. Released: 3/59 (U.S.: 4/60). Distributor: Governor Films. Director: Gerald Thomas. Screenplay: Norman Hudis, adapted from the play by Patrick Cargill, Jack Beale, *Ring for Catty.*

Catch-22 122 min. Technicolor. Released: 6/70. Distributor: Paramount. Screenplay: Buck Henry, based on the novel by Joseph Heller, *Catch-22* (New York: Simon and Schuster, 1961).

The Cavell Case 6 reels. B & W. Released: 10/27/18. Distributor: Select. Director: John G. Adolfi. Screenplay: Anthony Paul Kelly, based on his story.

Ceiling Zero 95 min. B & W. Reviewed: 12/24/35. Distributor: Warner Brothers. Producer: Harry Joe Brown. Director: Howard Hawks. Screenplay: Frank Wead, from the play by Frank Wead, *Ceiling Zero.*

Celeste of the Ambulance Corps 3 reels. B & W. Released: 1/8/16. Distributor: Edison.

Central Airport 70 min. B & W. Reviewed: 3/29/33. Distributor: Warner Brothers. Director: William A. Wellman. Screenplay: Rian James, James Seymour, adapted from the story by Jack Moffitt, "Hawk's Mate."

Cherry, Harry and Raquel 71 min. DeLuxe Color. Released: 11/26/69. Distributor: Eve Productions. Director: Russ Meyer. Screenplay: Tom Wolfe, Russ Meyer.

A Child Is Born 79 min. B & W. Released: 10/11/40. Distributor: Paramount. Director: Lloyd Bacon. Screenplay: Robert Rossen, from the book by Mary McDougal Axelson, *A Child is Born* (Caldwell, ID: Caxton Printers, 1939).

The Child Thou Gavest Me 61 min. B & W. Released: 8/20/21. Distributor: First National. Director: John M. Stahl. Scenario: Chester Roberts.

The Christian 80 min. B & W. Released: 1/14/23. Distributor: Vitagraph. Director: Maurice Tourneur. Scenario: Paul Bern.

Christmas in Connecticut 101 min. B & W. Released: 8/11/45. Distributor: Warner Brothers. Director: Peter Godfrey. Screenplay: Lionel Houser, Adele Commandini, from an original screen story by Aileen Hamilton.

City on Fire 101 min. Color. Released: 1980. Distributor: Avco Embassy. Director: Alvin Rakoff.

Coma 112 min. Metrocolor. Released: 1/78. Distributor: United Artists. Director: Michael Crichton. Screenplay: Michael Crichton, adapted from the novel by Robin Cook, *Coma* (Boston: Little, Brown, 1976).

Come to the Stable 94 min. B & W. Released: 9/49. Distributor: 20th Century-Fox. Director: Henry Koster. Screenplay: Oscar Millard, Sally Benson, adapted from a screen story by Clare Booth Luce.

Condemned Women 77 min. B & W. Released: 4/1/38. Distributor: RKO. Director: Lew Landers. Screenplay: Lionel Houser.

The Corpse Grinders 72 min. Eastman Color. Released: 1972. Distributor: Gemeni Films. Director: Ted V. Mikels. Screenplay: Arch Hall, Joseph L. Cranston.

The Country Doctor 110 min. B & W. Reviewed: 3/2/36. Distributor: 20th Century-Fox. Director: Henry King. Screenplay: Sonya Levien, from an original screen story by Charles Blake.

The Crazy World of Julius Vrooder 98 min. DeLuxe Color. Released: 10/74. Distributor: 20th Century-Fox. Director: Arthur Hiller. Screenplay: Daryl Henry.

Crime Doctor 66 min. B & W. Released: 6/22/43. Distributor: Columbia. Producer: Ralph Cohn. Director: Michael Gordon. Screenplay: Graham Baker, Louise Lantz, adapted from a screenplay based on the radio program by Max Marcin, *Crime Doctor.*

Crime Doctor's Strangest Case 68 min. B & W. Released: 12/9/43. Distributor: Columbia. Director: Eugene J. Forde. Screenplay: Eric Taylor, based on the radio program by Max Marcin, *Crime Doctor.*

Cross of Iron 133 min. Technicolor. Released: 5/77. Distributor: Avco Embassy. Director: Sam Peckinpah. Screenplay: Julius J. Epstein, Herbert Asmodi, adapted form the book by Willi Heinrich, *The Cross of Iron* (New York: Bobbs-Merrill, 1956).

Cross Red Nurse 2 reels. B & W. Released: 8/31/18. Distributor: World Film Corporation.

Cry Havoc 97 min. B & W. Reviewed: 11/9/43. Distributor: MGM. Director: Richard Thorpe. Screenplay: Paul Osborn, from the three-act drama by Allan R. Kenward, *Proof Through the Night.*

Dark Delusion 90 min. B & W. Released: 6/47. Distributor: MGM. Director: Willis Goldbeck. Screenplay: Jack Andrews, Harry Ruskin, based on a character created by Max Brand.

The Daughter: Or I A Woman, Part 3 (Denmark) 84 min. Movielab. Released (U.S.): 9/2/70. Distributor: Chevron. Director: Mac Ahlberg. Screenplay: Peer Guildbrandsen.

Dawn (Great Britain) 73 min. B & W. Released: 2/28. Distributor: British and Dominions Film Corporation. Director: Herbert Wilcox. Screenplay: Herbert Wilcox, Robert J. Cullen, adapted from the play by Reginald Berkeley, *Dawn.*

Death of a Champion 67 min. B & W. Released: 9/7/39. Distributor: Paramount. Director: Robert Florey. Screenplay: Stuart Palmer, Cortland Fitzsimmons, adapted from the short story by Frank Gruber, "Dog Show Murder."

Deep Throat 73 min. Color. Released: 6/72. Distributor: Aquarius. Director: Jerry Gerard. Writer: Jerry Gerard.

Deep Throat, Part 2 87 min. Color. Released: 2/74. Distributor: Bryanson. Director: Joe Sarno. Screenplay: Joe Sarno.

The Disorderly Orderly 90 min. Technicolor. Released: 12/16/64. Distributor: Paramount. Director: Frank Tashlin. Screenplay: Frank Tashlin, from an original story by Norm Liebmann and Ed Haas.

The Doctor and the Girl 98 min. B & W. Released: 9/49. Distributor: MGM. Direc-

tor: Curtis Bernhardt. Screenplay: Theodore Reeves, adapted from the book by Maxence van der Meersch, *Bodies and Souls* (London: William Kimber, 1950).

Doctor and the Woman 6 reels. B & W. Released: 2/5/18. Distributor: Universal. Director: Lois Weber, adapted from the novel by Mary Roberts Rinehart, *K* (Boston: Houghton Mifflin, 1915).

Doctor at Large (Great Britain) 98 min. Eastman Color. Released: 11/57. Distributor: Universal. Director: Ralph Thomas. Screenplay: Nicholas Phipps, adapted from the novel by Richard Gordon, *Doctor at Large* (New York: Harcourt, Brace, 1956).

Doctor Blood's Coffin (Great Britain) 92 min. Eastman Color. Released: 1/61 (U.S.: 4/26/61). Distributor: United Artists. Director: Sid Furie. Screenplay: Jerry Juran.

Dr. Broadway 67 min. B & W. Reviewed: 5/7/42. Distributor: Paramount. Director: Anton Mann. Screenplay: Art Arthur, adapted from a short story by Borden Chase.

Dr. Gillespie's Criminal Case 89 min. B & W. Released: 11/43. Distributor: MGM. Director: Willis Goldbeck. Screenplay: Martin Barkeley, Harry Ruskin, Lawrence P. Bachman, from a screenplay based on the character created by Max Brand.

Dr. Gillespie's New Assistant 87 min. B & W. Reviewed: 11/12/42. Distributor: MGM. Director: Willis Goldbeck. Screenplay: Harry Ruskin, Willis Goldbeck, Lawrence P. Bachmann, adapted from the character created by Max Brand.

Doctor in Distress (Great Britain) 103 min. Eastman Color. Released: 7/63. (U.S.: 7/7/64). Distributor: Governor. Director: Ralph Thomas. Screenplay: Nicholas Phipps, Ronald Scott Thorn, based on characters created by Richard Gordon.

Doctor in Love (Great Britain) 93 min. Eastman Color. Released: 7/60 (U.S.: 11/15/61). Distributor: Governor. Director: Ralph Thomas. Screenplay: Nicholas Phipps, adapted from the novel by Richard Gordon, *Doctor in Love* (New York: Harcourt, Brace, 1957).

Doctor in the House (Great Britain) 92 min. Technicolor. Released: 3/54. (U.S.: 2/2/55). Distributor: Republic-Rank. Producer: Betty E. Box. Director: Ralph Thomas. Screenplay: Nicholas Phipps, adapted from the book by Richard Gordon, *Doctor in the House* (New York: Harcourt, Brace, 1953).

Dr. Kildare Goes Home 78 min. B & W. Released: 9/6/40. Distributor: MGM. Director: Harold S. Bucquet. Screenplay: Harry Ruskin, Willis Goldbeck, from an

original screen story by Max Brand and Willis Goldbeck.

Dr. Kildare's Crisis 75 min. B & W. Released: 11/29/40. Distributor: MGM. Director: Harold S. Bucquet. Screenplay: Harry Ruskin, Willis Goldbeck, from an original screen story by Max Brand and Willis Goldbeck.

Dr. Kildare's Strange Case 76 min. B & W. Released: 4-12-40. Distributor: MGM. Director: Harold S. Bucquet. Screenplay: Harry Ruskin, Willis Goldbeck, from an original screen story by Max Brand and Willis Goldbeck.

Dr. Kildare's Victory 92 min. B & W. Reviewed: 12/3/41. Distributor: MGM. Director: W.S. Van Dyke II. Screenplay: Harry Ruskin, Willis Goldbeck, adapted from a short story by Joseph Harrington adapted from the character created by Max Brand.

Dr. Kildare's Wedding Day 82 min. B & W. Released: 8/22/41. Distributor: MGM. Director: Harold S. Bucquet. Screenplay: Willis Goldbeck, Harry Ruskin, adapted from a screen story by Ormond Ruthven based on the character created by Max Brand.

Dr. Monica 61 min. B & W. Reviewed: 6/22/34. Distributor: Warner Brothers. Director: William Keighley. Screenplay: Charles Kenyon, Laura Walker Mayer, from the play by Marja Morozowicz, *Dr. Monica.*

Dr. Neighbour 5 reels. B & W. Released: 5/6/16. Distributor: Universal. Director: L.B. Carleton. Screenplay: Agnes Hay.

A Doctor's Diary 71 min. B & W. Released: 1/5/37. Distributor: Paramount. Director: Charles Vidor. Screenplay: David Boehm, from a screenplay by Samuel Ornitz, Joseph Anthony.

Doctors' Wives 80 min. B & W. Released: 3/15/31. Distributor: Fox. Director: Frank Borzage. Screenplay: Maurine Watkins, adapted from a story by Henry Lieferant, Sylvia Lieferant.

Doctor's Wives 102 min. Color. Released: 11/7/71. Distributor: Columbia. Director: George Schaefer. Screenplay: Daniel Taradash, adapted from the novel by Frank G. Slaughter (Garden City, NY: Doubleday, 1967).

Doctor Zhivago 197 min. Metrocolor. Released: 12/22/65. Distributor: MGM. Director: David Lean. Screenplay: Robert Bolt, adapted from the novel by Boris Leonidovich Pasternak, *Doctor Zhivago* (New York: Pantheon, 1958).

Don Winslow of the Coast Guard (serial in 13 episodes) 260 min. B & W. Released: 3/30/43. Distributor: Universal. Director: Lewis D. Collins. Screenplay: Paul Huston, George H. Plympton, Griffin Joy, based on the comic strip owned and copyrighted by Lieutenant Commander Frank V. Martinek, U.S. Navy (retired).

Don Winslow of the Navy (serial in 15 episodes) 300 min. B & W. Released: 1942. Distributor: Universal. Directors: Ford Beebe, Ray Taylor.

Duffy of San Quentin 78 min. B & W. Released: 3/13/54. Distributor: Warner Brothers. Director: Walter Doniger. Screenplay: Berman Swarttz, Walter Doniger, adapted form the book by Clinton T. Duffy, *The San Quentin Story* (New York: Doubleday, 1950).

Ellery Queen and the Murder Ring 65 min. B & W. Released: 11/18/41. Distributor: Columbia. Director: James Hogan. Screenplay: Eric Taylor, Gertrude Purcell, adapted from the book by Ellery Queen, *The Dutch Shoe Mystery* (Toronto: Blue Ribbon Books, 1940).

Don't Go Near the Water 102 min. Metrocolor. Released: 12/57. Distributor: MGM. Director: Charles Walters. Screenplay: Dorothy Kingsley, George Wells, adapted from the novel by William Brinkley, *Don't Go Near the Water* (New York: Random House, 1956).

Emergency Call 65 min. B & W. Released: 6/24/33. Distributor: RKO. Director: Edward Cahn. Screenplay: John B. Clymer, Joseph L. Mankiewicz, from a story by John B. Clymer.

Emergency Hospital 62 min. B & W. Released: 7/53. Distributor: United Artists. Director: Lee Sholem. Screenplay: Don Martin.

Emergency Wedding 78 min. B & W. Released: 11/50. Distributor: Columbia. Director: Eddie Buzzell. Screenplay: Nat Perrin, Claude Binyon, adapted from a story by Dalton Trumbo (unpublished).

The Enemies of Women 105 min. B & W. Released: 4/15/23. Distributor: Goldwyn. Director: Alan Crosland. Scenario: John Lynch, from the book by Vicente Blasco-Ibanez, *Los Enemigos de la Mujer* (New York: E. P. Dutton, 1920).

Ensign Pulver 104 min. Technicolor. Released: 6/29/64. Distributor: Warner Brothers. Director: Joshua Logan. Screenplay: Joshua Logan, Peter S. Feibleman, from an original story by Joshua Logan and Thomas Heggen.

Escape from Zahrain 93 min. Technicolor. Released: 5/23/62. Distributor: Paramount. Director: Ronald Neame. Screenplay: Robin Estridge, adapted from the novel by Michael Barrett, *Appointment in Zahrain* (London: Michael Joseph, 1960).

Exodus 213 min. Technicolor. Released: 12/15/60. Distributor: United Artists. Director: Otto Preminger. Screenplay: Dalton Trumbo, adapted from the novel by Leon Uris, *Exodus* (Garden City, NY: Doubleday, 1958).

Experiment Alcatraz 58 min. B & W. Released: 11/23/50. Distributor: RKO. Director: Edward L. Cahn. Screenplay: Orville H. Hampton.

Eyewitness (Great Britain) 82 min. B & W. Released: 7/56. Distributor: Rank. Director: Muriel Box. Story: Janet Green.

A Farewell to Arms 80 min. B & W. Released: 12/10/32. Distributor: Paramount. Director: Frank Borzage. Screenplay: Benjamin Glazer, Oliver H.P. Garrett, Charles Lang, adapted from the novel by Ernest Hemingway, *A Farewell to Arms* (New York: Scribner's, 1929).

A Farewell to Arms 152 min. DeLuxe Color. Released: 12/57. Distributor: 20th Century-Fox. Director: Charles Vidor. Screenplay: Ben Hecht, adapted from the novel by Ernest Hemingway, *A Farewell to Arms* (New York: Scribner's, 1929).

Fear Strikes Out 100 min. B & W. Released: 3/57. Distributor: Paramount. Director: Robert Mulligan. Screenplay: Ted Berkman, Raphael Blau, adapted from a short story by James A. Piersall, Albert S. Hirschberg.

A Fight to the Finish 59 min. B & W. Released: 6/30/37. Distributor: Columbia. Director: C.C. Coleman. Screenplay: Harold Shumate.

Firefly of France 68 min. B & W. Released. 7/14/18. Distributor: Paramount. Director: Donald Crisp. Based on the novel by Marion Polk Angelloti (New York: Century, 1918).

Five Gates to Hell 98 min. B & W. Released: 10/59. Distributor: 20th Century-Fox. Director: James Clavell. Screenplay: James Clavell.

Five of a Kind 83 min. B & W. Released: 10/14/38. Distributor: 20th Century-Fox. Producer: Sol M. Wurtzel. Director: Herbert I. Leeds. Screenplay: Lou Breslow, John Patrick.

The Flame 97 min. B & W. Released: 11/24/47. Distributor: Republic. Director: John H. Auer. Screenplay: Lawrence Kimble, based on a story by Robert T. Shannon.

Flight 107 min. B & W. Released: 11/1/29. Distributor: Columbia. Director: Frank R. Capra. Scenario: Howard J. Green.

Flight Angels 74 min. B & W. Released: 5/18/40. Distributor: Warner Brothers. Director: Lewis Seiler. Screenplay: Maurice Leo, from an original screen story by Jerry Wald, Richard Macaulay.

Flight at Midnight 66 min. B & W. Released: 8/28/39. Distributor: Republic. Director: Sidney Salkow. Screenplay: Eliot Gibbons, adapted from an original screen story by Daniel Moore, Hugh King.

Flight Nurse 90 min. B & W. Released: 11/15/53. Distributor: Republic. Director: Allan Dwan. Screenplay: Alan LeMay.

Florence Nightingale 35 min. B & W. Released: 11/20/15. Distributor: Ideal. Director: Maurice Elvey. Screenplay: Eliot Stannard, adapted from the novel by Edward Cook, *The Life of Florence Nightingale* (New York: Macmillan, 1913).

Flying Hostess 70 min. B & W. Reviewed: 12/16/36. Distributor: Universal. Director: Murray Roth. Screenplay: Brown Holmes, Harvey Gates, Harry Clork, from an original screen story by George Sayre.

Flying Tigers 102 min. B & W. Released: 10/8/42. Distributor: Republic. Director: David Miller. Screenplay: Kenneth Gamet, Barry Trivers, from a screen story by Kenneth Gamet.

The Fog 67 min. B & W. Released: 6/18/23. Distributor: Metro. Director: Paul Powell. Scenario: Winifred Dunn, adapted from the book by William Dudley Pelley, *The Fog* (Boston: Little, Brown, 1921).

Forever After 63 min. B & W. Released: 10/24/26. Distributor: First National. Director: F. Harmon Weight. Scenario: Paul Gangelin, from the book by Owen Davis, *Forever After* (New York: Grosset and Dunlap, 1928).

Four Girls in White 70 min. B & W. Released: 1/27/39. Distributor: MGM. Director: S. Sylvan Simon. Screenplay: Dorothy Yost, from an original screen story by Nathalie Bucknall, Endre Bohem.

Francis 91 min. B & W. Reviewed: 12/13/49. Distributor: Universal. Director: Arthur Lubin. Screenplay: David Stern, adapted from the book by David Stern, *Francis* (New York: Farrar, Straus, 1946).

Francis in the Navy 80 min. B & W. Released: 8/55. Distributor: Universal. Director: Arthur Lubin. Screenplay: Devery Freeman, based on the character created by David Stern.

Fugitive in the Sky 58 min. B & W. Reviewed: 1/6/37. Distributor: Warner Brothers. Director: Nick Grinde. Screenplay: George Bricker.

The Garden Murder Case 62 min. B & W. Reviewed: 2/29/36. Distributor: MGM. Director: Edward L. Marin. Screenplay: Bertram Milhauser, from the book by S.S. Van Dine, *The Garden Murder Case* (New York: Scribner's, 1935).

The Gentle Touch (Great Britain) 86 min. Technicolor. Released: 8/57. Distributor: Rank. Director: Pat Jackson. Cinematography: Paul Beeson, adapted from the novel by Sheila McKay Russell, *The Lamp is Heavy* (Philadelphia: J.B. Lippincott, 1950).

Girl from God's Country 71 min. B & W. Released: 7/30/40. Distributor: Republic. Director: Sidney Salkow. Screenplay: Elizabeth Meehan, Robert Lee Johnson, from the short story by Ray Millholland, "Island Doctor."

Girl from Leningrad (Russia) 82 min. B & W. Released: 12/19/41. Distributor: Artkino. Director: Victor Eisimont. Screenplay: Sergei Mikhailov, Mikhail Rosenberg.

Girl in 419 62 min. B & W. Released: 5/20/33. Distributor: Paramount. Director: George Somnes, Alexander Hall. Screenplay: P.J. Wolfson, Allen Rivkin, Manuel Seff, from a story by Jules Furthman.

The Girl in the News (Great Britain) 77 min. B & W. Released: 1/31/41. Distributor: 20th Century-Fox. Director: Carol Reed. Screenplay: Sidney Gilliatt, adapted from the book by Roy Vickers, *Girl in the News* (London: Jenkins, Herbert, 1938).

The Girl in the Pullman 59 min. B & W. Released: 10/31/27. Distributor: Pathe. Director: Erle Kenton. Adaptation: F. McGrew Willis, from Wilson Collison's *The Girl in Upper C* (New York: R.M. McBride, 1926).

The Girl in White 93 min. B & W. Released: 5/23/52. Distributor: MGM. Director: John Sturgess. Screenplay: Irmegard Von Cube, Philip Stevenson, adapted from a novel by Emily Dunning Barringer, *Bowery to Bellevue* (New York: Norton, 1950).

Girls in White 16 min. B & W. Released: 1949. Distributor: RKO. Director: Harry W. Smith. Producer: Jay Bonafield. Story: Dudley Hale.

The Glorious Fool 54 min. B & W. Released: 1/15/22. Distributor: Goldwyn. Director: E. Mason Hopper. Adaptation: J.G. Hawks, from the stories by Mary Roberts Rinehart, "In the Pavilion" and "Twenty-Two."

The G-Men 85 min. B & W. Reviewed: 4/18/35. Distributor: Warner Brothers. Director: William Keighley. Screenplay: Seton I. Miller.

Golden Shackles 56 min. B & W. Released: 3/15/28. Distributor: Peerless. Director: Dallas M. Fitzgerald. Scenario: Ada McQuillan, Gladys Gordon.

Good Morning, Miss Dove 107 min. DeLuxe Color. Released: 11/55. Distributor: 20th Century-Fox. Director: Henry Koster. Screenplay: Eleanore Griffin, from the book by Frances Gary Patton, *Good Morning Miss Dove* (New York: Dodd, Mead, 1954).

Good Morning, Nurse 46 min. B & W. Released: 3/6/17. Distributor: Victor. Director: Allen Curtis. Screenplay: Maie B. Havey.

Good Night Nurse 12 min. B & W. Released: 8/9/13. Distributor: Essanay.

Good Night Nurse 17 min. B & W. Released: 5/26/16. Distributor: Universal. Story: Albert E. Christie.

Good Night Nurse 2 reels. B & W. Released: 7/8/18. Distributor: Paramount. Director/Writer: Roscoe Arbuckle.

Good Night Nurse 20 min. B & W. Released: 4/23/29. Distributor: Educational Film Exchanges. Director: Henry W. George.

The Great Hospital Mystery 59 min. B & W. Released: 5/14/37. Distributor: 20th Century-Fox. Director: James Tinling. Screenplay: Bass Meredyth, William Conselman, Jerry Cady, adapted from the story by Mignon Eberhart, *Dead Yesterday* (New York: Doubleday, Doran, 1933).

The Great Jewel Robber 91 min. B & W. Released: 7/15/50. Distributor: Warner Brothers. Director: Peter Godfrey. Screenplay: Borden Chase.

The Great Victory 5 reels. B & W. Released: 1/4/19. Distributor: Metro. Director: Charles Miller. Screenplay: June Mathis, A.S. LeVino.

Green for Danger (Great Britain) 93 min. B & W. Released: 9/13/47. Distributor: Eagle-Lion. Director: Sidney Gilliatt. Screenplay: Sidney Gilliatt, Claude Guerney, adapted from the novel by Christiana Brand, *Green for Danger* (New York: Dodd, Mead, 1944).

Green Light 85 min. B & W. Released: 2/20/37. Distributor: Warner Bros. Director: Frank Borzage. Screenplay: Milton Krims, from the book by Lloyd C. Douglas, *Green Light* (Boston: Houghton Mifflin, 1935).

Half Angel 77 min. Technicolor. Released: 6/51. Distributor: 20th Century-Fox. Director: Richard Sale. Screenplay: Robert Riskin, adapted from a story by Robert Hardy Andrews (unpublished).

The Hand that Rocks the Cradle 6 reels. B & W. Released: 1917. Distributor: Universal.

Harvey 104 min. B & W. Released: 10/13/50. Distributor: Universal. Director: Henry Koster. Screenplay: Mary C. Chase, Oscar Brodney, adapted from the play by Mary C. Chase, *Harvey.*

The Hasty Heart 99 min. B & W. Reviewed: 12/2/49. Distributor: Warner Brothers. Director: Vincent Sherman. Screenplay: Ronald MacDougall, adapted from the play by John Patrick, *The Hasty Heart.*

The Haunted House 58 min. B & W. Released: 11/4/28. Distributor: First National. Producer: Wid Gunning. Director: Benjamin Christensen. Scenario: Richard Bee, Lajos Biro, from the play by Owen David, *The Haunted House: An American Comedy in Three Acts.*

Heart of Humanity 9 reels. B & W. Released: 2/10/19. Distributor: Universal.

Director: Allen Holubar. Screenplay: Allen Holubar, Olga Scholl.

Hellcats of the Navy 82 min. B & W. Released: 5/57. Distributor: Columbia. Director: Nathan Juran. Screenplay: David Lang, Raymond Marcus, adapted from the novel by Charles Lockwood, Hans Christian Adamson, *Hellcats of the Sea* (New York: Greenberg, 1955).

Hemingway's Adventures of a Young Man 145 min. DeLuxe Color. Released: 7/18/62. Distributor: 20th Century-Fox. Director: Martin Ritt. Screenplay: A.E. Hotchner, adapted from short stories by Ernest Hemingway.

Her Double Life 6 reels. B & W. Released: 1916. Distributor: Fox. Director: J. Gordon Edwards. Screenplay: Mary Murillo, adapted from her story, "The New Magdalen."

High Anxiety 94 min. DeLuxe Color. Released: 12/77. Distributor: 20th Century-Fox. Director: Mel Brooks. Screenplay: Mel Brooks, Ron Clark, Rudy DeLuca, Barry Levinson.

High Barbaree 91 min. B & W. Released: 5/47. Distributor: MGM. Director: Jack Conways. Screenplay: Anne Morrison Chapin, Whitfield Cook, Cyril Hume, adapted from the novel by Charles Bernard Nordhoff, James Norman Hall, *High Barbaree* (Boston: Little, Brown, 1945).

The Highest Trump 5 reels. B & W. Released: 2/3/19. Distributor: Vitagraph. Director: James Young. Story: H. H. Van Loan, Earle Williams.

His Forgotten Wife 65 min. B & W. Released: 4/14/24. Distributor: Film Booking Offices of America. Director: William Seiter. Story/Screenplay: Will Lambert.

His Master's Voice 58 min. B & W. Released: 9/25. Distributor: Lumas Film. Director: Renaud Hoffman. Scenario: Henry McCarty.

Homecoming 113 min. B & W. Released: 5/28/48. Distributor: MGM. Director: Mervyn LeRoy. Screenplay: Paul Osborn, from an original story by Sidney Kingsley.

The Honeymoon Killers 106 min. B & W. Released: 2/70. Distributor: Cinerama. Director: Leonard Kastle. Screenplay: Leonard Kastle.

The Horizontal Lieutenant 90 min. Metrocolor. Released: 4/18/62. Distributor: MGM. Director: Richard Thorpe. Screenplay: George Wells, adapted from the novel by Gordon Gotler, *The Bottletop Affair* (New York: Simon and Schuster, 1959).

The Hospital 103 min. DeLuxe Color. Released: 12/71. Distributor: United Artists. Director: Arthur Hiller. Screenplay: Paddy Chayefsky.

A Hospital Hoax 10 min. B & W. Released: 9/28/12. Distributor: Kalem.

House Calls 98 min. Color. Released: 3/31/78. Distributor: Universal. Director: Howard Zieff. Screenplay: Max Shulman, Julius J. Epstein, Alan Mandel, Charles Shyer, from a story by Max Shulman and Julius J. Epstein.

House of Dracula 67 min. B & W. Released: 12/7/45. Distributor: Universal. Director: Erle C. Kenton. Screenplay: Edward T. Lowe.

The House of Youth 67 min. B & W. Released: 10/19/24. Distributor: Producers Distributing. Director: Ralph Ince. Scenario: C. Gardner Sullivan, from the book by Maude Radford Warren, *The House of Youth* (Indianapolis: Bobbs-Merrill, 1923).

I, A Woman (Denmark/Sweden) 90 min. B & W. Released: 1965 (U.S.: 10/11/66). Distributor: Audubon Films. Director: Mac Ahlberg. Screenplay: Peer Guldbrandsen, adapted from Siv Holm's *Jeg, en kvinde* (Copenhagen: Stig Vendelkaers Forlag, 1961).

I, A Woman Part 2 (Denmark/Sweden) 81 min. Eastman Color. Released: 1968 (U.S.: 3/14/69). Distributor: Chevron. Director: Mac Ahlberg. Screenplay: Peer Guldbrandsen, adapted from the novel by Siv Holm, *Jeg, en kvinde 2* (Copenhagen: Stig Vendelkaers Forlag, 1968).

Ice Cold in Alex (Great Britain) 129 min. B & W. Released. 7/58. Distributor: Associated British Picture Corporation. Director: J. Lee-Thompson. Screenplay: Christopher Landon, J. Lee-Thompson, adapted from a novel by Christopher Landon.

Impulse 45 min. B & W. Released: 7/15/22. Distributor: Arrow Films. Director: Norval MacGregor, from the story by Maude Woodruff Newell, "Her Unknown Knight."

I Never Promised You a Rose Garden 96 min. Color. Released: 7/77. Distributor: New World. Director: Anthony Page. Screenplay: Gavin Lambert.

In Harm's Way 165 min. B & W. Released: 4/6/65. Distributor: Paramount. Director: Otto Preminger. Screenplay: Wendell Mayes, adapted from the novel by James Bassett, *Harm's Way* (Cleveland: World Publishing Co., 1962).

In Love and War 111 min. DeLuxe Color. Released: 11/58. Distributor: 20th Century-Fox. Director: Philip Dunne. Screenplay: Edward Anhalt, adapted from the novel by Anton Myrer, *The Big War* (New York: Appleton, Century Crofts, 1957).

Internes Can't Take Money 77 min. B & W. Released: 4/9/37. Distributor: Paramount. Director: Alfred Santell. Screenplay: Rian James, Theodore Reeves, from a short story by Max Brand.

The Interns 120 min. B & W. Released: 8/8/62. Distributor: Columbia. Director: David Swift. Screenplay: Walter Newman, adapted from the novel by Richard Frede, *The Interns* (New York: Random House, 1960).

Island of Desire 103 min. Technicolor. Released: 7/4/52. Distributor: United Artists. Director: Stuart Heisler. Screenplay: Stephanie Nordli, adapted from the novel by Hugh Brooke, *Saturday Island* (New York: Doubleday, 1935).

It Happened at the World's Fair 105 min. Metrocolor. Released: 4/3/63. Distributor: MGM. Director: Norman Taurog. Screenplay: Si Rose, Seaman Jacobs.

It Happened in Brooklyn 105 min. B & W. Released: 3/22/47. Distributor: MGM. Director: Richard Whorf. Screenplay: Isobel Lennart, from an original story by John McGowan.

It's Only Money 84 min. B & W. Released: 11/21/62. Distributor: Paramount. Director: Frank Tashlin. Screenplay: John Fenton Murray.

I Walked with a Zombie 69 min. B & W. Reviewed: 3/17/43. Distributor: RKO. Producer: Val Lewton. Director: Jacques Tourneur. Screenplay: Curt Siodmak, Ardel Wray, from an original screen story by Inez Wallace.

I Want My Man 62 min. B & W. Released: 3/22/25. Distributor: First National. Director: Lambert Hillyer. Scenario: Joseph Poland, Earle Snell, from the book by Maxwell Struthers Burt, *The Interpreter's House* (New York: Scribner's, 1924).

I Was a Spy 85 min. B & W. Reviewed: 1/13/34. Distributor: Fox. Director: Victor Saville. Screenplay: W.P. Lipscomb, Ian Hay, adapted from the book by Martha McKenna, *I Was a Spy* (New York: McBride, 1933).

Jessica (United States/France/Italy; also titled *La Sage Femme, le Curé et le Bon Dieu*) 105 min. Technicolor. Released: 3/28/62 (United States); 6/62 (France); 2/62 (Italy). Distributor: United Artists. Director: Jean Negulesco, Oreste Palella. Screenplay: Edith Sommer, Ennio De Concini, adapted from Flora Sandstrom's, *The Midwife of Pont Clery* (New York: John Day Co., 1957).

Johnny Got His Gun 111 min. Color. Released: 8/71. Distributor: Cinemation. Director: Dalton Trumbo. Screenplay: Dalton Trumbo, adapted from his novel.

Jolson Sings Again 96 min. B & W. Reviewed: 8/12/49. Distributor: Columbia-Buchman. Producer/Screenplay: Sidney Buchman. Director: Henry Levin.

K: The Unknown 72 min. B & W. Released: 8/31/24. Distributor: Universal-Jewel. Director: Harry Pollard. Based on Mary Roberts Rinehart's novel, *K* (Boston: Houghton Mifflin, 1915).

The Killer that Stalked New York 79 min. B & W. Released: 12/50. Distributor: Columbia. Director: Earl McEvoy. Screenplay: Harry Essex, adapted from a magazine story by Milton Lehman.

King of Alcatraz 56 min. B & W. Released: 9/30/38. Distributor: Paramount. Director: Robert Florey. Screenplay: Irving Reis.

The Kiss Barrier 6 reels. B & W. Released: 5/31/25. Distributor: Fox. Director: R. William Neill. Scenario: E. Magnus Ingleton, from a story by Frederick Hatton, Fanny Hatton.

Kiss the Blood Off My Hands 79 min. B & W. Released: 11/48. Distributor: Universal-International-Hecht. Director: Norman Foster. Screenplay: Leonardo Bercovici, adapted from the novel by Gerald Butler, *Kiss the Blood Off My Hands* (London: Nicholson, 1940).

The Lady Takes a Flyer 94 min. Eastman Color. Released: 3/58. Distributor: Universal. Director: Jack Arnold. Screenplay: Danny Arnold, adapted from a short story by Edmund H. North (unpublished).

The Lady with the Lamp (Great Britain) 110 min. B & W. Released: 10/51. Distributor: BL. Director: Herbert Wilcox. Screenplay: Warren Chetham Strode, adapted from the play by Reginald Berkeley.

The Lamp Still Burns (Great Britain) 90 min. B & W. Released: 11/43. Distributor: General Film Distributors. Producer: Leslie Howard. Director: Maurice Elvey. Screenplay: Elizabeth Baron, Roland Pertwee, Major Neilson, adapted from the novel by Monica Dickens, *One Pair of Feet* (New York: Harper, 1942).

The Last Hour 67 min. B & W. Released: 1/1/23. Distributor: Mastodon Films. Director: Edward Sloman. From a story by Frank R. Adams, "Blind Justice."

The Last Man 5 reels. B & W. Released: 1916. Distributor: Vitagraph. Director: William Wolbert. Story: James Oliver Curwood.

The Left Hand of God 87 min. DeLuxe Color. Released: 9/55. Distributor: 20th Century-Fox. Director: Edward Dmytryk. Screenplay: Alfred Hayes, adapted from the book by William E. Barrett, *The Left Hand of God* (New York: Doubleday, 1951).

Lew Tyler's Wives 68 min. B & W. Released: 6/15/26. Distributor: Preferred Pictures. Director: Harley Knoles. Adaptation: Eugene Clifford, Arthur Hoerl, from the book by Wallace Irwin, *Lew Tyler's Wives: A Novel* (New York: G. P. Putnam's Sons, 1923).

Life Begins 71 min. B & W. Released: 10/1/32. Distributor: Warner Brothers. Director: James Flood. Screenplay: Earl Baldwin, adapted from the three-act play by Mary MacDougal Axelson, *Life Begins.*

Lifeboat 96 min. B & W. Released: 1/28/44. Distributor: 20th Century-Fox. Director: Alfred Hitchcock. Screenplay: Jo Swerling, adapted from a story by John Steinbeck (unpublished).

Life in Emergency Ward 10 (Great Britain) 86 min. B & W. Released: 3/59. Distributor: Eros. Director: Robert Day. Screenplay: Tessa Diamond, Hazel Adair, adapted from the TV serial by Tessa Diamond, *Emergency Ward 10.*

The Light 5 reels. B & W. Released: 1/12/19. Distributor: Fox. Director: J. Gordon Edwards. Screenplay: Adrian Johnson, Charles Kenyon. Story: Arthur Reed, Bret Page.

Little Accident 82 min. B & W. Released: 9/1/30. Distributor: Universal. Director: William James Craft. Screenplay: Anthony Brown, adapted from the play by Floyd Dell, Thomas Mitchell, *Little Accident.*

Little Wildcat 50 min. B & W. Released: 11/12/22. Distributor: Vitagraph. Director: David Divad. Scenario: Bradley J. Smollen.

The Love Doctor 55 min. B & W. Released: 10/5/29. Distributor: Paramount Famous Lasky Corp. Director: Melville Brown. Dialogue: Guy Bolton. Adaptation: Guy Bolton, J. Walter Ruben, from the play by Winchell Smith, Victor Mapes, *The Boomerang: Comedy in Three Acts.*

Love Takes Flight 73 min. B & W. Released: 8/13/37. Distributor: Grand National. Director: Conrad Nage. From a short story by Anne Morrison Chaplin.

Luxury Liner 68 min. B & W. Reviewed: 2/4/33. Distributor: Paramount. Director: Lothar Mendes. Screenplay: Gene Markey, Kathryn Scola, from the book by Gina Kaus, *Luxury Liner* (New York: R. Long and R. R. Smith, 1932).

Magnificent Obsession 112 min. B & W. Reviewed: 12/31/35. Distributor: Universal. Director: John M. Stahl. Screenplay: George O'Neil, Sarah Y. Mason, Victor Heerman, from the book by Lloyd C. Douglas, *Magnificent Obsession* (New York: Willett, Clark, 1933).

Magnificent Obsession 108 min. Technicolor. Released: 8/54. Distributor: Universal. Director: Douglas Sirk. Screenplay: Sarah Y. Mason, Victor Heerman, from the book by Lloyd C. Douglas, *Magnificent Obsession* (New York: Willett Clark, 1933)

Maimed in the Hospital 18 min. B & W. Released: 1/26/18. Distributor: Universal. Director/Writer: Craig Hutchinson.

Man and Maid 53 min. B & W. Released: 4/20/25. Distributor: Metro-Goldwyn. Director: Victory Schertzinger. Scenario: Elinor Glyn, from the book by Elinor Glyn, *Man and Maid* (Philadelphia: Lippincott, 1922).

Man in the Middle (United States/Great Britain) 94 min. B & W. Released: 1/29/64 (United States): 10/63 (Great Britain). Distributor: 20th Century-Fox. Director: Guy Hamilton. Screenplay: Keith Waterhouse, Willis Hall, adapted from the novel by Howard Melvin Fast, *The Winston Affair* (New York: Morrow, 1959).

A Man's World 60 min. B & W. Released: 9/14/42. Distributor: Columbia. Director: Charles Barton. Adapted from an original screen story by Jack Roberts, George Bricker.

A Man to Remember 80 min. B & W. Released: 10/14/38. Distributor: RKO. Director: Garson Kanin. Screenplay: Dalton Trumbo, from the short story by Katherine Haviland Taylor, "The Failure" in *Box Office* (New York: Ziff-Davis, 1943).

The Man Who Came to Dinner 112 min. B & W. Reviewed: 12/24/41. Distributor: Warner Brothers. Director: William Keighley. Screenplay: Joseph West, adapted from the book by George S. Kaufman, Moss Hart, *The Man Who Came to Dinner* (New York: Random House, 1939).

The Man Who Found Himself 67 min. B & W. Released: 4/2/37. Distributor: RKO. Director: Lew Landers. Screenplay: J. Robert Bren, Edmund L. Hartman, from an original screen story by Alice F. Curtis.

The Man Who Lived Again (Great Britain) 61 min. B & W. Reviewed: 12/16/36. Distributor: Gaumont British Productions. Director: Robert Stevenson. Screenplay: L. du Garde Peach, Sidney Gilliat.

The Market of Souls 5 reels. B & W. Released: 9/7/19. Distributor: Famous Players-Lasky. Director: Joseph De Grasse. Screenplay: C. Gardner Sullivan. Story: John Lynch.

The Martyrdom of Nurse Cavell (Australia) 29 min. B & W. Released: 1916. Director: C. Post Mason.

Mary Stevens, M.D. 72 min. B & W. Reviewed: 7/28/33. Distributor: Warner Brothers. Director: Lloyd Bacon. Screenplay: Rian James, from a story by Virginia Kellogg.

*M*A*S*H* 116 min. DeLuxe Color. Released: 1/70. Distributor: 20th Century-Fox. Director: Robert Altman. Screenplay: Ring Lardner Jr., from the novel by Richard Hooker.

*M*A*S*H*D* 75 min. Color. Released: 5/76. Distributor: Hudson. Director/Screenplay: Emton Smith.

Mayor of Hell 85 min. B & W. Reviewed: 9/15/33. Distributor: Warner Brothers. Director: Archie Mayo. Screenplay: Ed Sullivan, from a story by Islin Auster.

Medium Cool 110 min. Technicolor. Released: 8/27/69. Distributor: Paramount. Director: Haskell Wexler. Screenplay: Haskell Wexler, adapted from the novel by Jack Couffer, *The Concrete Wilderness* (New York: Hawthorn, 1967).

The Men 85 min. B & W. Released. 9/8/50. Distributor: United Artists. Director: Fred Zinnemann. Screenplay: Glenn Tryon, from an original story by Carl Foreman.

Men in White 80 min. B & W. Reviewed: 3/28/34. Distributor: MGM. Director: Richard Boleslavsky. Screenplay: Waldemar Young, adapted from the play by Sidney Kingsley, *Men in White.*

Men Must Fight 72 min. B & W. Released: 3/11/33. Distributor: MGM. Director: Edgar Selwyn. Screenplay: C. Gardner Sullivan, adapted from the play by Reginald Lawrence, S.K. Lauren, *Men Must Fight.*

Mine Own Executioner (Great Britain) 103 min. B & W. Released: 7/48. Distributor: 20th Century-Fox. Director: Anthony Kimmins. Screenplay: Nigel Balchin, adapted from the novel by Nigel Balchin, *Mine Own Executioner* (London: Collins, 1945).

Mission Batangas 100 min. Technicolor. Released: 11/68. Distributor: Manson Distributing Corporation. Director: Keith Larsen. Screenplay: Lew Antonio, from an original story by Keith Larsen.

Mission Over Korea 85 min. B & W. Released: 8/53. Distributor: Columbia. Director: Fred F. Sears. Screenplay: Jesse Lasky Jr., Eugene Ling, Martin M. Goldsmith, from a screen story by Richard Tregaskis.

Miss Pinkerton 66 min. B & W. Released: 7/30/32. Distributor: Warner Brothers. Director: Lloyd Bacon. Screenplay: Lillian Hayward, Nevin Bush, adapted from the book by Mary Roberts Rinehart, *Miss Pinkerton* (New York: Farrar and Rinehart, 1932).

Miss Susie Slagle's 88 min. B & W. Reviewed: 12/13/45. Distributor: Paramount. Director: John Berry. Screenplay: Anne Froelich, Hugo Butler, from the novel by Augusta Tucker, *Miss Susie Slagle's* (New York: Harper, 1939).

Mr. Belvedere Rings the Bell 87 min. B & W. Released: 8/51. Distributor: 20th Century-Fox. Director: Henry Koster. Screenplay: Ronald MacDougall, based on the character created by Gwen Davenport and on the play by Robert McEnroe, *The Silver Whistle.*

Mister Roberts 123 min. Warner-Color. Released: 7/30/55. Distributor: Warner Brothers. Directors: John Ford, Mervyn LeRoy. Screenplay: Frank Nugent, Joshua Logan, adapted from the play by Thomas Heggen, Joshua Logan, *Mr. Roberts.*

The Mob 87 min. B & W. Released: 10/51. Distributor: Columbia. Director: Robert Parrish. Screenplay: William Bowers, adapted from the novel by Ferguson Findley, *Waterfront* (New York: Macmillan, 1934).

Murder by an Aristocrat 60 min. B & W. Reviewed: 6/13/36. Distributor: Warner Brothers. Director: Frank McDonald. Screenplay: Luci Ward, Roy Chanslor, from the book by Mignon G. Eberhart, *Murder by an Aristocrat* (New York: Doubleday, Doran, 1932).

The Murder of Dr. Harrigan 66 min. B & W. Reviewed: 1/21/36. Distributor: Warner Brothers. Director: Frank McDonald. Screenplay: Peter Milne, Sy Bartlett, Charles Belden, from the book by Mignon G. Eberhart, *From This Dark Stairway* (Garden City, NY: Doubleday, Doran, 1931).

My Brother Jonathan (Great Britain) 102 min. B & W. Released: 6/1/49. Distributor: Allied Artists-Associated British. Director: Harold French. Screenplay: Leslie Landau, Adrian Alington, from the book by Francis Brett Young, *My Brother Jonathan* (New York: Knopf, 1928).

Mystery House 61 min. B & W. Released: 5/21/38. Distributor: Warner Brothers. Director: Noel Smith. Screenplay: Sherman Lowe, Robertson White, from the book by Mignon G. Eberhart, *Mystery of Hunting's End* (Garden City, NY: Doubleday, Doran, 1930).

Mystery of the White Room 58 min. B & W. Released: 3/17/39. Distributor: Universal. Director: Otis Garrett. Screenplay: Alex Gottlieb.

The Naked Kiss 93 min. B & W. Released: 5/4/64. Distributor: Allied Artists. Director: Samuel Fuller. Screenplay: Samuel Fuller.

The National Health 97 min. Color. Released: 4/29/72. Distributor: Warners. Director: Jack Gold. Screenplay: Peter Nichols, based on his stage play.

Naughty Nurses 85 min. Color. Released: 1973. Distributor: Target. Director: Don Edmonds. Screenplay: Don Edmonds.

Navy Nurse 20 min. B & W Released: 3/16/45. Distributor: Vitaphone. Director: D. Ross Lederman.

The Navy vs. The Night Monster 87 min. DeLuxe Color. Released: 6/8/66. Distributor: Realart Pictures. Director: Michael A. Hoey. Screenplay: Michael A. Hoey,

adapted from a novel by Murray Leinster, *Monster from the Earth's End* (Greenwich, CT: Fawcett, 1959).

Navy Wife 69 min. B & W. Reviewed: 9/17/35. Distributor: Fox. Director: Allan Dwan. Screenplay: Sonya Levien, from the book by Kathleen Norris, *Beauty's Daughter* (New York: Doubleday, Doran, 1935).

The New Commandment 70 min. B & W. Released: 11/1/25. Distributor: First National. Director: Howard Higgin. Adaptation: Sada Cowan, Howard Higgin, from the book by Frederick Palmer, *Invisible Wounds* (New York: Dodd, Mead, 1925).

The New Interns 123 min. B & W. Released: 8/19/64. Distributor: Columbia. Director: John Rich. Screenplay: Wilton Schiller, based on characters created by Richard Frede.

Nick Carter—Master Detective 60 min. B & W. Released: 12/15/39. Distributor: MGM. Director: Jacques Tourneur. Screenplay: Bertram Millhauser, from an original screen story by Bertram Millhauser, Harold Buckley.

Nifty Nurses 18 min. B & W. Released: 10/10/34. Distributor: Educational Productions. Director/Story: Leigh Jason.

Night and Day 128 min. B & W. Released: 8/3/46. Distributor: Warner Brothers. Director: Michael Curtiz. Screenplay: Charles Hoffman, Leo Townsend, William Bowers, based on the career of Cole Porter.

Night Angel 86 min. B & W. Released: 7/18/31. Distributor: Paramount. Director: Edmund Goulding. Screenplay: Edmund Goulding.

Night Call Nurses 85 min. Metrocolor. Released: 6/15/72. Distributor: New World. Director: Jonathan Kaplan. Screenplay: George Armitage.

Night Nurse 72 min. B & W. Released: 8/8/31. Distributor: Warner Brothers. Director: William A. Wellman. Screenplay: Oliver H.P. Garett, Charles Kenyon, suggested by the book by Dora Macy, *Night Nurse* (New York: Brentano's, 1930).

Night Work 84 min. B & W. Released: 8/3/30. Distributor: Pathe. Director: Russell Mack. Screenplay: Walter De Leon, from an original story by Walter De Leon.

Nobody's Baby 65 min. B & W. Released: 4/23/37. Distributor: MGM. Director: Gus Meins. Screenplay: Harold Law, Hal Yates, Pat C. Flick.

Nobody's Perfect 103 min. Technicolor. Released: 1/68. Distributor: Universal. Director: Alan Rafkin. Screenplay: John D.F. Black, adapted from the novel by Allan R. Bosworth, *The Crows of Edwina Hill* (New York: Harper, 1961).

No Place Like Homicide (Great Britain; originally titled *What a Carve Up!*) 87 min. B & W. Released: 7/61 (U.S.: 6/13/62). Distributor: Embassy. Director: Pat Jackson. Screenplay: Ray Cooney, Tony Hilton, adapted from Frank King's *The Ghoul* (London: G.H. Watt, 1928).

North West Mounted Police 125 min. Technicolor. Released: 12/27/40. Distributor: Paramount. Director: Cecil B. DeMille. Screenplay: Alan Le May, Jessie Lasky Jr., C. Gardner Sullivan, adapted from the novel by R.C. Fetherstonhaugh, *Royal Canadian Mounted Police* (New York: Carrick and Evans, 1938).

Not as a Stranger 135 min. B & W. Released: 7/55. Distributor: United Artists. Director: Stanley Kramer. Screenplay: Edna Anhalt, Edward Anhalt, adapted from the book by Morton Thompson, *Not as a Stranger* (New York: Scribner's, 1954).

No Time for Tears (Great Britain) 86 min. Eastman Color. Released: 8/57. Distributor: Associated British. Director: Cyril Frankel. Story: Anne Burnaby.

Not of This Earth 67 min. B & W. Released: 2/10/57. Distributor: Allied Artists. Producer/Director: Roger Corman. Screenplay: Charles Griffith, Mark Hanna.

The Notorious Landlady 123 min. B & W. Released: 6/27/62. Distributor: Columbia. Director: Richard Quine. Screenplay: Larry Gelbart, Blake Edwards, adapted from a short story by Margery Sharp, "Notorious Tenant."

Not With My Wife, You Don't! 118 min. Technicolor. Released: 11/2/66. Distributor: Warner Brothers. Director: Norman Panama. Screenplay: Norman Panama, Larry Gelbart, Peter Barnes, from an original story by Norman Panama, Melvin Frank.

Numbered Woman 6 min. B & W. Released: 5/22/38. Distributor: Monogram. Director: Karl Brown. Screenplay: John T. Neville.

The Nun's Story 149 min. Technicolor. Released: 7/4/59. Distributor: Warners. Director: Fred Zinneman. Screenplay: Robert Anderson, adapted from the novel by Kathryn Hulme, *The Nun's Story* (Boston: Little, Brown, 1956).

The Nurse 10 min. B & W. Released: 2/17/12. Distributor: Edison.

Nurse and Martyr (Great Britain) 30 min. B & W. Released: 1915. Distributor: Midland. Director: Percy Moran. Story: Edgar Wallace, Percy Moran, Cora Lee.

The Nurse and The Counterfeiter 10 min. B & W. Released: 4/18/14. Distributor: Kalem.

The Nurse at Mulberry Bend 10 mins. B & W. Released: 1/18/13. Distributor: Kalem.

Nurse Edith Cavell 95 min. B & W. Released: 9/29/39. Distributor: RKO. Director: Herbert Wilcox. Screenplay: Michael Hogan, adapted from the book by Reginald Berkeley, *Dawn* (New York: J.H. Sears, 1928).

Nurse From Brooklyn 67 min. B & W. Released: 4/15/38. Distributor: Universal. Director: S. Sylvan Simon. Screenplay: Roy Chanslor, from the story by Steve Fisher, "If You Break My Heart."

Nurse Marjorie 52 min. B & W. Released: 3/28/20. Distributor: Realart. Director: William D. Taylor. Screenplay: Julia Crawford Ivers. Story: Israel Zargwill.

Nurse! Nurse! (Great Britain) 20 min. B & W. Released: 1916. Distributor: Moss. Director: Alexander Butler. Story: Reuben Gilmer.

The Nurse of An Aching Heart 2 reels. B & W. Released: 9/22/17. Distributor: L-Ko Motion Pictures. Director: Archie Mayo.

Nurse on Wheels (Great Britain) 86 min. B & W. Released: 6/63 (U.S.: 11/63). Distributor: Janus Films. Director: Gerald Thomas. Screenplay: Norman Hudis, adapted from the novel by Joanna Jones, *Nurse Is a Neighbour* (London: Joseph, 1958).

The Nurses 71 min. Eastman Color. Released: 1979. Distributor: Sherpix. Producer/Director: Terry Sullivan.

Nurses Attending the Wounded (Great Britain) 1 min. B & W. Released: 12/1899. Production Company: R.W. Paul. Director: Sir Robert Ashe.

The Nurse's Brother (Great Britain) 1 min. B & W. Released: 7/1900. Production Company: Mitchell and Kenyon.

A Nurse's Devotion (Great Britain) 10 min. B & W. Released: 1912. Production Company: Brighton and County Films. Director: Walter Speer.

Nurses For Sale 84 min. Eastman Color. Released: 7/77. Distributor: Independent-International. Director: Rolf Olson.

Nurse Sherri 88 min. Eastman Color. Released: 8/78. Distributor: Independent International. Director: Al Adamson. Screenplay: Michael Bockman, Gregg Tittinger.

A Nurse's Sacrifice 16 min. B & W. Released: 1/2/17. Distributor: Nordisk Films.

The Nurse's Secret 65 min. B & W. Released: 5/24/41. Distributor: Warner Brothers. Director: Noel M. Smith. Screenplay: Anthony Coldeway, adapted from the novel by Mary Roberts Rinehart, *Miss Pinkerton* (New York: Farrar and Rinehart, 1932).

Nurse to You 20 min. B & W. Released: 9/2/35. Distributor: MGM. Director: Charles Parrott, Jeff Moffitt.

Oh, Doctor! 66 min. B & W. Released: 10/27/26. Distributor: Universal. Director: Harry A. Pollard. Adaptation/Continuity: Harvey Thew, from the novel by Harry Leon Wilson, *Oh Doctor!* (New York: Cosmopolitan Book Corporation, 1923).

Oh, Doctor 70 min. B & W. Released: 5/16/37. Distributor: Universal. Director: Ray McCarey. Screenplay: Harry Clork, Brown Holmes, from the book by Harry Leon Wilson, *Oh, Doctor!* (New York: Cosmopolitan Book Corporation, 1923).

Oh, Nursie 20 min. B & W. Released: 3/16/23. Distributor: Universal.

Oh, Oh Nursie 10 min. B & W. Released: 9/9/19. Distributor: Universal. Writer/Director: Lyons and Moran.

Oh, What a Nurse! 69 min. B & W. Released: 3/20/26. Distributor: Warner Brothers. Director: Charles Reisner. Adaptation: Darryl Francis Zanuck, from the story by Robert Emmet Sherwood, Bertram Bloch, "Oh, What a Nurse!" (publication undetermined).

Once to Every Woman 70 min. B & W. Reviewed: 3/24/34. Distributor: Columbia. Director: Lambert Hillyer. Screenplay: Jo Swerling, from the book by Archibald Joseph Kronin, *Kaleidoscope in K* (Berlin: P. Zeolnun, 1939).

One Flew Over the Cuckoo's Nest 129 min. Color. Released: 11/75. Distributor: United Artists. Director: Milos Forman. Screenplay: Lawrence Hauben, Bo Goldman, based on the novel by Ken Kesey, *One Flew over the Cuckoo's Nest* (New York: New American Library, 1962).

One Hysterical Night 53 min. B & W. Released: 10/6/29. Distributor: Universal. Director: William J. Craft. Scenario: Earl Snell.

One Increasing Purpose 77 min. B & W. Released: 1/2/27. Distributor: Fox. Director: Harry Beaumont. Scenario: Bradley King, from the book by Arthur Stuart-Menteth Hutchinson, *One Increasing Purpose* (Boston: Little, Brown, 1925).

One Sunday Afternoon 70 min. B & W. Reviewed: 9/2/33. Distributor: Paramount. Director: Stephen Roberts. Screenplay: Grover Jones, William. Slavens McNutt, adapted from the play by James Hagan, *One Sunday Afternoon.*

One Sunday Afternoon 90 min. B & W. Reviewed: 12/14/48. Distributor: Warner Brothers. Director: Raoul Walsh. Screenplay: Robert L. Richards, adapted from the play by James Hagan, *One Sunday Afternoon.*

Operation Mad Ball 105 min. B & W. Released: 11/57. Distributor: Columbia. Director: Richard Quine. Screenplay: Arthur Carter, adapted from the play by Arthur Carter, *Operation Mad Ball.*

Operation Pacific 111 min. B & W. Released: 1/27/51. Distributor: Warner Brothers. Director: George Waggner. Screenplay: George Waggner.

Operation Petticoat 124 min. Eastman Color. Released: 12/59. Distributor: Universal. Director: Blake Edwards. Screenplay: Stanley Shapiro, Maurice Richlin, adapted from a short story by Paul King, Joseph Stone (unpublished).

Our Little Girl 63 min. B & W. Reviewed: 6/7/35. Distributor: Fox. Director: John Robertson. Screenplay: Stephen Avery, Allen Rivkin, Jack Yellen, from the short story by Florence Leighton, "Heaven's Gate."

Out All Night 68 min. B & W. Reviewed: 4/8/33. Distributor: Universal. Director: Sam Taylor. Screenplay: William Anthony McGuire, from a story by Tim Whelan.

Outside the Law 66 min. B & W. Reviewed: 10/26/38. Distributor: Columbia. Director: Lewis D. Collins. Screenplay: Gordon Rigby, from an original screen story by Gordon Rigby, Carlton Sand.

Outside the Wall 80 min. B & W. Released: 3/50. Distributor: Universal. Director: Crane Wilbur. Screenplay: Crane Wilbur, from an original story by Edward Helseth.

Pacific Liner 76 min. B & W. Released: 1/6/39. Distributor: RKO. Director: Lew Landers. Screenplay: John Twist, from an original screen story by Anthony Coldeway, Henry Robert Symonds.

Parachute Nurse 65 min. B & W. Released: 6/18/42. Distributor: Columbia. Director: Charles Barton. Screenplay: Rian James, adapted from an original screen story by Elizabeth Meehan.

Paranoiac (Great Britain) 80 min. B & W. Released: 9/63 (U.S.: 5/15/63). Distributor: Universal. Director: Freddie Francis. Screenplay: Jimmy Sangster.

The Patent Leather Kid 120 min. B & W. Released: 9/1/27. Distributor: First National. Producer/Director: Alfred Santell. Scenario: Winifred Dunn, from the story by Rupert Hughes, "Patent Leather Kid," in *Patent Leather Kid and Several Others* (New York: Grosset and Dunlap, 1927).

The Patient in Room 18 60 min. B & W. Released: 1/8/38. Distributor: Warner Brothers. Director: Bobby Connolly, Crane Wilbur. Screenplay: Eugene Solow, Robertson White, from the book by Mignon G. Eberhart, *Patient in Room 18* (Garden City, NY: Doubleday, Doran, 1929).

Patrick (Australia) 96 min. Color. Released: 1979. Distributor: Filmways. Director: Richard Franklin. Writer: Everett de Roche.

Patriotism 47 min. B & W. Released: 6/16/18. Distributor: Paralta. Director: Raymond B. West. Screenplay: R.B. Kidd, Jane Holly.

The People vs. Dr. Kildare 78 min. B & W. Released: 5/2/41. Distributor: MGM. Director: Harold S. Bucquet. Screenplay: Willis Goldbeck, Harry Ruskin, adapted from the book by Max Brand, *Dr. Kildare's Trial* (Toronto: Dodd, 1942).

Percy 100 min. B & W. Released: 4/71. Distributor: MGM. Director: Ralph Thomas. Screenplay: Hugh Leonard, adapted from the novel by Raymond Hitchcock.

Period of Adjustment 112 min. B & W. Released: 10/31/62. Distributor: MGM. Director: George Roy Hill. Screenplay: Isobel Lennart, adapted from the play by Tennessee Williams, *High Point over a Cavern.*

Persona (Sweden) 81 min. B & W. Released: 10/66 (U.S.: 3/6/67). Distributor: Lopert Pictures. Director: Ingmar Bergman. Screenplay: Ingmar Bergman.

Pinky 102 min. B & W. Released: 11/49. Distributor: 20th Century-Fox. Director: Elia Kazan. Screenplay: Philip Dunne, Dudley Nichols, from the novel by Cid Ricketts Summer, *Quality* (London: Dymock, n.d.).

Police Nurse 64 min. B & W. Released: 5/63. Distributor: 20th Century-Fox. Director: Maury Dexter. Screenplay: Harry Spalding.

Possessed 108 min. B & W. Released: 10/25/47. Distributor: Warner Brothers. Director: Curtis Bernhardt. Screenplay: Silvia Richards, Ranald MacDougall, adapted from a short story by Rita Weiman, *"One Man's Secret."*

Prison Nurse 65 min. B & W. Released: 3/4/38. Distributor: Republic. Director: James Cruze. Screenplay: Earl Fenton, Sidney Salkow, from the book by Dr. Louis Berg, *Prison Nurse* (New York: Macaulay, 1934).

Prison Without Bars (Great Britain) 80 min. B & W. Released: 10/38. Distributor: United Artists. Director: Brian Desmond Hurst. Screenplay: Hans Wilhelm, Margaret Kennedy, adapted from the play by Gina Kaus, E. Eis, O. Eis, Hilde Koveloff, *Prison Sans Barreaux.*

Private Duty Nurses 80 min. Metrocolor. Released: 1971. Distributor: New World. Director: George Armitage. Screenplay: George Armitage.

The Private Navy of Sgt. O'Farrell 92 min. Technicolor. Released: 5/8/68. Distributor: United Artists. Director: Frank Tashlin. Screenplay: Frank Tashlin, from an original story by John L. Greene, Robert M. Fresco.

Private Nurse 60 min. B & W. Released: 8/22/41. Distributor: 20th Century-Fox.

Director: David Burton. Screenplay: Samuel G. Engel.

Private Worlds 84 min. B & W. Reviewed: 3/9/35. Distributor: Paramount. Director: Gregory LaCava. Screenplay: Lynn Starling, adapted from the book by Phyllis Bottome, *Private Worlds* (Boston: Houghton Mifflin, 1934).

The Promise Land 3 reels. B & W. Released: 6/7/16. Distributor: Essanay.

Rear Window 112 min. Technicolor. Released: 9/54. Distributor: Paramount. Director: Alfred Hitchcock. Screenplay: John Michael Hayes, from the short story by Cornell Woolrich, "Rear Window" in *After Dinner Story* (Philadelphia: J.B. Lippincott, 1944).

Recompense 74 min. B & W. Released: 4/26/25. Distributor: Warner Brothers. Director: Harry Beaumont. Scenario: Dorothy Farnum, from the book by Robert Keable, *Recompense: A Sequel to "Simon Called Peter"* (New York: G.P. Putnam's Sons, 1924).

A Red Cross Martyr 14 min. B & W. Released: 12/30/11. Production Company: Vitagraph. Director: Larry Trimble. Screenplay: Marguerite Bertsch.

The Red Cross Nurse 3 reels, B & W. Released: 10/10/14. Production Company: Columbus.

The Red Tent 121 min. Technicolor. Released: 7/71. Distributor: Paramount. Director: Mickail K. Kalatozov. Screenplay: Ennio De Concini, Richard Adams.

The Regeneration of Margaret 3 reels. B & W. Released: 7/1/16. Distributor: Essanay.

Registered Nurse 62 min. B & W. Reviewed: 6/1/34. Distributor: Warner Brothers. Director: Robert Florey. Screenplay: Lillie Hayward, Peter Milne, adapted from the play by Florence Johns, Wilton Lackaye, *Miss Benton, R.N.*

Remedy for Riches 60 min. B & W. Released: 11/29/40. Distributor: RKO. Director: Erle C. Kenton. Screenplay: Lee Loeb.

Reunion 80 min. B & W. Reviewed: 11/13/36. Distributor: 20th Century-Fox. Director: Norman Taurog. Screenplay: Sam Hellman, Gladys Lehman, Sonya Levien, from a story by Bruce Gould (unpublished).

Revelation 7 reels. B & W. Released: 3/18. Distributor: Metro. Director: George D. Baker, based on the novel by Mabel Wagnalls.

Reward Unlimited 10 min. B & W. Released: 1944. Production supervised by David O. Selznick.

Rhino! 91 min. Metrocolor. Released: 5/20/64. Distributor: MGM. Director: Ivan Thors. Screenplay: Art Arthur, Arthur Weiss.

The Right to Live 75 min. B & W. Reviewed: 2/16/35. Distributor: Warner Brothers. Director: William Keighley. Screenplay: Ralph Block, from the book by William Somerset Maugham, *The Sacred Flame* (New York: Doubleday, 1928).

Ringside 63 min. B & W. Released: 7/49. Distributor: Screen Guild. Director: Frank McDonald. Screenplay: Daniel B. Ullman.

The Road to Glory 95 min. B & W. Reviewed: 6/2/36. Distributor: 20th Century-Fox. Director: Howard Hawks. Screenplay: Joel Sayre, William Faulkner.

Rosie Dixon—Night Nurse (Great Britain) 88 min. Color. Released: 2/19/78. Distributor: Columbia. Director: Justin Cartwright. Screenplay: Christopher Wood, Justin Cartwright, adapted from the novel by Rosie Dixon, *Rosie Dixon—Night Nurse.*

Ruling Passions 5 reels. B & W. Released: 2/29/18. Distributor: Schomer. Director/Writer: Abraham S. Schomer.

The Sacred Flame 61 min. B & W. Released: 11/24/29. Distributor: Warner Brothers. Director: Archie L. Mayo. Scenario/Dialoguer: Harvey Thew, from the play by William Somerset Maugham, *The Sacred Flame: A Play in Three Acts.*

A Sanitarium Scramble 2 reels. B & W. Released: 1/22/16. Distributor: American. Director: Reaves Easton.

Scream and Scream Again (Great Britain) 95 min. Movielab. Released: 2/70. Distributor: American-International. Director: Gordon Hessler. Screenplay: Christopher Wicking, from the novel by Peter Saxon, *Disoriented Man* (New York: Paperback Library, 1970).

Secret of Dr. Kildare 84 min. B & W. Released: 11/24/39. Distributor: MGM. Director: Harold S. Bucquet. Screenplay: Willis Goldbeck, Harry Ruskin, from the book by Max Brand, *The Secret of Dr. Kildare* (New York: Dodd, Mead, 1940).

Secrets of a Nurse 69 min. B & W. Released: 12/9/38. Distributor: Universal. Director: Arthur Lubin. Screenplay: Tom Lennon, Lester Cole, from a short story by Quentin Reynolds, "West Side Miracle."

She Goes to War 95 min. B & W. Partial sound. Also 84 min. B & W. Silent. Released: 6/8/29. Distributor: United Artists. Director: Henry King. Scenario: Howard Estabrook, from a story by Rupert Hughes in *She Goes to War and Other Stories* (New York: Grosset and Dunlap, 1929).

Shining Victory 80 min. B & W. Released: 6/7/41. Distributor: Warner Brothers. Director: Irving Rapper. Screenplay: Howard Koch, Anne Froelick, adapted from the play by Archibald

Joseph Cronin, *Jupiter Laughs* (Boston: Little, Brown, 1940).

Shock 70 min. B & W. Released: 2/46. Distributor: 20th Century-Fox. Director: Alfred Werker. Screenplay: Eugene Ling, from an original story by Albert Demond.

The Shrike 88 min. B & W. Released: 9/55. Distributor: Universal. Director: Jose Ferrer. Screenplay: Ketti Frings, from the play by Joseph Kramm, *The Shrike.*

Sick Abed 5 reels. B & W. Released: 6/27/20. Distributor: Paramount. Director: Sam Wood. Screenplay: Clara G. Kennedy. Story: Ethel W. Mumford.

Since You Went Away 172 min. B & W. Released: 7/20/44. Distributor: United Artists. Director: John Cromwell. Screenplay: David O. Selznick, adapted from the novel by M.A. Wilder, *Since You Went Away: Letters from a Soldier to His Wife* (New York: McGraw-Hill, 1943).

The Sins of Rachel Cade 124 min. Technicolor. Released: 3/29/61. Distributor: Warners. Director: Gordon Douglas. Screenplay: Edward Anhalt, adapted from the novel by Charles E. Mercer, *Rachel Cade* (New York: Putnam's, 1956).

Sister Kenny 116 min. B & W. Released: 7/17/46. Distributor: RKO. Director: Dudley Nichols. Screenplay: Dudley Nichols, Alexander Knox, Mary McCarthy, adapted from the novel by Elizabeth Kenny in collaboration with Martha Ostenso, *And They Shall Walk* (New York: Dodd, Mead, 1943).

The Sleeping City 85 min. B & W. Released: 9/50. Distributor: Universal. Director: George Sherman. Screenplay: Jo Eisinger, from an original story by Jo Eisinger.

Slim 85 min. B & W. Released: 6/12/37. Distributor: Warner Bros. Director: Ray Enright. Screenplay: William Wister Haines, from his book, *Slim* (Boston: Little, Brown, 1934).

The Snake Pit 108 min. B & W. Reviewed: 11/3/48. Distributor: 20th Century-Fox. Director: Anatole Litvak. Screenplay: Frank Partos, Millen Brand, adapted from the novel by Mary Jane Ward, *The Snake Pit* (New York: Random House, 1946).

Society Doctor 63 min. B & W. Released: 2/3/35. Distributor: Metro. Director: George B. Seitz. Screenplay: Michael Fessier, Samuel Marx, adapted from the play by Theodore Reeves, *The Harbor.*

Some Nurse 2 reels. B & W. Released: 4/16/17. Distributor: Universal. Director: Allen Curtis. Story: J. Cunningham.

Some Nurse 20 min. B & W. Released: 10/23/23. Distributor: Grand-Asher. Director: Arvid Gillstrom.

So Proudly We Hail 126 min. B & W. Reviewed: 6/22/43. Distributor: Paramount. Director: Mark Sandrich. Screenplay: Allan Scott.

Souls in Pawn 6 reels. B & W. Released: 8/6/17. Distributor: Mutual. Director: Henry King. Based on the story by Julius Grinnel Furthman.

South Pacific 171 min. Technicolor. Reviewed: 3/20/58. Distributor: Magna Theater. Director: Joshua Logan. Screenplay: Paul Osborn, adapted from the book by James A. Michener, *Tales of the South Pacific* (New York: Macmillan, 1947).

South to Karanga 59 min. B & W. Released: 8/2/40. Distributor: Universal. Director: Harold Schuster. Screenplay: Edmond L. Hartmann, Stanley Rubin.

The Spirit of the Red Cross 25 min. B & W. Released: 4/28/18. Distributor: The American Red Cross. Director: Jack Eaton. Screenplay: James Montgomery Flagg.

The Splendid Sinner 73 min. B & W. Released: 3/24/18. Distributor: Goldwyn. Director: Hogo Balin. Story: Kate Jordan.

The Sporting Lover 66 min. B & W. Released: 6/17/26. Distributor: First National. Director: Alan Hale. Adaptation: Carey Wilson, from the play by Seymour Hicks, Ian Hay, *Good Luck.*

The Storm 75 min. B & W. Released: 10/28/38. Distributor: RKO. Director: Harold Young. Screenplay: Theodore Reeves, Daniel Moore, Hugh King, from an original screen story by Daniel Moore, Hugh King.

The Story of Dr. Wassell 140 min. Technicolor. Released: 4/26/44. Distributor: Paramount. Director: Cecil B. DeMille. Screenplay: Alan LeMay, Charles Bennett, adapted from the novel by James Hilton, *Story of Dr. Wassell* (Boston: Little, Brown, 1943).

The Story of Seabiscuit 93 min. B & W. Released: 11/20/49. Distributor: Warner Brothers. Director: David Butler. Screenplay: John Taintor Foote.

The Strange Case of Dr. Meade 68 min. B & W. Released: 10/26/38. Distributor: Columbia. Director: Lewis D. Collins. Story: Gordon Rigby, Carlton Sand. Screenplay: Gordon Rigby.

The Strawberry Blonde 97 min. B & W. Released: 2/22/41. Distributor: Warner Brothers. Director: Raoul Walsh. Screenplay: Julius J. Epstein, Philip G. Epstein, adapted from the play by James Hagan, *One Sunday Afternoon.*

The Stripper 95 min. B & W. Released: 6/19/63. Distributor: 20th Century-Fox. Director: Franklin Schaffner. Screenplay: Meade Roberts, adapted from the play by William Inge, *A Loss of Roses.*

Student Nurses. 85 min. Movielab. Released: 1970. Distributor: New World. Director: Stephanie Rothman. Screenplay: Don Spencer.

Suddenly, Last Summer 114 min. B & W. Reviewed: 12/16/59. Distributor: Columbia. Director: Joseph L. Mankiewicz. Screenplay: Gore Vidal. Based on the play by Tennessee Williams, *Suddenly Last Summer*

Tammy and The Doctor 88 min. Eastman Color. Released: 5/29/63. Distributor: Universal. Director: Harry Keller. Screenplay: Oscar Brodney, based on the characters created by Cid Ricketts Sumner.

Tell It to The Marines 88 min. B & W. Released: 12/23/26. Distributor: MGM. Director: George Hill. Story/Scenario: E. Richard Schayer.

They Gave Him a Gun 94 min. B & W. Released: 5/14/37. Distributor: MGM. Director: S.W. Van Dyke. Screenplay: Cyril Hume, Richard Maibaum, Maurice Rapf, from the book by William Joyce Cowen, *They Gave Him a Gun* (New York: H. Smith and Robert Haas, 1936).

They Were Expendable 135 min. B & W. Released: 12/45. Distributor: MGM. Director: John Ford. Screenplay: Lieutenant Commander Frank Wead, from the book by William Lindsay White, *They Were Expendable* (New York: Harcourt, Brace, 1942).

Three Men in White 85 min. B & W. Released: 6/44. Distributor: MGM. Director: Willis Goldbeck. Screenplay: Martin Berkeley, Harry Ruskin, based on a character created by Max Brand.

Three Russian Girls 80 min. B & W. Released: 12/30/43. Distributor: United Artists. Director: Fedor Ozep, Henry Kesler. Screenplay: Aben Kandel, Dan James, adapted by Maurice Clark, Victor Trivas from the original screenplay, *The Girl from Leningrad.*

Thunderbirds 98 min. B & W. Released: 11/27/52. Distributor: Republic. Director: John H. Auer. Screenplay: Mary McCall Jr., from an original story by Kenneth Gamet.

To The Shores of Tripoli 86 min. B & W. Released: 4/10/42. Distributor: 20th Century-Fox. Director: Bruce Humberstone. Screenplay: Lamar Trotti, adapted from an original screen story by Steve Fisher.

The Tragedy of Ambition 20 min. B & W. Released: 3/7/14. Distributor: Selig. Director: Colin Campbell. Based on the story by Lanier Bartlett.

The Trial (France/Italy/West Germany) 118 min. B & W. Released: 12/62 (France); 9/63 (Italy); 4/63 (West Germany); 2/20/63 (United States). Distributor: Astor Pictures. Director: Orson Welles. Screenplay: Orson Welles, adapted from the novel by Franz Kafka, *The Trial* (New York: Knopf, 1925).

Troopship (Great Britain; titled *Farewell Again* in the United States) 83 min. B & W. Reviewed: 4/27/38. Distributor: United Artists. Producer: Erich Pommer. Director: Tim Whelan. Screenplay: From an original story by Wolfgang Wilhelm.

Twice Round the Daffodils (Great Britain) 89 min. B & W. Released: 2/62. Distributor: Anglo-Amalgamated. Producer: Peter Rogers. Director: Gerald Thomas. Screenplay: Norman Hudis, adapted from the play by Patrick Cargill, Jack Beale, *Ring for Catty*.

The Unexpected Father 71 min. B & W. Released: 1/3/32. Distributor: Universal. Director: Thornton V. Freeland. Screenplay: Robert Keith, Max Lief, Dale Van Every.

Untamed 83 min. Technicolor. Released: 7/2/40. Distributor: Paramount. Director: George Archainbaud. Screenplay: Frederick Hazlitt Brennan, Frank Butler, from the book by Sinclair Lewis, *Mantrap* (New York: American Mercury, 1938).

The Unwritten Code 61 min. B & W. Released: 10/26/44. Distributor: Columbia. Director: Herman Rotsten. Screenplay: Leslie T. White, Charles Kenyon, from an original story by Charles Kenyon, Robert Wilmont.

Up in Arms 106 min. Technicolor. Released: 3/44. Distributor: RKO. Director: Elliott Nugent. Screenplay: Don Hartman, Allen Boretz, Robert Pirosh, adapted from the play by Owen Davis, *The Nervous Wreck*.

Vacation from Marriage (Great Britain; titled *Perfect Strangers* in the United States) 111 min. B & W. Released: 11/45. Distributor: MGM. Director: Sir Alexander Korda. Screenplay: Clemence Dane, Anthony Pelissier, adapted from an original screen story by Clemence Dane.

Vendetta 6 reels. B & W. Released: 12/19/21. Distributor: Commonwealth. Director: George Jacoby. Story: George Jacoby, Leo Lasko.

Victory and Peace (Great Britain) 80 min. B & W. Released: 1918. Production Company: National War Aims Committee. Director: Herbert Brenon. Story: Hall Caine.

Vigil in the Night 96 min. B & W. Released: 2/9/40. Distributor: RKO. Director: George Stevens. Screenplay: Fred Guiol, P.J. Wolfson, Rowland Leigh, from the book by Archibald Joseph Cronin, *Vigil in the Night* (Boston: Little, Brown, 1938).

Violent Saturday 91 min. DeLuxe Color. Released: 4/55. Distributor: 20th Century-Fox. Director: Richard Fleischer.

Screenplay: Sydney Boehm, from the book by William L. Heath, *Violent Saturday* (New York: Harper and Row, 1955).

Vive La France! 5 reels. B & W. Released: 9/15/18. Distributor: Paramount. Director: R. William Neill. Screenplay: C. Gardner Sullivan. Author: H.H. Van Loan.

A Voice in the Dark 43 min. B & W. Released: 3/26/21. Distributor: Goldwyn. Director: Frank Lloyd. Scenario: Arthur F. Statter, from the play by Ralph E. Dyar, *A Voice in the Dark*.

Voice of the Whistler 60 min. B & W. Released: 1/16/46. Distributor: Columbia. Director: William Castle. Screenplay: Wilfred H. Pettit, William Castle, adapted from a story by Allan Rader suggested by the CBS radio program *The Whistler* (unpublished).

Wanted, a Nurse 2 reels. B & W. Released: 1915. Distributor: Vitagraph. Director: Sidney Drew. Author: A. Maude Hendrickson.

War Nurse 80 min. B & W. Released: 11/22/30. Distributor: MGM. Director: Edgar Selwyn. Screenplay: Becky Gardiner, Joe Farnham, adapted from the book by an anonymous author, *War Nurse: The True Story of a Woman Who Lived, Loved and Suffered on the Western Front* (New York: Cosmopolitan Book Corporation, 1930).

West Point Widow 63 min. B & W. Released: 6/20/41. Distributor: Paramount. Director: Sol C. Siegel. Associate Producer: Colbert Clark. Director: Robert Siodmak. Screenplay: F. Hugh Herbert, Hans Kraly, adapted from the short story by Anne Wormser, "The Baby's Had a Hard Day."

When a Woman Sins 7 reels. B & W. Released: 9/15/18. Distributor: Fox. Director: J. Gordon Edwards. Screenplay: E. Lloyd Sheldon. Story: Betta Breuil.

Where Danger Lives 84 min. B & W. Released: 7/14/50. Distributor: RKO. Director: John Farrow. Screenplay: Charles Bennett, from an original story by Leo Rosten.

Where Does it Hurt? 90 min. Eastman Color. Released: 9/72. Distributor: Cinerama. Director: Rod Amateau. Screenplay: Rod Amateau, Bud Robinson, adapted from their unpublished novel, *The Operator.*

Where's Poppa? 87 min. Color. Released: 11/70. Distributor: United Artists. Director: Carl Reiner. Screenplay: Robert Klane, based on his novel *Where's Poppa?* (New York: Random House, 1970).

Whiffs 90 min. Color. Released: 11/75. Distributor: 20th Century-Fox. Director: Ted Post. Screenplay: Malcolm Marmorstein.

While the Patient Slept 67 min. B & W. Reviewed: 3/2/35. Distributor: Warner Brothers. Director: Ray Enright. Screenplay: Robert N. Lee, Eugene Solow, Brown Holmes, from the book by Mignon G. Eberhart, *While the Patient Slept* (New York: Doubleday, 1930).

The White Angel 75 min. B & W. Reviewed: 6/2/36. Distributor: Warner Brothers. Director: William Dieterle. Screenplay: Michel Jacoby, Mordaunt Shairp, adapted from the chapter "Florence Nightingale" of the novel by Giles Lytton Strachey, *Eminent Victorians* (New York: Putnam, 1918).

White Corridors 102 min. B & W. Released: 7/15/52. Distributor: Rank. Director: Pat Jackson. Screenplay: Jan Read, Pat Jackson, adapted from a novel by Helen Ashton, *Yeomans Hospital* (New York: Viking, 1945).

The White Desert 65 min. B & W. Released: 5/4/25. Distributor: MGM. Director: Reginald Barker. Scenario: L.B. Rigby, from the book by Courtney Ryley Cooper, *The White Desert* (Boston: Little, Brown, 1922).

The White Parade 90 min. B & W. Reviewed: 10/22/34. Distributor: Fox. Director: Irving Cummings. Screenplay: Rian James, Sonya Levien, Ernest Pascal, Jesse L. Lasky, Jess Lasky Jr., adapted from the book by Rian James, *The White Parade* (New York: A.H. King, 1934).

The White Sister 6 reels. B & W. Released: 6/26/15. Distributor: Essanay. Director: Fred E. Wright. Screenplay: E.H. Calvert, adapted from the novel by Francis Marion Crawford, *The White Sister* (New York: Macmillan, 1909).

The White Sister 101 min. B & W. Released: 9/5/23. Also 94 min. Released: 4/17/24. Distributor: Metro. Director: Henry King. Scenario: George V. Hobart, Charles E. Whittaker, from the book by Francis Marion Crawford, *The White Sister* (New York: Macmillan, 1909).

The White Sister 101 min. B & W. Released: 2/24/33. Distributor: Metro. Director: Victor Fleming. Screenplay: Donald Ogden Stewart, adapted from the novel by Francis Marion Crawford, *The White Sister* (New York: Macmillan, 1909).

White Sister 96 min. Technicolor. Released: 1971. Distributor: Columbia-Warner. Director: Alberto Lattuada. Producer: Carlo Ponti. Screenplay: Iaia Fiastri, Alberto Lattuada, Tonino Gherra, Ruggerio Maccari, from a story by Tonino Gherra, Ruggerio Maccari.

White Witch Doctor 96 min. Technicolor. Released: 7/53. Distributor: 20th Century-Fox. Producer: Otto Lang. Director: Henry Hathaway. Screenplay: Ivan Goff, Ben Roberts, from the book by Louise A. Stinetorf, *White Witch Doctor* (Philadelphia: Westminster Press, 1950).

Why Germany Must Pay 5 reels. B & W. Released: 1/19/19. Distributor: Metro. Director: Charles Miller. Screenplay: June Mathis, A.S. Le Vino.

Why Worry? 55 min. B & W. Released: 9/16/23. Distributor: Pathe. Director: Fred Newmeyer, Sam Taylor. Story: Sam Taylor.

Wife, Doctor and Nurse 86 min. B & W. Released: 9/17/37. Distributor: 20th Century-Fox. Director: Walter Lang. Screenplay: Kathryn Scola, Darrell Ware, Lamar Trotti, from an original screen story by Kathryn Scola, Darrell Ware.

The Wild Blue Yonder 98 min. B & W. Released: 12/5/51. Distributor: Republic. Director: Allan Dwan. Screenplay: Richard Tregaskis, from an original story by Andrew Geer, Charles Grayson.

The Winding Stair 61 min. B & W. Released: 10/25/25. Distributor: Fox. Director: John Griffith Wray. Scenario: Julian La Mothe, from the book by Alfred Edward Woodley Mason, *The Winding Stair* (New York: George H. Doran, 1923).

Windom's Way (Great Britain) 108 min. Eastman Color. Released: 12/58. Distributor: Rank. Director: Ronald Neame. Screenplay: Jill Craigie, adapted from the novel by James Ramsey Ullman, *Windom's Way* (Philadelphia: J.B. Lippincott, 1952).

With a Song in My Heart 117 min. Technicolor. Released: 4/52. Distributor: 20th Century-Fox. Director: Walter Lang. Screenplay: Lamar Trotti.

Without Orders 64 min. B & W. Reviewed: 9/25/36. Distributor: RKO. Director: Lew Landers. Screenplay: J. Robert Bren, Edmund L. Cartman, from a short story by Peter B. Kyne.

Witness for the Prosecution (Great Britain) 114 min. B & W. Reviewed: 11/27/57. Distributor: United Artists. Director: Billy Wilder. Screenplay: Billy Wilder, Harry Kurnitz, adapted by Larry Marcus from the play by Agatha Christie, *Witness for the Prosecution*.

Woman of Straw (Great Britain) 120 min. Eastman Color. Released: 4/64 (U.S.: 9/9/64). Distributor: United Artists. Director: Basil Dearden. Screenplay: Robert Muller, Stanley Mann, Michael Relph, adapted from the novel by Catherine Arley, *Woman of Straw* (New York: Random House, 1958).

The Woman the Germans Shot 6 reels. B & W. Released: 1916. Distributor: Select. Director: John G. Adolfi. Screenplay: Anthony Paul Kelly, based on his story.

Women in War 71 min. B & W. Released: 6/6/40. Distributor: Republic. Associate Producer: Sol C. Siegel. Director: John H. Auer. Screenplay: F. Hugh Herbert, Doris Anderson.

Women Love Diamonds 64 min. B & W. Released: 2/12/27. Distributor: MGM. Director/Story: Edmund Goulding. Scenario: Lorna Moon, Waldemar Young.

Women Men Love 6 reels. B & W. Released: 1/29/21. Distributor: Bradley. Director: Samuel R. Bradley. Scenario: Charles T. Dazey, Frank Dazey, from the story by Charles T. Dazey, "Women Men Love" (publication undetermined).

Women Who Dare 66 min. B & W. Released: 3/31/28. Distributor: Excellent. Director: Burton King. Adaptation: Adrian Johnson, from a story by Langdon McCormick.

Yanks Ahoy 55 min. B & W. Released: 8/6/43. Distributor: United Artists-Roach.

Yellow Jack 83 min. B & W. Released: 5/27/38. Distributor: MGM. Director: George B. Seitz. Screenplay: Edward Chodorov, adapted from the play by Sidney Howard, Paul De Kruif, *Yellow Jack*.

You For Me 71 min. B & W. Released: 8/8/52. Distributor: MGM. Director: Don Weis. Screenplay: William Roberts.

Young Dr. Kildare 81 min. B & W. Released: 10/14/38. Distributor: MGM. Director: Harold S. Bucquet. Screenplay: Willis Goldbeck, Harry Ruskin, from the book by Max Brand, *Young Doctor Kildare* (New York: Dodd, Mead, 1941).

The Young Doctors 100 min. B & W. Released: 8/23/61. Distributor: United Artists. Director: Phil Karlson. Screenplay: Joseph Hayes, adapted from the novel by Arthur Hailey, *The Final Diagnosis* (Garden City, NY: Doubleday, 1959).

The Young Nurses 77 min. Metrocolor. Released: 3/73. Distributor: New World. Director: Clinton Kimbro. Screenplay: Howard R. Cohen.

Yours, Mine and Ours 111 min. DeLuxe. Released: 4/24/68. Distributor: United Artists. Director: Melville Shavelson. Screenplay: Melville Shavelson, Mort Lachman, based on the novel by Helen Beardsley, *Who Gets the Drumstick* (New York: Random House, 1965).

Youth Will Be Served 66 min. B & W. Released: 11/22/40. Distributor: 20th Century-Fox. Director: Otto Brower. Screenplay: Wanda Tuchock. Story: Ruth Fasken, Hilda Vincent.

TELEVISION SERIES

A.E.S. Hudson Street (30 min., Comedy) ABC. March 17, 1978, to April 20, 1978. 5 episodes. Nurses in regular cast: Nurse Rosa Santiago (Rosana Soto); Nurse Rhoda Todd (Julienne Wells); Nurse Newton (Ray Stewart).

Amanda Fallon (60 min., Medical-Drama Pilot) NBC. March 5, 1972. 1 episode. Nurse in regular cast: Nurse Crawford (Lillian Lehman).

Annie Flynn (60 min., Comedy Pilot) CBS. Jan. 21, 1978. 1 episode. Nurse in regular cast: Annie Flynn (Barrie Youngfellow).

Ben Casey (60 min., Medical Drama) ABC. Oct. 2, 1961, to March 21, 1966. 153 episodes. Nurse in regular cast: Nurse Wills (Jeanne Bates).

The Black Sheep Squadron (60 min., Adventure) NBC. Dec. 14, 1977, to Sept. 1, 1978 (as *Baa Baa Black Sheep* Sept. 21, 1976, to Aug. 30, 1977). 34 episodes. Nurses in regular cast (The Fighting Angels): Nancy Gilmore (Nancy Conrad); Samantha Greene (Denise DuBarry); Captain Dottie Dickson (Katherine Cannon); Ellie Farrell (Kathy McCullem); Sue Webster (Brianne Leary); Anne Wilson (Leslie Charleson); Cheryl (Sharon Ullrick).

The Bob Crane Show (30 min., Comedy) NBC. March 6, 1975, to June 19, 1975. 14 episodes. No regular nurse characters.

The Bold Ones: The Doctors (60 min., Medical Drama) NBC. Sept. 14, 1969, to June 23, 1973. 44 episodes. No regular nurse characters.

Breaking Point (60 min., Medical Drama) ABC. Sept. 16, 1963, to Sept. 7, 1964. 30 episodes. No regular nurse characters.

Calling Dr. Storm, M.D. (30 min., Comedy Pilot) NBC. Aug. 25, 1977. 1 episode. No regular nurse characters.

City Hospital (30 min., Medical Drama) CBS. March 25, 1952, to Oct. 1, 1953. 72 episodes. No regular nurse characters.

Cutter to Houston (60 min., Medical Drama) CBS. Oct. 1, 1983, to Dec. 31, 1983. 11 episodes. Nurses in regular cast: Nurse Connie (K. Callan); Nurse Patty (Susan Styles).

Doc (30 min., Comedy) CBS. Sept. 13, 1975, to Aug. 14, 1976. 23 episodes. Nurse in regular cast: Beatrice Tully (Mary Wickes).

Doc (30 min., Comedy) CBS. Sept. 25, 1976, to Oct. 30, 1976. 6 episodes. Nurse in regular cast: Janet Scott ("Scotty") (Audra Lindley).

Doc Elliott (60 min., Medical Drama) ABC. Oct. 10, 1973, to Aug. 14, 1974. 15 episodes. No regular nurse characters.

The Doctor (30 min., Medical Anthology) NBC. Aug. 24, 1952, to June 28, 1953. 36 episodes. No regular nurse characters.

Doctor Christian (30 min., Medical Drama) Syndicated. 1956. 39 episodes. Nurses in regular cast: Nurse (Jan Shepard); Nurse (Cynthia Baer); Nurse (Kay Faylen).

Dr. Hudson's Secret Journal (30 min., Medical Drama) Syndicated. 1955–57. 78 episodes. Nurse in regular cast: Nurse Ann Talbot (Frances Mercer).

Dr. Kildare (60 min., Medical Drama) NBC. Sept. 27, 1961, to Aug. 29, 1966. 190 episodes. Nurses in regular cast: Nurse Zoe Lawton (Lee Kurty); Nurse Conant (Jo Helton).

The Doctors (30 min., Drama) NBC. Premiered April 1, 1963. 5,000-plus episodes. Nurses in regular cast: Nurse Kathy Ryker (Nancy Barrett, Holly Peters); Carolee Aldrich (Carolee Campbell, Jada Rowland); Laurie James (Marie Thomas); Nurse (Susan Adams); Nurse Brown (Dorothy Blackburn), Nurse M.J. Carroll (Kathy Glass).

Doctors Hospital (60 min., Medical Drama) NBC. Sept. 10, 1975, to Jan. 14, 1976. (The 2-hour pilot film, *One of Our Own*, aired on NBC May 5, 1975.) 12 episodes. Nurses in regular cast: Nurse Connie Kimbrough (Elisabeth Brooks); Heather Stanton, admissions nurse (Adrian Ricard); Nurse Forester (Barbara Darrow); Nurse Wilson (Elaine Church).

Doctor Simon Locke (30 min., Medical Drama) Syndicated. 1971. 39 episodes. Nurse in regular cast: Nurse Louise Wynn (Nuala Fitzgerald).

Doctor's Private Lives (60 min., Medical Drama) ABC. March 5, 1979, to April 26, 1979. (The 2-hour pilot film aired on ABC March 20, 1978.) 4 episodes. Nurse in regular cast: Nurse Diane Curtis (Eddie Benton).

The Donna Reed Show (30 min., Comedy) ABC. Sept. 24, 1958, to Sept. 3, 1966. 274 episodes. Nurse in regular cast: Donna Stone (Donna Reed).

The Eleventh Hour (60 min., Medical Drama) NBC. Oct. 3, 1962, to Sept. 9, 1964. 62 episodes. No regular nurse characters.

Emergency! (60 min., Medical Drama) NBC. Jan. 22, 1972, to Sept. 3, 1977. 115 episodes. Nurses in regular cast: Nurse Dixie McCall (Julie London); Nurse Carol Williams (Lillian Lehman); Nurse (Deidre Hall); Nurse (Ginny Golden).

E/R (30 min., Comedy) CBS. Sept. 25, 1984 to March 6, 1985. 22 episodes. Nurses in regular cast: Nurse Thor (Conchata Ferrell); Nurse Julie (Lynne Moody).

The First 36 Hours of Dr. Durant (90 min., Medical Drama Pilot) ABC. May 13, 1975. 1 episode. Nurses in regular cast: Nurse Katherine Gunther (Katherine Helmond); Nurse Olive Olin (Karen Carlson).

The Flying Doctor (30 min., Adventure) Syndicated. 1959. 39 episodes. Nurse in regular cast: Mary (Jill Adams).

General Hospital (30 min., April 1, 1963, to July 23, 1976; 45 min., July 26, 1976, to Jan. 13, 1978; 60 min., Jan. 16, 1978 to date; Drama) ABC. Premiered April 1, 1963. 5,000-plus episodes. Nurses in regular cast: Nurse Audrey March (Rachel Ames); Nurse Iris Fairchild (Peggy McCay); Nurse Jesse Brewer (Lois Kibbee, Emily McLaughlin, Aneta Corsaut); Nurse Kendell Jones (Joan Tompkins); Nurse Lucille March (Lucille Wall); Nurse Linda Cooper (Linda Cooper); Bobbi (Jackie Zeman-Kaufman).

Handle with Care (30 min., Comedy Pilot) CBS. May 9, 1977. 1 episode. Nurses in regular cast: Liz Baker (Marlyn Mason); Jackie Morse (Didi Conn); Major Hinkley (Mary Jo Catlett); Shirley "Scoop" Nichols (Betsey Slade); Turk (Jeannie Wilson).

Hennesey (30 min., Comedy/Drama) CBS. Sept. 28, 1959, to Sept. 17, 1962. 92 episodes. Nurse in regular cast: Martha Hale (Abby Dalton).

House Calls (30 min., Comedy) CBS. Dec. 17, 1979, to Sept. 13, 1982. 79 episodes. Nurses in regular cast: Head Nurse Bradley (Aneta Corsaut); The Admissions Nurse (Sharon DeBord); Nurse (Peggy Frees); Nurse (Terri Berland); Nurse (Georgia Jeffries).

The Interns (60 min., Medical Drama) CBS. Sept. 18, 1970, to Sept. 10, 1971. 24 episodes. Nurse in regular cast: Nurse (Jenny Blackton).

Janet Dean, Registered Nurse (30 min., Drama) Syndicated. 1953–55. 39 episodes. Nurse in regular cast: Janet Dean (Ella Raines).

Julia (30 min., Comedy) NBC. Sept. 17, 1968, to May 25, 1971. 86 episodes. Nurses in regular cast: Nurse Julia Baker (Diahann Carroll); Hannah Yarby, head nurse (Lurene Tuttle).

Julie Farr, M.D. (Having Babies) (60 min., Medical Drama) ABC. March 28, 1978, to April 18, 1978; June 12, 1979, to June 26, 1979; March 7, 1978, to March 21, 1978. 8 episodes. Nurse in regular cast: Nurse (Deborah Green).

The Lazarus Syndrome (60 min., Medical Drama) ABC. Sept. 11, 1979, to Oct. 9, 1979. 6 episodes. Nurse in regular cast: The Admissions Nurse (Christine Alvila).

Lifeline (60 min., Medical Documentary) NBC. Oct. 8, 1978, to Dec. 30, 1978. 10 episodes. No regular nurse characters.

The Little People (30 min., Comedy) NBC. Sept. 15, 1972, to Sept. 7, 1973 (as *The Brian Keith Show* Sept. 21, 1973, to Aug. 30, 1974). 48 episodes. Nurse in regular cast: Puni (Victoria Young).

The March of Medicine (30 min., Documentary) ABC. July 8, 1958, to July 29,

1958. 3 episodes. No regular nurse characters.

Marcus Welby, M.D. (60 min., Medical Drama) ABC. Sept. 23, 1969, to May 11, 1976. 172 episodes. Nurses in regular cast: Consuelo Lopez (Elena Verdugo); Nurse Kathleen Faverty (Sharon Gless).

M*A*S*H (30 min., Comedy/Drama) CBS. Sept. 17, 1972, to Feb. 28, 1983. 250 episodes. Nurses in regular cast: Major Margaret "Hot Lips" Houlihan (Loretta Switt); Nurse (Lt.) Maggie Dish (Karen Philipp); Nurse (Lt.) Ginger Ballis (Odessa Cleveland); Nurse (Lt.) Leslie Scorch (Linda Meiklejohn); Nurse (Lt.) Jones (Barbara Brownell); Nurse Louise Anderson (Kelly Jean Peters); Nurse Maggie Cutler (Marcia Strassman, Lynnette Metty); Nurse Bigelow (Enid Kent); Nurse Abel (Judy Farrell); Nurse Baker (Jean Powell, Lynne Marie Stewart, Linda Kelsey); Nurse Mary Jo Walsh (Mary Jo Catlett); Nurse Gaynor (Carol Locatell); Nurse Preston (Patricia Sturges); Nurse (Shari Saba); Nurse Memdenhal (Shelly Long); Nurse (Jennifer Davis); Nurse (Gwen Farrell); Nurse (Connie Izay).

Matt Lincoln (60 min., Medical Drama) ABC. Sept. 24, 1970, to Jan. 14, 1971. 15 episodes. No regular nurse characters.

Medic (30 min., Medical Drama) NBC. Sept. 1954 to Nov. 1956. 60 episodes. No regular nurse characters.

Medical Center (60 min., Medical Drama) CBS. Sept. 24, 1969, to Sept. 6, 1976. 169 episodes. Nurses in regular cast: Nurse Chambers (Jayne Meadows); Nurse Holmby (Barbara Baldavin); Nurse Courtland (Chris Huston); Nurse Higby (Catherine Ferrar); Nurse Murphy (Jane Dulo); Nurse Wilcox (Audrey Totter); Nurse Crawford (Virginia Hawkins); Nurse Bascomb (Louise Fitz); Nurse Loring (Nancy Priddy).

Medical Horizons (30 min., Public Affairs) ABC. Sept. 12, 1955, to March 5, 1956. 26 episodes. No regular nurse characters.

Medical Story (60 min., Anthology) NBC. Sept. 4, 1975, to Jan. 8, 1976. 11 episodes. No regular nurse characters.

Mr. Peepers (30 min., Comedy) NBC. July 3, 1952, to June 12, 1955. 96 episodes. Nurse in regular cast: Nancy Remington (Patricia Benoit).

Mother and Me, M.D. (30 min., Comedy Pilot) NBC. June 14, 1979. 1 episode. Nurse in regular cast: Lil Brenner (Rue McClanahan).

The New Healers (60 min., Medical Drama Pilot) ABC. March 27, 1972. 1 episode. Nurse in regular cast: Nurse Michelle Johnson (Kate Jackson).

The New Operation Petticoat (30 min., Comedy) ABC. Sept. 25, 1978, to Oct. 19,

1978; June 1, 1979, to Aug. 3, 1979. 9 episodes. Nurses in regular cast: Lt. Dolores Crandall (Melinda Naud); Lt. Catherine O'Hara (Jo Ann Pflug); Lt. Betty Wheeler (Hilary Thompson).

Nurse (60 min., Medical Drama) CBS. April 2, 1981 to May 21, 1982. 23 episodes. Nurses in regular cast: Nurse Mary Benjamin (Michael Learned); Nurse Toni (Hatti Winston); Nurse Penny (Bonnie Hellman); Nurse Betty LaSada (Hortensia Colorado); Nurse Bailey (Clarice Taylor).

The Nurses (The Doctors and The Nurses) (60 min., Medical Drama) CBS. Sept. 27, 1962, to Sept. 17, 1964; as *The Doctors and The Nurses* Sept. 22, 1964, to Sept. 7, 1965. 103 episodes. Nurses in regular cast: Nurse Liz Thorpe (Shirl Conway); Nurse Gail Lucas (Zina Bethune); Nurse Ayres (Hilda Simms).

The Nurses (30 min., Serial) ABC. Sept. 27, 1965, to March 31, 1967. 390 episodes. Nurses in regular cast: Liz Thorpe (Mary Fickett); Gail Lucas (Melinda Plank); Brenda (Patricia Hyland); Nurse Dorothy Warner (Leonie Norton).

Operating Room (60 min., Comedy Pilot) NBC. Oct. 4, 1979. 1 episode. No regular nurse characters.

Operation Petticoat (30 min., Comedy) ABC. Sept. 17, 1977, to Aug. 25, 1978. 22 episodes. Nurses in regular cast: Major Edna Hayward (Yvonne Wilder); Lt. Dolores Crandall (Melinda Naud); Lt. Barbara Duran (Jamie Lee Curtis); Lt. Ruth Colfax (Dorrie Thompson); Lt. Claire Reid (Bond Gideon).

Police Surgeon (30 min., Crime Drama) Syndicated. 1972. 76 episodes. No regular nurse characters.

The Practice (30 min., Comedy) NBC. Jan. 30, 1976, to Aug. 6, 1976; Oct. 13,

1976, to Jan. 20, 1977. 22 episodes. Nurse in regular cast: Molly Gibbons (Dena Dietrich).

Quincy, M.E. (60 min., Crime Drama) NBC. Feb. 4, 1977, to Sept. 5, 1983. 176 episodes. No regular nurse characters.

Rafferty (60 min., Medical Drama) CBS. Sept. 5, 1977, to Nov. 28, 1977. 10 episodes. Nurses in regular cast: Vera Wales (Millie Slavin); Beryl Kaynes (Joan Pringle).

The Rookies (60 min., Crime Drama) ABC. Sept. 11, 1972, to June 15, 1976. 68 episodes. Nurse in regular cast: Jill Danko (Kate Jackson).

St. Elsewhere (60 min., Medical Drama) NBC. Oct. 26, 1982, to Sept. 24, 1986. 92 episodes. Nurses in regular cast: Nurse Helen Rosenthal (Christina Pickles); Nurse Shirley Daniels (Ellen Bry).

Scalpels (30 min., Comedy Pilot) NBC. Oct. 26, 1980. 1 episode. Nurse in regular cast: Connie Primble (Kimberly Beck).

The Specialist (90 min., Medical Drama Pilot) NBC. Jan. 6, 1975. 1 episode. No regular nurse characters.

Stat! (30 min., Medical Drama Pilot) CBS. July 31, 1973. 1 episode. Nurse in regular cast: Nurse Ellen Quayle (Marian Collier).

Temperatures Rising (30 min., Comedy) ABC. Sept. 12, 1972, to Aug. 29, 1974. 42 episodes. Nurses in regular cast: Nurse Ann Carlisle (Joan Van Ark); Nurse Mildred MacInerney (Reva Rose); Nurse Ellen Turner (Nancy Fox); Wendy Winchester (Jennifer Darling); Miss Tillis (Barbara Cason); Nurse Kelly (Barbara Rucker).

Three's Company (30 min., Comedy) ABC. March 15, 1977, to April 21, 1977; Aug. 11, 1977, to Sept. 20, 1984. 154 epi-

sodes. Nurse in regular cast: Terri Alden (Priscilla Barnes).

Trapper John, M.D. (60 min., Medical Drama) CBS. Sept. 23, 1979, to Sept. 23, 1986. 161 episodes. Nurses in regular cast: Nurse "Starch" Willoughby (Mary McCarty); Nurse Gloria "Ripples" Brancusi (Christopher Norris); Nurse (Jennifer Davis); Nurse (Brenda Elder); Scrub Nurse Ernestine Shoop (Madge Sinclair).

Trauma Center (60 min., Medical Drama) ABC. Sept. 22, 1983, to Dec. 8, 1983. 11 episodes. Nurses in regular cast: Nurse Decker (Eileen Heckart); Nurse Hooter (Jayne Modean).

The Waltons (60 min., Drama) CBS. Sept. 14, 1972, to March 27, 1981. 208 episodes. Nurses in regular cast: Mary Ellen Walton (Judy Norton-Taylor); Nora, the county nurse (Kaiulani Lee).

Westside Medical (60 min., Medical Drama) ABC. March 15, 1977, to April 14, 1977. 5 episodes. No regular nurse characters.

Where's Poppa? (30 min., Comedy Pilot) ABC. July 17, 1979. 1 episode. Nurse in regular cast: Louise Hamelin (Judith-Marie Bergen).

Women in White (60 and 120 min., Drama) NBC. Feb. 8, 1979, to Feb. 22, 1979. 3 episodes. Nurses in regular cast: Nurse Cathy Payson (Patty Duke Astin); Nurse Lisa Gordon (Sheree North); Nurse (Gloria Delaney); Nurse Jane Robinson (June Witney Taylor); Admitting Nurse (Janet Winter).

Young Doctor Kildare (30 min., Medical Drama) Syndicated. 1972. 24 episodes. Nurses in regular cast: Nurse Marsha Lord (Marsha Mason); Nurse Ferris (Dixie Marquis); Nurse Newell (Olga James).

INDEXES

NAME INDEX

TITLE INDEX

SUBJECT INDEX